Your *Clinics* subscription just got better!

You can now access the FULL TEXT of this publication online at no additional cost! Activate your online subscription today and receive...

- Full text of all issues from 2002 to the present
- Photographs, tables, illustrations, and references
- Comprehensive search capabilities
- Links to MEDLINE and Elsevier journals

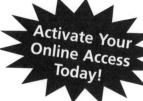

Activate Your Online Access Today!

Plus, you can also sign up for E-alerts of upcoming issues or articles that interest you, and take advantage of exclusive access to bonus features!

To activate your individual online subscription:

1. Visit our website at **www.TheClinics.com**.

2. Click on "Register" at the top of the page, and follow the instructions.

3. To activate your account, you will need your subscriber account number, which you can find on your mailing label (note: the number of digits in your subscriber account number varies from six to ten digits). See the sample below where the subscriber account number has been circled.

This is your subscriber account number

```
*****************************
FEB00  J0167  C7   123456-8
J.H. DOE, MD
531 MAIN ST
CENTER CITY, NY  10001-001
```

D1417237

4. That's it! Your online access to the most trusted source for clinical reviews is now available.

the**clinics**.com

ELSEVIER

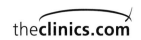

PEDIATRIC CLINICS
OF NORTH AMERICA

Pediatric Rheumatology

GUEST EDITOR
Ronald M. Laxer, MD, FRCPC

April 2005 • Volume 52 • Number 2

SAUNDERS

An Imprint of Elsevier, Inc.
PHILADELPHIA   LONDON   TORONTO   MONTREAL   SYDNEY   TOKYO

W.B. SAUNDERS COMPANY
A Division of Elsevier Inc.

The Curtis Center • Independence Square West • Philadelphia, Pennsylvania 19106

http://www.theclinics.com

THE PEDIATRIC CLINICS OF NORTH AMERICA   Volume 52, Number 2
April 2005   ISSN 0031-3955
Editor: Carin Davis   ISBN 1-4160-2749-1

The ideas and opinions expressed in *The Pediatric Clinics of North America* do not necessarily reflect those of the Publisher. The Publisher does not assume any responsibility for any injury and/or damage to persons or property arising out of or related to any use of the material contained in this periodical. The reader is advised to check the appropriate medical literature and the product information currently provided by the manufacturer of each drug to be administered to verify the dosage, the method and duration of administration, or contraindications. It is the responsibility of the treating physician or other health care professional, relying on independent experience and knowledge of the patient, to determine drug dosages and the best treatment for the patient. Mention of any product in this issue should not be construed as endorsement by the contributors, editors, or the Publisher of the product or manufacturers' claims.

The Pediatric Clinics of North America (ISSN 0031-3955) is published bi-monthly by W.B. Saunders Company, Corporate and Editorial offices: 1600 JFK Boulevard, Suite 1800, Philadelphia, PA 19103-2822. Accounting and Circulation offices: 6277 Sea Harbor Drive, Orlando, FL 32887-4800. Periodicals postage paid at Orlando, FL 32862, and additional mailing offices. Subscription prices are $135.00 per year (US individuals), $246.00 per year (US institutions), $177.00 per year (Canadian individuals), $320.00 per year (Canadian institutions), $200.00 per year (international individuals), $320.00 per year (international institutions), $68.00 per year (US students), $100.00 per year (Canadian students), and $100.00 per year (foreign students). To receive student/resident rate, orders must be accompanied by name of affiliated institution, date of term, and the signature of program/residency coordinator on institution letterhead. Orders will be billed at individual rate until proof of status is received. Foreign air speed delivery is included in all Clinics subscription prices. All prices are subject to change without notice. POSTMASTER: Send address changes to *The Pediatric Clinics of North America*, W.B. Saunders Company, Periodicals Fulfillment, Orlando, FL 32887-4800. **Customer Service: 1-800-654-2452 (US). From outside of the US, call 1-407-345-4000.** E-mail: hhspcs@harcourt.com.

The Pediatric Clinics of North America is also published in Spanish by McGraw-Hill Inter-americana Editores S.A., Mexico City, Mexico; in Portuguese by Reichmann and Affonso Editores, Rua Comandante Coelho 1085, CEP 21250, Rio de Janeiro, Brazil; and in Greek by Althayia SA, Athens, Greece.

The Pediatric Clinics of North America is covered in *Index Medicus, Excerpta Medica, Current Contents, Current Contents/Clinical Medicine, Science Citation Index, ASCA, ISI/BIOMED,* and *BIOSIS.*

Printed in the United States of America.

GUEST EDITOR

RONALD M. LAXER, MD, FRCPC, Professor, Pediatrics and Medicine, University of Toronto; Vice President, Clinical and Academic Affairs, The Hospital for Sick Children, Toronto, Ontario, Canada

CONTRIBUTORS

KELLY K. ANTHONY, PhD, Clinical Associate, Division of Medical Psychology, Department of Psychiatry and Behavioral Sciences, Duke University Medical Center, Durham, North Carolina

PAUL BABYN, MDCM, Radiologist in Chief, Hospital for Sick Children; Associate Professor, Medical Imaging, University of Toronto, Toronto, Ontario, Canada

SUSANNE M. BENSELER, MD, Division of Rheumatology, Department of Pediatrics, The Hospital for Sick Children, Toronto, Ontario, Canada

DAVID A. CABRAL, MBBS, Clinical Associate Professor in Pediatrics, Division of Pediatric Rheumatology, British Columbia Children's Hospital, Vancouver, British Columbia, Canada

SANDRINE COMPEYROT-LACASSAGNE, MD, Clinical Fellow, Division of Rheumatology, The Hospital for Sick Children, Toronto, Canada

FATMA DEDEOGLU, MD, Assistant in Medicine, Program in Rheumatology, Division of Immunology, Children's Hospital; Instructor in Pediatrics, Harvard Medical School, Boston, Massachusetts

ANDREA S. DORIA, MD, MSc, PhD, Staff Radiologist, Hospital for Sick Children; Assistant Professor, Medical Imaging, University of Toronto, Toronto, Ontario, Canada

CIARÁN M. DUFFY, MB, BCh, MSc, FRCPC, Director, Division of Paediatric Rheumatology, Montreal Children's Hospital; McGill University Health Centre; Associate Professor of Pediatrics, McGill University, Montreal, Quebec, Canada

BRIAN M. FELDMAN, MD, MSc, FRCPC, Associate Professor of Pediatrics, Health Policy Management and Evaluation, and Public Health Sciences, University of Toronto; Division of Rheumatology, The Hospital for Sick Children, Toronto, Canada

NORMAN T. ILOWITE, MD, Professor of Pediatrics, Albert Einstein College of Medicine, New York; Chief, Division of Pediatric Rheumatology, Schneider Children's Hospital, New Hyde Park, New York

ALBERTO MARTINI, MD, Professor and Department Head, Department of Pediatrics, University of Genova; Pediatria II, Istituto di Ricovero e Cura a Carattere Scientifico G. Gaslini, Genoa, Italy

SHAI PADEH, MD, Senior Lecturer, Pediatric Rheumatology, Edmond & Lily Safra Children Hospital, The Chaim Sheba Medical Center, Tel Hashomer; Sackler School of Medicine, Tel-Aviv University, Tel Aviv, Israel

ANGELO RAVELLI, MD, Dirigente Medico, Pediatria II, Istituto di Ricovero e Cura a Carattere Scientifico G. Gaslini, Genoa, Italy

LAURA E. SCHANBERG, MD, Associate Professor, Division of Pediatric Rheumatology, Department of Pediatrics, Duke University Medical Center, Durham, North Carolina

EARL D. SILVERMAN, MD, FRCP, Division of Rheumatology, Department of Pediatrics, The Hospital for Sick Children, Toronto, Ontario, Canada

KATHLEEN E. SULLIVAN, MD, PhD, Associate Professor of Pediatrics, University of Pennsylvania School of Medicine, Division of Allergy and Immunology, Children's Hospital of Philadelphia, Philadelphia, Pennsylvania

ROBERT P. SUNDEL, MD, Director of Rheumatology and Assistant in Medicine, Children's Hospital; Associate Professor of Pediatrics, Harvard Medical School, Boston, Massachusetts

LORI B. TUCKER, MD, Clinical Associate Professor in Pediatrics, Division of Pediatric Rheumatology, Centre for Community Child Health Research, British Columbia Children's Hospital, Vancouver, British Columbia, Canada

JENNIFER E. WEISS, MD, Fellow, Division of Pediatric Rheumatology, Schneider Children's Hospital, New Hyde Park, New York

FRANCESCO ZULIAN, MD, Pediatric Rheumatology Unit, Department of Pediatrics, University of Padova, Padua, Italy

CONTENTS

Inflammation evolved to aid in the clearance of microorganisms. In pediatric arthritides, the inflammation persists and causes damage to the joint. The contribution of the innate immune system to inflammation is significant and can be exploited therapeutically. Although cells of the adaptive immune system such as T cells and B cells participate in the disease process, many of the features of arthritis are directly attributable to inflammatory mediators. Recent advances in the understanding of these processes have led to dramatic improvements in treatment.

Several groups have undertaken research on health status, functional status, and quality of life in the pediatric rheumatic diseases, particularly juvenile idiopathic arthritis (JIA) and juvenile rheumatoid arthritis. This article highlights the principles involved in this type of measurement, discusses the measures that have been developed for JIA, and describes the outcomes determined from recent retrospective and prospective longitudinal outcome studies. These studies suggest that although there has been improvement in overall outcomes, significant numbers of individuals persist with active disease into adulthood and have significant damage, reduced functional ability, and disability.

describes a recent patient who presented with typical JDM and uses her case to discuss aspects of the childhood inflammatory myopathies.

FORTHCOMING ISSUES

RECENT ISSUES

PEDIATRIC CLINICS OF NORTH AMERICA APRIL 2005

GOAL STATEMENT

The goal of *Pediatric Clinics of North America* is to keep practicing physicians and residents up to date with current clinical practice in pediatrics by providing timely articles reviewing the state-of-the-art in patient care.

ACCREDITATION

The *Pediatric Clinics of North America* is planned and implemented in accordance with the Essential Areas and Policies of the Accreditation Council for Continuing Medical Education (ACCME) through the joint sponsorship of the University of Virginia School of Medicine and Elsevier. The University of Virginia School of Medicine is accredited by the ACCME to provide continuing medical education for physicians.

The University of Virginia School of Medicine designates this educational activity for a maximum of 90 category 1 credits per year, 15 category 1 credits per issue, toward the AMA Physician's Recognition Award. Each physician should claim only those credits that he/she actually spent in the activity.

The American Medical Association has determined that physicians not licensed in the US who participate in this CME activity are eligible for AMA PRA category 1 credit.

Category 1 credit can be earned by reading the text material, taking the CME examination online at http://www.theclinics.com/home/cme, and completing the evaluation. After taking the test, you will be required to review any and all incorrect answers. Following completion of the test and evaluation, your credit will be awarded and you may print your certificate.

FACULTY DISCLOSURE

Disclosure of faculty financial affiliations: As a provider accredited by the Accreditation Council for Continuing Medical Education (ACCME), the Office of Continuing Medical Education of the University of Virginia School of Medicine must ensure balance, independence, objectivity, and scientific rigor in all its individually sponsored or jointly sponsored educational activities. All authors/editors participating in a sponsored activity are expected to disclose to the readers any significant financial interest or other relationship (1) with the manufacturer(s) of any commercial product(s) and/or provider(s) of commercial services discussed in an educational presentation and (2) with any commercial supporters of the activity (significant financial interest or other relationship can include such things as grants or research support, employee, consultant, stock holder, member of speakers bureau, etc.) The intent of this disclosure is not to prevent authors/editors with a significant financial or other relationship from writing an article, but rather to provide readers with information on which they can make their own judgments. It remains for the readers to determine whether the author's/editor's interest or relationships may influence the article with regard to exposition or conclusion.

The authors/editors listed below have identified no professional or financial affiliations related to their presentation: Kelly K. Anthony, PhD; Paul Babyn, MDCM; Susanne M. Benseler, MD; David A. Cabral, MBBS; Sandrine Compeyrot-Lacassagne, MD; Fatma Dedeoglu, MD; Andrea S. Doria, MD, MSc, PhD; Ciaran M. Duffy, MB, ChB, MSc, FRCPC; Brian M. Feldman, MD, MSc, FRCPC; Alberto Martini, MD; Shai Padeh, MD; Angelo Ravellii, MD; Laura E. Schanberg, MD; Earl Silverman, MD, FRCPC; Kathleen E. Sullivan, MD, PhD; Robert P. Sundel, MD; Lori B. Tucker, MD; Jennifer E. Weiss, MD; and, Francesco Zulian, MD.

The authors listed below have identified the following professional or financial affiliation related to their presentations:
Norman T. Ilowite, MD has received grant support and is on the speakers' bureau for Amgen, is on the Wyeth speakers' bureau, and has received honoraria from Abbott.

Disclosure of Discussion of non-FDA approved uses for pharmaceutical products and/or medical devices: The University of Virginia School of Medicine, as an ACCME provider, requires that all authors identify and disclose any "off label" uses for pharmaceutical and medical device products. The University of Virginia School of Medicine recommends that each physician fully review all the available data on new products or procedures prior to instituting them with patients.

All authors who provided disclosures have indicated that they will not be discussing off-label uses except the following:
Kelly K. Anthony, PhD will dicuss the use of nortriptyline and amitriptyline for generalized chronic pain associated with sleep disturbance.
Susanne M. Benseler, MD and Earl Silverman, MD report that many of the drugs mentioned are not indicated for use in Pediatric SLE although some have indications for SLE while others have other pediatric indications. Azathioprine has no indication for pediatrics or SLE. Most NSAIDs do not have pediatric indications, except naproxen but it has no indication for SLE. Cyclophosphamide has no indication for SLE but appears to have some for pediatric tumors.
Sandrine Compeyrot-Lacassagne, MD and Brian M. Feldman, MD, MSc, FRCPC will discuss the use of corticosteroid, methotrexate, intravenous immunoglobulin, cyclophosphamide, hydroxychloroquine, and, cyclosporine A: for the treatment of juvenile myositis.
Norman T. Ilowite, MD will discuss the off-label use of sulfasalazine, infliximuab, anakinra, adalimumab, MRA for the treatment of JIA.
Laura E. Schanberg, MD serotonin reuptake inhibitors and Tricyclic antidepressants to treat pain.
Robert P. Sundel, MD will discuss the treatment of vasculitis in children using biologic response modifiers, including TNF inhibitors, abciximab, and rituximab.
Jennifer E. Weiss, MD will discuss the use of the following for the treatment of JIA: Anit- iL6 (MRA), leflunomide, adalimumab, infliximab, diclofenac, indomethacin, anakinra, and rituximab.

TO ENROLL

To enroll in the *Pediatric Clinics of North America* Continuing Medical Education program, call customer service at **1-800-654-2452** or visit us online at www.theclinics.com/home/cme. The CME program is available to subscribers for an additional fee of $195.00.

PEDIATRIC CLINICS

OF NORTH AMERICA

ELSEVIER
SAUNDERS

Pediatr Clin N Am 52 (2005) xi–xii

Preface

Pediatric Rheumatology

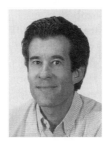

Ronald M. Laxer, MD, FRCPC
Guest Editor

It has been a decade since the *Pediatric Clinics of North America* devoted an issue to pediatric rheumatology. The advances in the areas of basic science, diagnostic tools, and therapeutics have changed the field remarkably over that time. And although it is not possible to cover all the progress that has been made, this issue provides an excellent overview of the more common pediatric rheumatic diseases.

Kathleen Sullivan starts this issue off by describing some of the basic mechanisms involved in the inflammatory process of juvenile idiopathic arthritis (JIA). Understanding these mechanisms has allowed for the development of much more effective therapies, as described by Jennifer Weiss and Norm Ilowite. These therapies will no doubt result in better health status and long-term outcomes for our patients. Ciaran Duffy provides an excellent overview of the outcome measures that have been used and will be used to determine that these therapies are effective, and also describes the rationale for the use of these measures.

The classification of chronic arthritis in childhood has been a confusing area for many years. Recent efforts to establish a unified classification scheme under the term JIA had been undertaken by the International League of Associations for Rheumatology. This new scheme is covered by Weiss and Ilowite (elsewhere in this issue) with an overview of the different subtypes, their complications, and outcomes. In addition, exciting new therapies are described.

The use of diagnostic imaging has expanded greatly over the last decade. Paul Babyn and Andrea Doria describe how the use of new techniques, such as color

0031-3955/05/$ – see front matter © 2005 Elsevier Inc. All rights reserved.
doi:10.1016/j.pcl.2005.02.003   *pediatric.theclinics.com*

Doppler ultrasonography, and well-established techniques for newer indications (such as CT scanning for interstitial pulmonary fibrosis) have improved our ability to diagnose and therefore treat rheumatic diseases and their complications. They also describe how imaging can help in the differential diagnosis of arthritis.

We have only recently come to appreciate the importance of pain in arthritis, and how the treatment of pain (in addition to the inflammatory component itself) can help children with JIA. In addition, idiopathic pain syndromes are common in children, and the treating practitioner must be aware of these and not treat them as an inflammatory rheumatic disease. This area is well-covered by Kelly Anthony and Laura Schanberg.

Adolescents with chronic disease face a difficult time leaving the world of pediatric care and moving to the world of adult care. This transition is often done poorly and in a disorganized fashion, leading to a situation in which patients frequently stop receiving appropriate care. Lori Tucker and David Cabral highlight the issues that must be addressed when planning to send the adolescent with a chronic rheumatic disease to an adult rheumatologist, and describe a model which has worked very successfully in their program. This model can be used for many other chronic diseases.

One of the most exciting areas in rheumatology has been the study of the periodic fever syndromes. A great deal of order has now been given to what was previously a group of poorly defined disorders through the use of molecular genetic studies. Not only have the genes been identified for many of these syndromes, but understanding of the mechanisms involved in disease pathogenesis has allowed for successful treatment in many cases. This area is covered extensively by Shai Padeh.

Advances in the classic inflammatory disorders, including systemic lupus erythematosus (Susanne Benseler and Earl Silverman), juvenile dermatomyositis (Sandrine Compeyrot-Lacassagne and Brian Feldman), scleroderma (Francesco Zulian) and vasculitis (Fatma Dedeoglu and Rob Sundel) are covered by experts in the respective areas. The anti-phospholipid antibody syndrome—relevant to so many pediatric specialties, including hematology, neurology and dermatology—is reviewed by Angelo Ravelli and Alberto Martini.

My role as Guest Editor was made easy because of the skill and expertise of each of the authors, who I thank sincerely for their tremendous efforts in making this such an outstanding issue. I am particularly proud that this issue has taken on an international flavor. In addition, I am grateful for the help and support provided by Carin Davis at Elsevier for making the editorial process go so smoothly.

Ronald M. Laxer, MD, FRCPC
Department of Pediatrics and Medicine
University of Toronto
The Hospital for Sick Children
555 University Avenue
Toronto, ON M5G 1X8, Canada
E-mail address: ronald.laxer@sickkids.ca

ELSEVIER
SAUNDERS

PEDIATRIC CLINICS
OF NORTH AMERICA

Pediatr Clin N Am 52 (2005) 335–357

Inflammation in Juvenile Idiopathic Arthritis

Kathleen E. Sullivan, MD, PhD

*University of Pennsylvania School of Medicine, Division of Allergy and Immunology,
Children's Hospital of Philadelphia, 34th Street and Civic Center Boulevard,
Philadelphia, PA 19104, USA*

The pediatric arthritides encompass the seven types of juvenile idiopathic arthritis (JIA) (formerly known as juvenile rheumatoid arthritis and juvenile chronic arthritis) as well as granulomatous arthritis caused by pediatric sarcoid, or by Blau syndrome. Many of the recent studies on pathogenesis have simply divided patients into three categories: oligoarthritis, polyarthritis, and systemic arthritis. Where the existing data allow, this article uses the approved Durban criteria (Box 1) [1]. In many cases, however, the older data do not reflect the more recent understanding of the clinical subsets.

Pediatric arthritides are both similar and distinct from adult-onset arthritides. For example, spondyloarthropathies and rheumatoid arthritis may present in childhood. The course of rheumatoid factor–positive JIA proceeds in childhood in a manner similar to rheumatoid arthritis seen in adults [2], whereas the spondyloarthropathies have a course that is marked by increased extra-axial symptoms and modest sacroiliitis compared with adults [3]. The other types of JIA are unique to children. Recent studies have begun to expose the distinct types of inflammation occurring in these disorders.

The basics of inflammation

Inflammation is nearly always defined as the presence of redness, pain, warmth, and swelling. Inflammation is considered deleterious in the setting of autoimmune disease, but it exists to defend optimally against infection. As such, a variety of mediators and cells participate. Cells and mediators of the innate

E-mail address: sullivak@mail.med.upenn.edu

doi:10.1016/j.pcl.2005.01.002
pediatric.theclinics.com

Box 1. Juvenile idiopathic arthritis

1. Systemic arthritis
2. Oligoarthritis
    A. Persistent
    B. Extended
3. Polyarthritis (rheumatoid factor–negative)
4. Polyarthritis (rheumatoid factor–positive)
5. Psoriatic arthritis
6. Enthesitis-related arthritis (spondyloarthropathies)
7. Other
    A. Does not meet any criteria for JIA
    B. Meets the criteria for more than one type of JIA

---

immune system, such as neutrophils, monocytes, mast cells, tumor necrosis factor α (TNFα), interleukin (IL)-1, and IL-12, often play a role in the early stages of inflammation. These cells are programmed to respond to foreign antigens and do not require DNA recombination to recognize a threat. Chronic inflammation is generally accompanied by cells and mediators of the adaptive immune system such as T cells, B cells, IL-2, IL-4, and γ-interferon. This distinction is not absolute, and inflammation requires intricate cell–cell communication at all stages. Although several of the early mediators causing inflammation have been known for decades, the complex choreography between the various mediators has only recently become appreciated. These features can occur in the absence of infection or elements of the adaptive immune system, but sustaining a response and initiation of an aberrant autoimmune inflammatory response requires cells of both the innate and adaptive immune response.

The role of the innate immune system in arthritis

The most elemental inflammatory response is caused by tissue damage, which leads to the activation of the kinin system, which ultimately leads to bradykinin production (Fig. 1). Bradykinin is responsible for vascular permeability and pain, which, although unpleasant to experience, lead to the efflux of useful plasma proteins from the bloodstream to the site of tissue damage [4]. These proteins (complement proteins, coagulation factors, and antibodies) amplify the response and perform surveillance for pathogens. Trauma activates Hageman factor, which is the driving force behind the activation of the clotting cascade, production of bradykinin, and activation of the complement cascade [5]. Thus, all the features of inflammation may be induced simply through trauma and the cascade of mediators activated by Hageman factor. Anyone who has experienced a burn or crush injury can attest to the immediate erythema, warmth, swelling, and ten-

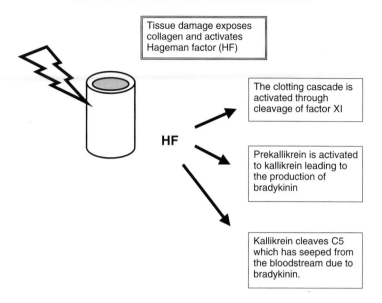

Fig. 1. Early mediators of inflammation. Trauma (*lightning bolt*) exposes collagen and damages blood vessels. Hageman factor is activated and initiates activation of the clotting cascade, the production of bradykinin, and activation of the complement pathway.

derness as a result of these mediators. These elemental inflammatory processes are undoubtedly active in a joint that is red, warm, swollen, and tender. In fact, elevated kininogen and kallikrein have been directly demonstrated in inflamed joints [6].

Subsequent to the clotting cascade, complement activation, and production of bradykinin, platelets become enmeshed in the clot produced at the site of trauma (Fig. 2). Although direct and obvious trauma infrequently contributes to the inflammatory process in JIA, TNFα produced locally induces endothelial cell activation, which in turn activates tissue factor leading to thrombin and fibrin deposition. Entrapment of platelets in the fibrin and adherence to the endothelium leads to platelet activation and release of chemokines CCL5 and CXCR4. These chemokines facilitate neutrophil and monocyte recruitment into the area [7,8]. In this complex response, platelets also release phospholipase A2 leading to the production of arachidonic acid and thromboxane A2. Mast cells that are in the area may also be directly activated through trauma but are more frequently activated after the production of tissue proteases or activation of the complement cascade [9]. Mast cells are notable for their release of preformed mediators such as histamine and leukotrienes [10]. When activated, they also release substantial TNFα, IL-4, IL-5, IL-6, and IL-8. TNFα and IL-8 are important mediators of neutrophil recruitment.

Leukotrienes and other metabolites of arachidonic acid are often the forgotten inflammatory mediators. They are unquestionably important, and the fact that the mainstay of therapy for JIA remains nonsteroidal anti-inflammatory

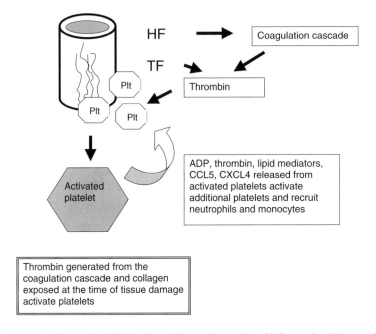

Fig. 2. Platelets (Plt) are technically the first cells to arrive at a site of inflammation. Hageman factor (HF) initiates the clotting cascade leading to generation of thrombin, which activates platelets. Activated platelets in turn release lipid mediators and ADP, which further enhances activation of surrounding platelets. These early steps in inflammation are important in slowing blood flow (clot formation) and increasing vascular permeability (bradykinin), allowing useful plasma proteins, such as complement factors, immunoglobulins, and additional coagulation factors, to enter into the site. Subsequently, cell-dependent processes, such as the release of TNFα from mast cells or monocytes/macrophages, lead to influx of inflammatory cells. TF, tissue factor.

agents (NSAIDs) testifies to the importance of this set of pathways (Fig. 3) [11]. They are not often discussed or studied because they are remarkably difficult to measure using standard laboratory techniques. Their short half-life also discourages study. Nevertheless, these agents have potent proinflammatory activities and are typically considered the late mediators of inflammation. Table 1 describes certain well-described activities of these lipid mediators. Notice that up until this point in the inflammatory process, there is little cell involvement. All the facets of inflammation induced by these early and late mediators are designed primarily to enhance egress of cells and proteins from the blood stream. The vasodilatation, vascular permeability, clot formation, and smooth muscle contraction all lead to slow blood flow and the optimal conditions for neutrophil and monocyte emigration from the bloodstream to the site of damage [12].

The cell-dependent phase of inflammation relies on the directed migration of neutrophils and monocytes to the site of tissue injury. Cellular migration to the site uses complement cleavage products, particularly C5a, as well as the leukotrienes, IL-8, and platelet-activating factor produced locally [13,14]. Mast cell release of TNFα leads to increased expression of endothelial cell adhesion

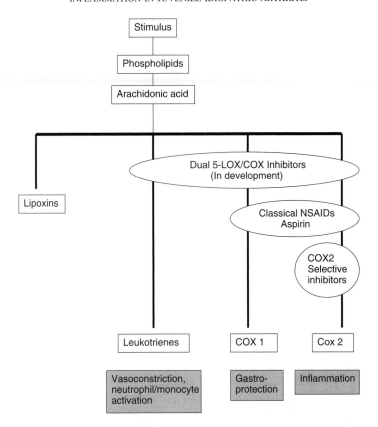

Fig. 3. Lipid mediators are often exploited therapeutically but are poorly understood. These short-lived molecules are released from cells after appropriate activation. Current therapeutics (NSAIDs and aspirin) target cyclooxygenase (COX) 1– and COX 2–mediated processes. The selective COX 2 inhibitors elicit the desired effects on inflammation without the loss of gastroprotective effects mediated by COX 1. Dual lipoxygenase/COX inhibitors are in development and may be more potent because of additional effects on myeloid cells.

molecules, which direct neutrophil rolling [15,16]. Subsequent steps lead to diapedesis of the neutrophils and chemotaxis toward the site of tissue damage. The egress of cells from the bloodstream is exceedingly inefficient in the absence of infection or other stimuli. Bacteria provide a danger signal that is important in directing cells toward a perceived threat. In arthritis, this signal is believed to be provided by activated T cells and stromal cells. In addition to the hematologic and stromal cells participating in the inflammatory process, neural input is also critical. Substance P, bradykinin, serotonin, and prostaglandins are released in response to nociceptor stimulation. These agents enhance inflammation [17]. Thus, local or epidural anesthesia is superior to general anesthesia in preventing thrombosis in the neighborhood of the surgical procedure, because nociceptive responses include the release of plasminogen activators that inhibit fibrinolysis [18]. Lidocaine inhibits platelet activation and neutrophil diapedesis as well,

Table 1
Functions of lipid mediators

Function	Mediator
Pyrogenic	Prostaglandin E2
Vasoconstriction	Thromboxane A2
Vasodilation	Prostaglandins I2, E2, D2, F2
Vascular permeability	Leukotrienes C4, D4, E4
Chemotaxis of phagocytes	Leukotriene B4, 5-hydroxyeicosatetraenoic acid, platelet-activating factor
Platelet aggregation	Thromboxane A2, platelet-activating factor

further dampening the early inflammatory response. Rheumatologists have recognized that in adults, rheumatoid arthritis does not develop in a paralyzed limb [19]. Thus, appropriate analgesia is not simply the humane act of the caregiver, it directly affects the inflammatory process.

This innate phase of inflammation is common to the various forms of arthritis and to inflammation caused by allergic responses, immune complex deposition, and infection. What separates the various types of inflammation are the inciting agent and the character of the cellular infiltrate. Most inflammatory processes involve a mixed cellular infiltrate with neutrophils, monocytes, T cells, B cells, and plasma cells. In JIA, both lymphocytes and myeloid cells are seen easily in the synovial fluid. Neutrophils are nearly always the dominant cell, suggesting that the inflammation is largely produced by cells of the innate immune system. Neutrophils are activated to secrete destructive proteases by TNFα, IL-1, IL-6, and lipoxins, and evidence of neutrophil activation is common in JIA [20,21]. Synovial T cells are the next most common cell type; they are predominantly activated memory cells with a predominance of CD4 T cells, although CD8 T cells constitute a significant minority [22–24]. There are differences between the various subtypes of JIA. Oligoarthritis is associated with the highest level of CD8 T-cell activation but with the lowest relative percentage of infiltrating CD8 T cells [25]. Polyarthritis of both types is associated with overall lower T-cell activation but markedly higher CD4 T-cell infiltration than the other types. The infiltrating T cells are nearly always of a T-helper 1 phenotype [26,27]. This mixed cellular infiltrate is not unique to JIA, nor should the synovial fluid be considered the only manifestation of inflammation. The synovial tissue becomes engorged with new blood vessels, which enhance the migration of inflammatory cells into both the joint space and the synovial tissue [28]. Aggregates of B cells are sometimes seen, a feature common to adult rheumatoid synovium [25,29].

The role of the adaptive immune system in arthritis

The control of cell migration relies on the expression of various adhesion molecules that are either organ-specific or general. Fig. 4 demonstrates the se-

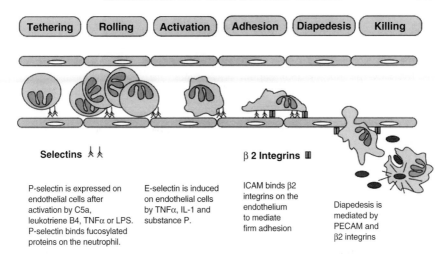

Fig. 4. Adhesion molecules mediate neutrophil migration into the joint. Selectins mediate the early rolling of the cells on the endothelium. Complex conformational changes in adhesion molecules are induced upon activation of the neutrophil and allow slowing of the neutrophil motion. Induction of expression of E-selectin also participates in the slowing of the motion. Actual adhesion to the endothelium is mediated by another class of adhesion molecules, the integrins. Finally, exit from the bloodstream into the tissue requires the joint use of integrins and platelet endothelial cell adhesion molecules (PECAM). Chemotaxis toward the identified threat is usually mediated by chemokines, bacterial cell wall products, or complement component C5a. In JIA, complement and chemokines seem to be the dominant forces leading to influx of neutrophils, monocytes, and lymphocytes. Monocytes and lymphocytes also rely on a similar choreography of adhesion molecules and chemotactic factors to mediate influx into the joint, but the specifics of the molecular events are not as well understood. ICAM, intracellular adhesion molecule; LPS, lipopolysaccharide.

quence of events that controls the migration of neutrophils into the joint. The relative contributions of TNFα, leukotriene B4, and substance P in JIA are not known. In some models of inflammation in JIA, an infectious trigger initially drives the inflammatory processes. T cells, following neutrophils into the inflamed joint, cross-react with host antigens, and the process becomes self-perpetuating as the autoreactive lymphocytes provide additional inflammatory signals [30]. There is little direct evidence for this hypothesis, but it has several attractive features. This section discusses the role of the adaptive immune system.

Both T cells and B cells participate in inflammation. In JIA, specifically, the role of the T cell is much better understood than the role of the B cell. T cells are unusual in that they can recognize antigen only in the context of a major histocompatibility complex (MHC) molecule on an antigen-presenting cell. Not all cells are competent to present antigen; dendritic cells and macrophages most commonly perform that function. The first important distinction is between MHC class I and MHC class II. MHC class I antigens present peptides derived from intracellular proteins. For example, viruses are almost uniformly presented to a T cell in the context of MHC class I. In contrast, MHC class II molecules present peptides from antigens that have been ingested from the extracellular space. These antigens could include bacteria, shed viral antigens, and self proteins (Fig. 5).

The initial data suggesting that T cells are involved in the etiopathogenesis of JIA was the finding that certain HLA types are associated with disease. Specifically, oligoarticular JIA is associated with HLA-A2, -B27, -B35, DR5, and DR8 [31–36]. In these early studies, oligoarthritis likely to represent a spondyloarthropathy was not differentiated from other oligoathritides, and this confounding variable is probably reflected in the association with HLA-B27. Oligoarthritis is also associated with specific DQ antigens, and these can confer a risk of iridocyclitis [37,38]. Thus, patients with DRB1*0801, DRB1*1301,

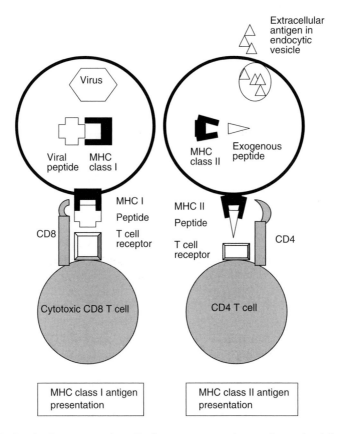

Fig. 5. MHC molecules present antigen. T-cell receptors cannot detect antigen unless it is processed and presented in the context of an MHC molecule. Intracellular antigens are presented primarily to CD8 T cells in the context of MHC class I. Extracellular antigens are presented primarily to CD4 T cells in the context of MHC class II. The molecule CD4 acts as a coreceptor for the T-cell receptor in MHC class II antigen presentation. The CD8 molecule performs a similar function for the T-cell receptor in MHC class I antigen presentation. In the absence of other molecules that signal the T cell that the antigen has been taken up in an inflammatory environment, the T cell will not react. In fact, the T cell often dies or becomes anergic. When the antigen is taken up in an inflammatory environment, the antigen-presenting cell expresses costimulatory molecules that instruct the T cell to become activated.

DR11, DQA1*0401, DQA1*0501, and DQA1*0601 have a higher risk of iridocyclitis. In contrast, polyarticular JIA that is associated with rheumatoid factor is strongly associated with DRB1*04, just as seen in rheumatoid factor–positive adult disease. Early-onset polyarticular disease that is rheumatoid factor–negative is associated with DRB1*0801 and DRB1*11 [39]. In contrast, systemic JIA is not strongly associated with specific HLA types, perhaps suggesting it is not antigen driven [40,41].

These data have a number of implications for the understanding of the disease processes. They certainly validate the current subset definitions of JIA. With different HLA associations, it is likely that the initiating factors are different for each subset of JIA. HLA associations assume the presence of distinct antigens, because each HLA type is optimal for presenting different peptides. Thus, it is believed that JIA associations with MHC class II antigens support the hypothesis that the stimulatory antigen is an exogenous antigen. This hypothesis is tenable but far from certain. There are also JIA–MHC class I associations, and the linkage disequilibrium within the MHC region makes such easy interpretations suspect. In addition, as described later, the MHC can influence immune responses in the absence of antigen presentation.

From the perspective of the antigen-presenting cell, uptake, processing, and presentation of antigens proceed in the same way regardless of whether it is self-protein intended to induce tolerance (an inability to respond to a given antigen) or a foreign protein that is intended to induce an active T-cell response. The different responses are regulated by the presence of a danger signal that the antigen-presenting cell delivers to the T cell at the time of antigen presentation [42]. In the absence of this danger signal, which is typically the expression of costimulatory molecules, presentation of antigen to a T cell results in tolerance or anergy. When a protein is recognized as foreign through opsonization with antibody, engagement of toll-like receptors (innate receptors for pathogens), or the concomitant recognition of inflammatory cytokines, costimulatory molecules such as B7 on the antigen-presenting cell are induced to signal the responding T cell that the threat requires an active response. In the case of JIA, an antigen presented in an inflamed joint would have a ready danger signal.

Although the association of MHC alleles with autoimmune diseases has been recognized for many years, the specific mechanism underlying the association is still not fully understood. There are several hypotheses regarding the role of specific MHC molecules in the predisposition to JIA [43–48].

1. A specific MHC molecule presents the self-protein less effectively than non–disease-related MHC. Inefficient presentation of the self-protein allows the escape of autoreactive T cells to the periphery (ie, inefficient tolerance).
2. A specific MHC molecule may have decreased stability. These unstable molecules present very few peptides, allowing the escape of autoreactive T-cell clones.
3. All the DR types associated with rheumatoid arthritis have a conserved amino acid sequence. The conserved amino acid sequence, or shared

epitope, is LLEQ(K/R)RAA at position 67–74 of the DRB1 chain. These DR antigens select for a very specific population of T cells that are able to present the autoantigen. In rheumatoid arthritis, as in most autoimmune diseases, the specific autoantigen is not known.

4. In another model, the shared epitope of rheumatoid arthritis constitutes the antigen.

5. For the spondyloarthropathies, HLA-B27 may act independently of antigen presentation by altering immune responses. This alteration may relate to the high rate of protein misfolding that occurs with HLA-B27, which could allow the B27 itself to be an antigen or to bind peptides aberrantly.

Data supporting the role of these specific MHC types implicated in JIA as involving antigen comes from the study of the T cells infiltrating the synovial space. Studies have generally concluded that the infiltrating T cells are oligoclonal (derived from one specific family of T cells), supporting the view that a specific antigen drives the process. Although the antigen in each case remains mysterious, it is clear that the synovial T cells have predominantly a memory phenotype, suggesting that they have responded to an antigen, and each subtype of JIA has a distinct cohort of oligoclonal resident T cells.

T cells that have engaged antigen proliferate and release cytokines unless they engaged antigen in the absence of a costimulatory signal (tolerance). Again, each subtype of JIA is associated with T-cell responses of a different character [49–51]. Table 2 describes the cytokines that have been detected in the synovial fluid of patients with different types of JIA.

The consequences of the activated T cells are being defined. Myeloid cytokines and myeloid cells predominate in the synovial fluid, but T cells are thought to be integral to the process for several reasons. B cells are generally incapable of producing IgG antibody in the absence of T-cell help [52]. Additionally, activated T cells can provide signals to antigen-presenting cells that modify their function. Specifically, they are thought to activate monocytes, macrophages, and synovial fibroblasts [53]. These cells then release IL-1, IL-6, and TNFα. These powerful inflammatory mediators drive adhesion molecule expression to recruit additional cells, stimulate matrix metalloproteinases that destroy cartilage, and induce chemokine expression that also participates in cell recruitment and activation [54]. Neutrophil proteases also play an important role in cartilage destruction. The resident T cells act on osteoclasts through osteoprotegerin to stimulate bone resorption. One general model of joint inflammation that addresses the notion of T-cell participation is shown in Fig. 6. This inflammation involves all structures of the joint, including synoviocytes and endothelial cells, which are often considered merely structural. These cells play a role in the inflammation through the regulation of cell migration, elaboration of inflammatory mediators, and production of proteases.

B cells have recently been shown to be active participants in adult rheumatoid arthritis. Their role in JIA is much less clear, however. The few published reports of synovial biopsies of patients with JIA have shown that there are B-cell ag-

Table 2
Synovial cytokines and chemokines in juvenal idiopathic arthritis

JIA type	Mediators	Producing cell type	Effects
Oligoarticular	TNFα	T cells, macrophages, endothelium	acute-phase response, fever, adhesion molecules, chemokines, apoptosis; activates macrophages
	γ-IFN	T cells, NK cells	
	IL-1α/β	macrophages	acute-phase proteins, adhesion molecules, fever, chemokine activation
	IL-6	macrophages, T cells, endothelial cells, stromal cells	acute-phase proteins, B-cell growth
	IL-8/ MCP-1	Many cells	chemotaxis, neutrophil activation, angiogenesis
Spondyloarthropathies/ enthesitis-related arthritis	IL-2	Activated T cells	T-cell apoptosis and stimulation
	TNFα/β	T cells, macrophages, endothelium	acute-phase response, fever, adhesion molecules, chemokines, apoptosis; activates macrophages
	γ-IFN	T cells, NK cells	
	IL-10	macrophages, T cells	inhibits macrophages
RF – Polyarticular	TNFα	T cells, macrophages, endothelium	acute-phase response, fever, adhesion molecules, chemokines, apoptosis
	IL-1α	macrophages	acute-phase proteins, adhesion molecules, fever, chemokine activation
	IL-8/MCP-1	many cells	chemotaxis, neutrophil activation, angiogenesis
RF + polyarticular	TNFα	T cells, macrophages, endothelium	acute-phase response, fever, adhesion molecules, chemokines, apoptosis
	IL-1α	macrophages	acute-phase proteins, adhesion molecules, fever, chemokine activation
	IL-6	macrophages, T cells, endothelial cells, stromal cells	acute-phase proteins, B-cell growth
	IL-8/MCP-1	many cells	chemotaxis, neutrophil activation, angiogenesis
Systemic arthritis	IL-6 (extremely high)	macrophages, T cells, endothelial cells, stromal cells	Acute-phase proteins, B-cell growth
	IL-8/MCP-1	many cells	chemotaxis, neutrophil activation, angiogenesis
	TNFβ (LTα)	many cells	Induction of inflammatory mediators, adhesion molecules, proliferation of fibroblasts
	macrophage migration inhibitory factor	macrophages, pituitary, thymus, others	promotes Th1 T cell development, inhibits hematopoietic development, antagonizes steroid effects

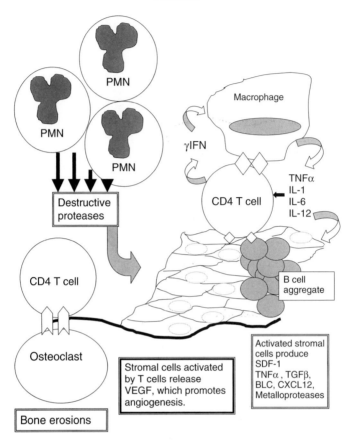

Fig. 6. A simplified view of the many cellular interactions arising in an inflamed joint. The neutrophils are activated by TNFα, IL-1, and other mediators to release destructive proteases such as elastase, collagenase, and myeloperoxidase. These agents can directly destroy synovium and cartilage. T-cell interactions with osteoclasts through receptor activator of NFκB (RANK) can locally activate the osteoclasts to resorb bone and induce erosions. The balance of osteoprotegerin and RANK ligand dictate the outcome of this interaction, and T-cell production of RANK ligand tips the balance toward bone loss. Other T-cell interactions with macrophages and stromal cells lead to the release of other mediators. In this diagram, CD4 T cells are shown; however, CD8 T cells may also participate in similar processes. In particular, activated stromal cell release of vascular endothelial growth factor (VEGF) leads to angiogenesis. Activated stromal cells also produce a variety of chemokines, which mediate cell migration into the joint, the formation of B-cell aggregates, and the release of metalloproteinases. Activation of macrophages by T cells leads to the release of TNFα, IL-1, IL-6, and IL-12. These agents act on the neutrophils and on additional T cells to promote differentiation and activation. This presentation is greatly simplified, because there are many interactions that are cell-contact dependent and many chemokine effects that are poorly characterized. BLC, B-lymphocyte chemoattractant; γIFN, interferon gamma; PMN, polymorphonuclear; SDF-1, stromal derived factor-1; TGFβ, transforming growth factor beta.

gregates in the synovium similar to those seen in adult rheumatoid arthritis [25,29]. This finding suggests that B cells are driven by local production of lymphotoxinα (TNFβ), B-lymphocyte chemoattractant, and T-cell signals. These agents are sufficient to induce B-cell aggregates experimentally [55]. In adult rheumatoid arthritis, the production of rheumatoid factor had suggested B-cell involvement, but there was a strong sense that this observation might represent an epiphenomenon. Recent studies showing improvement in patients with rheumatoid arthritis treated with a monoclonal antibody that depletes B cells have argued forcefully for a more central role for B cells in synovial inflammation [56]. Additionally, animal models demonstrating that a certain type of arthritis can be transferred from animal to animal by injections of cell-free serum have also led to renewed interest in the role of the B cell [56,57]. Oligoarticular JIA is associated with an expansion of B1 cells, a type of B cell independent of T-cell help [58]. The success of a B-cell–depleting antibody has raised as many questions as it has answered, because it achieves its beneficial effect before there is a significant effect on rheumatoid factor titers or on plasma cells that produce the bulk of the antibody. Hypotheses regarding the role of the B cell in light of these findings include B cells acting as antigen-presenting cells and B cells acting as sources of inflammatory mediators.

Consequences of inflammation

Inflammation of a joint is obviously associated with pain and disuse. The usual goal of treatment is to diminish the joint inflammation and restore the child's ability to function normally. This section addresses certain consequences of inflammation that are less obvious.

In adult-onset rheumatoid arthritis, chronic inflammation leads to an increased risk of cardiovascular disease [60]. Although pediatricians do not see the long-term results of therapeutic interventions, they must plan for the entire life of the patient, not just for the pediatric years. To provide insight into the possible long-term consequences of JIA, the lessons of rheumatoid arthritis are useful. It is generally agreed that cardiovascular risk is increased among patients with rheumatoid arthritis [60–62]. Renal disease and malignancies also seem to be increased [61,63]. The renal disease is often caused by vasculitis or amyloidosis, entities that are rare in JIA. The lymphoreticular malignancies may be a consequence of therapy or may be caused by chronic inflammation. At a minimum, the treatment of JIA should attempt to address prolonged systemic inflammation that could put the child at risk for premature coronary artery disease or stroke. In patients with rheumatoid arthritis, the use of methotrexate is associated with reduced risk for cardiovascular disease in spite of its potential to elevate homocysteine [64]. This association is often cited as a strong rationale for aggressive anti-inflammatory therapy for rheumatoid arthritis and supports the use of folic acid supplementation, which somewhat mitigates the increased homocysteine caused by methotrexate. A recent study on the use of statin drugs, typically used to lower cholesterol, found that the use of statins improves lipid parameters in patients with rheumatoid arthritis and improves joint inflammation [65]. No comparable studies have been performed in patients with JIA, but it is certainly imperative to address the long-term cardiac risk factors in patients with JIA and other chronic inflammatory diseases of childhood.

One important pediatric study attempted to define whether cardiovascular disease is an issue for patients with JIA. Aortic stiffness was measured by phase-contrast MRI in 31 JIA patients [66]. Increased aortic stiffness was seen in JIA patients with increasing age. There was no correlation with any specific type of JIA. Another study demonstrated that JIA patients have an elevated level of plasma homocysteine [67], which is known to be an independent risk factor for coronary artery disease. These data suggest that early vascular changes are occurring in children with JIA.

One surprise from recent outcome studies of JIA is that disability and active disease are common in adults who had JIA as children [2,68]. A significant percentage of affected adults had rheumatoid factor–positive JIA, which represents a pediatric onset of rheumatoid arthritis. Thus, it is no surprise that those patients continue to have active disease and accrue disability over time. What is surprising is that joint inflammation persists in so many other JIA patients well into adulthood (more than 40% in one study). Uveitis and glaucoma were also seen with distressing frequency in adults who had JIA as children. These studies are a testament that JIA can be a lifelong disorder in spite of its name. Therapeutic efforts should be targeted to limit irreversible joint damage, not just for the short term but over decades. The lessons of rheumatoid arthritis also suggest that therapy should address the systemic inflammation that can increase the risk of cardiovascular disease.

Other long-term issues relate to ongoing inflammation in patients with JIA. Osteopenia is common: approximately 40% of patients with JIA are osteopenic [69]. Longer disease duration and increased disability are risk factors for osteopenia, as one would expect [70]. Osteopenia is not specific to any one type of JIA. Although lack of weight bearing certainly contributes, the association of longer disease duration with osteopenia suggests that there is a direct effect from inflammation. Data supporting a role for TNFα in enhancing osteoclast activity support the idea that inflammation has a effect on general bone metabolism, not merely within the affected joint space. The implications of this finding again force pediatricians to consider the long-term effects of their actions. The role of bisphosphonates in JIA has not been adequately studied, but certainly maximizing the intake of calcium and vitamin D, encouraging weight-bearing exercises, and controlling disease activity should all be attempted to prevent the development of osteopenia [70].

Another possible consequence of JIA is decreased fertility. There is no comparable finding in adult rheumatoid arthritis, although there have not been any detailed studies, and the relationship to inflammation is uncertain. Inflammation could theoretically affect fertility. Specifically, TNFα seems to affect fertility for both men and women [71,72]. Only one study has directly addressed fertility in

JIA, but the findings are surprising and remarkable enough that the potential for fertility issues should be discussed with patients [73]. Women with a history of JIA were recruited. Nearly half had persistently active arthritis. Premature ovarian failure unrelated to medication use was seen in 3.4% of the patients. Additional patients had premature ovarian failure caused by chlorambucil use. This percentage is significantly higher than in the general population, in which premature ovarian failure is typically seen in 1%. Although a delay in first pregnancy could be caused by chronic illness, women with a history of JIA had their first child at an average of 27 years of age, compared with 23 years of age for the general population. Whether the phenomenon results from illness or from difficulty conceiving, the importance of this delayed childbearing is that 2% of the patients in this study experienced premature ovarian failure before 30 years of age.

The most dramatic systemic inflammation is seen in patients with systemic JIA. This disorder is somewhat different from the other forms of JIA. Fewer data support a role for T-cell and antigen-specific responses, and many of the manifestations seem to be caused by the overproduction of IL-6 (Fig. 7) [74]. This situation is in contrast to polyarticular and oligoarticular JIA, in which most of the manifestations are thought to be caused by TNFα. Many patients with systemic JIA have a self-limited course and require therapy for a relatively short period of time. A minority of patients with systemic JIA have extremely troubling disease. The joint disease is aggressive, and there is typically significant failure to thrive. The fevers are not merely draining: they are ruinous to the child. Evidence of myeloid activation dominates [75]. Hepatosplenomegaly, adenopathy, rash, and anemia are frequent. These patients seldom respond adequately to TNFα inhibitors, and the dose of steroid required to control the disease is often untenable for the long term. This subset of patients can develop amyloidosis as the result of chronic inflammation [76]. In addition to amyloidosis, which can be fatal, some children develop an entity called "macrophage activation syndrome" or, more properly, "hemophagocytic lymphohistiocytosis" (HLH) [77].

HLH can be caused by an inherited immunodeficiency, malignancy, or an underlying autoimmune disease. Rarely, it may occur in a previously healthy person. Systemic JIA is the autoimmune disease with the highest frequency of HLH. It is often precipitated by a viral infection. The pathologic sequence of events is that the viral infection is poorly controlled by natural killer cells and cytotoxic T cells, which nevertheless attempt to contain the infection through the secretion of inflammatory cytokines [78–80]. These cytokines activate macrophages systemically, which ingest hematopoietic cells and cause progressive pancytopenia. The treatment for HLH in this setting typically addresses the cytokine release through the use of cyclosporine and high doses of steroids.

The management of severe systemic-onset JIA typically requires the aggressive use of anti-inflammatory agents and surveillance for HLH. Neither methotrexate nor TNFα inhibitors seem to be as effective in this type of JIA as in other patients with polyarticular JIA. Early trials of an IL-6 inhibitor are extremely promising, suggesting IL-6 production participates in the pathologic processes [74,81]. Patients with this progressive form of systemic JIA suffer

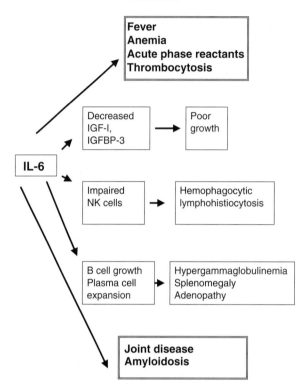

Fig. 7. IL-6 is an important mediator in all forms of JIA, but it is extremely elevated in systemic JIA and may mediate the features unique to systemic JIA. This subset of JIA is associated with high spiking fevers, anemia, rash, growth failure, expansion of secondary lymphoid organs, and a predisposition to a complication known as hemophagocytic lymphohistiocytosis. Not all of these features are directly attributable to IL-6. IL-6 can directly induce fever, acute-phase reactants, and anemia. It is also thought to incite inflammation in the joint directly through effects on the myeloid compartment. Systemic JIA is associated more strongly than the other subsets with neutrophil and monocyte activation and is less associated with T-cell activation. IL-6, through effects on insulin-like growth factor (IGF-1) and insulin like growth factor binding protein (IGFBP-3), can decrease linear growth. IL-6 at high levels decreases natural killer (NK) cell function, which is thought to be a prerequisite for hemophagocytic lymphohistiocytosis. IL-6 also acts as a B-cell growth factor, which may explain the expansion of the secondary lymphoid structures.

nearly all the consequences of prolonged inflammation. They have osteopenia, growth failure, anemia, and anorexia. Over the long term, they are at risk for amyloidosis. Cardiovascular risk has not been assessed in this population.

Implications for therapy

Many patients with JIA are successfully treated with NSAIDs or a combination of NSAIDs and intra-articular steroids. Unfortunately, recent studies of adults with a history of JIA have clearly shown that nearly half the patients continue to have active disease into adulthood [68]. This prolonged inflammation requires long-term strategies. Although NSAIDs still have a role, methotrexate is usually added when the child does not respond to NSAIDs [59]. Methotrexate in high doses has a cytotoxic and antiproliferative effect from the inhibition of dihydrofolate reductase. At lower doses it acts primarily as an anti-inflammatory through effects on adenosine and TNFα. The central role of TNFα in joint inflammation (Fig. 8) is the underlying explanation for the efficacy of methotrexate and TNFα inhibitors [82].

Another agent often used in patients who do not respond to NSAID therapy is sulfasalazine. This agent impairs phagocytic cell migration and impairs IL-8 secretion [83]. It has a beneficial effect on gut inflammation and for this reason often is used for spondyloarthropathies, which often have subclinical gut

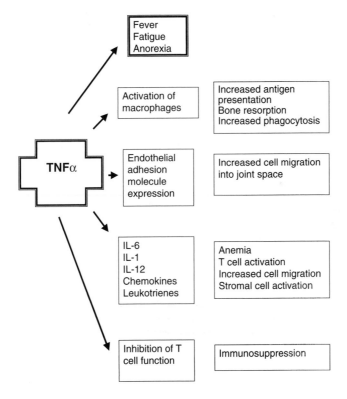

Fig. 8. TNFα is the cytokine that seems to mediate many of the effects seen in oligoarticular and polyarticular JIA. It directly induces fever, fatigue, anorexia, and the production of acute-phase reactants. Indirectly, it mediates cell influx into the joint space through its ability to induce the expression of adhesion molecules. TNFα is also critical for macrophage and dendritic cell activation. These cells present antigen, and their activation by TNFα provides the signal to the T cells that the antigen is dangerous and a proliferative T-cell response is required. TNFα also has many distal effects arising from its ability to stimulate a wide variety of other cells to release chemokines and other inflammatory mediators. Therefore, TNFα inhibitors address systemic signs of inflammation and the cellular influx into the joint that leads to joint destruction.

involvement. Sulfasalazine also impairs the production of IL-1 and TNFα, both of which are known to have important effects in the joint space [84].

The major advance in the treatment of JIA has also been the major advance in the treatment of rheumatoid arthritis. The use of cytokine inhibitors has led to improvement in symptoms and has arrested the progression of bone erosion [85,86]. Fig. 8 demonstrates the major functions of TNFα. TNFα inhibition is associated with decreased cellularity of the synovial fluid because migration is inhibited in the absence of TNFα-mediated adhesion molecule expression. The inflammatory mediators within the joint are also inhibited, thus accounting for the rapid decrease in pain. Over the long term, TNFα inhibition is associated with restoration of normal T-cell function [87]. Active systemic inflammation is associated with acquired T-cell dysfunction and immunologic compromise. The most worrisome adverse events associated with inhibition of TNFα are lymphoma and infections with intracellular organisms [88,89]. The mechanism underlying the predisposition to lymphoma (which has not been conclusively established) is not completely understood. The mechanism underlying the predisposition to intracellular organisms is the role of TNFα in the activation of macrophage intracellular killing and the formation of granulomas.

Summary

Inflammation in JIA results from the interaction of myeloid, lymphoid, and stromal cells, cartilage destruction, bone erosion, and debility These cells and the mediators they release cause cartilage destruction, bone erosion, and debility. Neutrophils are thought to mediate much of the actual destruction within a joint; however, many cases of JIA are not associated with boney erosions, but there is significant inflammation caused by the cellular infiltrate and the proliferation of synoviocytes. NSAIDs address many of the non–cell-dependent aspects of inflammation. Disease-modifying drugs are required for resistant or progressive disease. These agents are effective in modifying the cellular interactions that perpetuate inflammation. In particular, TNFα inhibitors impair cell migration into the joint and reduce macrophage functions.

References

[1] Petty RE, Southwood TR, Baum J, Bhettay E, Glass DN, Manners P, et al. Revision of the proposed classification criteria for juvenile idiopathic arthritis: Durban, 1997. J Rheumatol 1998;25:1991–4.

[2] Ravelli A. Toward an understanding of the long-term outcome of juvenile idiopathic arthritis. Clin Exp Rheumatol 2004;22:271–5.

[3] Burgos-Vargas R. Juvenile onset spondyloarthropathies: therapeutic aspects. Ann Rheum Dis 2002;61(Suppl 3):iii33–9.

[4] Hargreaves KM, Roszkowski MT, Swift JQ. Bradykinin and inflammatory pain. Agents Actions Suppl 1993;41:65–73.

[5] Kaplan AP. Hageman factor-dependent pathways: mechanism of initiation and bradykinin formation. Fed Proc 1983;42:3123–7.

[6] Volpe-Junior N, Donadi EA, Carvalho IF, Reis ML. Augmented plasma and tissue kallikrein like activity in synovial fluid of patients with inflammatory articular diseases. Inflamm Res 1996;45:198–202.

[7] Sambrano GR, Weiss EJ, Zheng YW, Huang W, Coughlin SR. Role of thrombin signalling in platelets in haemostasis and thrombosis. Nature 2001;413:74–8.

[8] Wagner DD, Burger PC. Platelets in inflammation and thrombosis. Arterioscler Thromb Vasc Biol 2003;23:2131–7.

[9] Paterson NA, Wasserman SI, Said JW, Austen KF. Release of chemical mediators from partially purified human lung mast cells. J Immunol 1976;117:1356–62.

[10] Dvorak AM, Schleimer RP, Lichtenstein LM. Human mast cells synthesize new granules during recovery from degranulation. In vitro studies with mast cells purified from human lungs. Blood 1988;71:76–85.

[11] Kulas DT, Schanberg L. Juvenile idiopathic arthritis. Curr Opin Rheumatol 2001;13:392–8.

[12] Edens HA, Parkos CA. Neutrophil transendothelial migration and alteration in vascular permeability: focus on neutrophil-derived azurocidin. Curr Opin Hematol 2003;10:25–30.

[13] Kruse-Elliott KT. Pulmonary and neutrophil responses to priming effects of platelet-activating factor in pigs. Am J Vet Res 1997;58:1386–91.

[14] Schmidt S, Haase G, Csomor E, Lutticken R, Peltroche-Llacsahuanga H. Inhibitor of complement, Compstatin, prevents polymer-mediated Mac-1 up-regulation of human neutrophils independent of biomaterial type tested. J Biomed Mater Res 2003;66A:491–9.

[15] Gibbs BF, Wierecky J, Welker P, Henz BM, Wolff HH, Grabbe J. Human skin mast cells rapidly release preformed and newly generated TNF-alpha and IL-8 following stimulation with anti-IgE and other secretagogues. Exp Dermatol 2001;10:312–20.

[16] Mattila P, Majuri ML, Mattila PS, Renkonen R. TNF alpha-induced expression of endothelial adhesion molecules, ICAM-1 and VCAM-1, is linked to protein kinase C activation. Scand J Immunol 1992;36:159–65.

[17] MacGregor RR, Thorner RE, Wright DM. Lidocaine inhibits granulocyte adherence and prevents granulocyte delivery to inflammatory sites. Blood 1980;56:203–9.

[18] Hahnenkamp K, Theilmeier G, Van Aken HK, Hoenemann CW. The effects of local anesthetics on perioperative coagulation, inflammation, and microcirculation [see comment]. Anesth Analg 2002;94:1441–7.

[19] Baerwald CG, Panayi GS. Neurohumoral mechanisms in rheumatoid arthritis. Scand J Rheumatol 1997;26:1–3.

[20] Foell D, Wittkowski H, Hammerschmidt I, Wulffraat N, Schmeling H, Frosch M, et al. Monitoring neutrophil activation in juvenile rheumatoid arthritis by S100A12 serum concentrations. Arthritis Rheum 2004;50:1286–95.

[21] Jarvis JN, Tang Y, Dozmorov I, Jiang K, Frank B, Chen Y, et al. Gene expression arrays reveal chronic intrinsic activation of neutrophils in children with polyarticular JRA. Is JRA primarily a neutrophil disorder? [abstract]. Arthritis Rheum 2004;50(Suppl):1114.

[22] Silverman ED, Isacovics B, Petsche D, Laxer RM. Synovial fluid cells in juvenile arthritis: evidence of selective T cell migration to inflamed tissue. Clin Exp Immunol 1993;91:90–5.

[23] Sediva A, Hoza J, Nemcova D, Pospisilova D, Bartunkova J, Vencovsky J. Immunological investigation in children with juvenile chronic arthritis. Med Sci Monit 2001;7:99–104.

[24] Thompson SD, Luyrink LK, Graham TB, Tsoras M, Ryan M, Passo MH, et al. Chemokine receptor CCR4 on CD4 + T cells in juvenile rheumatoid arthritis synovial fluid defines a subset of cells with increased IL-4:IFN-gamma mRNA ratios. J Immunol 2001;166:6899–906.

[25] Murray KJ, Luyrink L, Grom AA, Passo MH, Emery H, Witte D, et al. Immunohistological characteristics of T cell infiltrates in different forms of childhood onset chronic arthritis. J Rheumatol 1996;23:2116–24.

[26] Wedderburn LR, Robinson N, Patel A, Varsani H, Woo P. Selective recruitment of polarized T cells expressing CCR5 and CXCR3 to the inflamed joints of children with juvenile idiopathic arthritis. Arthritis Rheum 2000;43:765–74.

[27] Huang JL, Kuo ML, Hung IJ, Wu CJ, Ou LH, Cheng JH. Lowered IL-4-producing T cells and decreased IL-4 secretion in peripheral blood from subjects with juvenile rheumatoid arthritis. Chang Gung Med J 2001;24:77–83.

[28] Shahin AA, Shaker OG, Kamal N, Hafez HA, Gaber W, Shahin HA. Circulating interleukin-6, soluble interleukin-2 receptors, tumor necrosis factor alpha, and interleukin-10 levels in juvenile chronic arthritis: correlations with soft tissue vascularity assessed by power Doppler sonography. Rheumatol Int 2002;22:84–8.

[29] Gregorio A, Gerloni V, Ferlito F, Parafioriti A, Gregorio S, Viola S, et al. Lymphoid neogenesis in the synovial tissue of patients with JIA. Arthritis Rheum 2004;50(Suppl):873.

[30] Blair PJ, Riley JL, Harlan DM, Abe R, Tadaki DK, Hoffmann SC, et al. CD40 ligand (CD154) triggers a short-term CD4(+) T cell activation response that results in secretion of immunomodulatory cytokines and apoptosis. J Exp Med 2000;191:651–60.

[31] Prahalad S, Ryan MH, Shear ES, Thompson SD, Giannini EH, Glass DN. Juvenile rheumatoid arthritis: linkage to HLA demonstrated by allele sharing in affected sibpairs. Arthritis Rheum 2000;43:2335–8.

[32] Moroldo MB, Donnelly P, Saunders J, Glass DN, Giannini EH. Transmission disequilibrium as a test of linkage and association between HLA alleles and pauciarticular-onset juvenile rheumatoid arthritis. Arthritis Rheum 1998;41:1620–4.

[33] Howard JF, Sigsbee A, Glass DN. HLA genetics and inherited predisposition to JRA. J Rheumatol 1985;12:7–12.

[34] Giannini EH, Malagon CN, Van Kerckhove C, Taylor J, Lovell DJ, Levinson JE, et al. Longitudinal analysis of HLA associated risks for iridocyclitis in juvenile rheumatoid arthritis. J Rheumatol 1991;18:1394–7.

[35] Fraser PA, Stern S, Larson MG, Marcus-Bagley D, Awdeh Z, Glass DN, et al. HLA extended haplotypes in childhood and adult onset HLA-DR4-associated arthropathies. Tissue Antigens 1990;35:56–9.

[36] Alsaeid KM, Haider MZ, al-Awadhi AM, Srivastva BS, Ayoub EM. Role of human leukocyte antigen DRB1*0307 and DRB1*0308 in susceptibility to juvenile rheumatoid arthritis. Clin Exp Rheumatol 2003;21:399–402.

[37] Ihle J, Fleckenstein B, Terreaux C, Beck H, Albert ED, Dannecker GE. Differential peptide binding motif for three juvenile arthritis associated HLA-DQ molecules. Clin Exp Rheumatol 2003;21:257–62.

[38] Miller ML, Fraser PA, Jackson JM, Larson MG, Petersen RA, Chylack Jr LT, et al. Inherited predisposition to iridocyclitis with juvenile rheumatoid arthritis: selectivity among HLA-DR5 haplotypes. Proc Natl Acad Sci U S A 1984;81:3539–42.

[39] van Kerckhove C, Luyrink L, Taylor J, Melin-Aldana H, Balakrishnan K, Maksymowych W, et al. HLA-DQA1*0101 haplotypes and disease outcome in early onset pauciarticular juvenile rheumatoid arthritis. J Rheumatol 1991;18:874–9.

[40] Glass DN, Litvin DA. Heterogeneity of HLA associations in systemic onset juvenile rheumatoid arthritis. Arthritis Rheum 1980;23:796–9.

[41] Miller ML, Aaron S, Jackson J, Fraser P, Cairns L, Hoch S, et al. HLA gene frequencies in children and adults with systemic onset juvenile rheumatoid arthritis. Arthritis Rheum 1985;28:146–50.

[42] Gallucci S, Matzinger P. Danger signals: SOS to the immune system. Curr Opin Immunol 2001;13:114–9.

[43] McDevitt HO. The role of MHC class II molecules in susceptibility and resistance to autoimmunity. Curr Opin Immunol 1998;10:677–81.

[44] Baum H, Davies H, Peakman M. Molecular mimicry in the MHC: hidden clues to autoimmunity? Immunol Today 1996;17:64–70.

[45] Scofield RH, Warren WL, Koelsch G, Harley JB. A hypothesis for the HLA-B27 immune dysregulation in spondyloarthropathy: contributions from enteric organisms, B27 structure, peptides bound by B27, and convergent evolution. Proc Natl Acad Sci U S A 1993;90:9330–4.

[46] Colbert RA. HLA-B27 misfolding: a solution to the spondyloarthropathy conundrum? Mol Med Today 2000;6:224–30.

[47] Gregersen PK, Silver J, Winchester RJ. The shared epitope hypothesis. An approach to understanding the molecular genetics of susceptibility to rheumatoid arthritis. Arthritis Rheum 1987;30:1205–13.

[48] McColl GJ, Szer J, Kohaska H, Wicks IP. High dose chemotherapy and syngeneic progenitor cell transplantation for severe adult onset Still's disease. Arthritis Rheum 1998;41:1703.

[49] Murray KJ, Grom AA, Thompson SD, Lieuwen D, Passo MH, Glass DN. Contrasting cytokine profiles in the synovium of different forms of juvenile rheumatoid arthritis and juvenile spondyloarthropathy: prominence of interleukin 4 in restricted disease. J Rheumatol 1998;25: 1388–98.

[50] Mangge H, Schauenstein K. Cytokines in juvenile rheumatoid arthritis (JRA). Cytokine 1998; 10:471–80.

[51] Muzaffer MA, Dayer JM, Feldman BM, Pruzanski W, Roux-Lombard P, Schneider R, et al. Differences in the profiles of circulating levels of soluble tumor necrosis factor receptors and interleukin 1 receptor antagonist reflect the heterogeneity of the subgroups of juvenile rheumatoid arthritis. J Rheumatol 2002;29:1071–8.

[52] Cook MC, Basten A, Fazekas de St Groth B. Rescue of self-reactive B cells by provision of T cell help in vivo. Eur J Immunol 1998;28:2549–58.

[53] Wu Y, Liu Y. Viral induction of co-stimulatory activity on antigen-presenting cells bypasses the need for CD4 + T-cell help in CD8 + T-cell responses. Curr Biol 1994;4:499–505.

[54] Choy EH, Panayi GS. Cytokine pathways and joint inflammation in rheumatoid arthritis. N Engl J Med 2001;344:907–16.

[55] Buckley CD. Why does chronic inflammatory joint disease persist? Clin Med 2003;3:361–6.

[56] Edwards JC, Szczepanski L, Szechinski J, Filipowicz-Sosnowska A, Emery P, Close DR, et al. Efficacy of B-cell-targeted therapy with rituximab in patients with rheumatoid arthritis. N Engl J Med 2004;350:2572–81.

[57] Ji H, Ohmura K, Mahmood U, Lee DM, Hofhuis FM, Boackle SA, et al. Arthritis critically dependent on innate immune system players. Immunity 2002;16:157–68.

[58] Wouters CH, Ceuppens JL, Stevens EA. Different circulating lymphocyte profiles in patients with different subtypes of juvenile idiopathic arthritis. Clin Exp Rheumatol 2002;20: 239–48.

[59] Manners PJ. State of the art: Juvenile idiopathic arthritis. APLAR J Rheumatol 2002;5:29–34.

[60] Goodson N. Coronary artery disease and rheumatoid arthritis. Curr Opin Rheumatol 2002; 14:115–20.

[61] Thomas E, Symmons DP, Brewster DH, Black RJ, Macfarlane GJ. National study of cause-specific mortality in rheumatoid arthritis, juvenile chronic arthritis, and other rheumatic conditions: a 20 year followup study. J Rheumatol 2003;30:958–65.

[62] Watson DJ, Rhodes T, Guess HA. All-cause mortality and vascular events among patients with rheumatoid arthritis, osteoarthritis, or no arthritis in the UK General Practice Research Database. J Rheumatol 2003;30:1196–202.

[63] Sihvonen S, Korpela M, Mustonen J, Laippala P, Pasternack A. Renal disease as a predictor of increased mortality among patients with rheumatoid arthritis. Nephron Clin Pract 2004; 96:c107–14.

[64] Choi HK, Hernan MA, Seeger JD, Robins JM, Wolfe F. Methotrexate and mortality in patients with rheumatoid arthritis: a prospective study. Lancet 2002;359:1173–7.

[65] McCarey DW, McInnes IB, Madhok R, Hampson R, Scherbakov O, Ford I, et al. Trial of Atorvastatin in Rheumatoid Arthritis (TARA): double-blind, randomised placebo-controlled trial [see comment]. Lancet 2004;363:2015–21.

[66] Argyropoulou MI, Kiortsis DN, Daskas N, Xydis V, Mavridis A, Efremidis SC, et al. Distensibility and pulse wave velocity of the thoracic aorta in patients with juvenile idiopathic arthritis: an MRI study. Clin Exp Rheumatol 2003;21:794–7.

[67] Huemer M, Fodinger M, Huemer C, Sailer-Hock M, Falger J, Rettenbacher A, et al. Hyperhomocysteinemia in children with juvenile idiopathic arthritis is not influenced by methotrexate treatment and folic acid supplementation: a pilot study. Clin Exp Rheumatol 2003;21:249–55.

[68] Packham JC, Hall MA. Long-term follow-up of 246 adults with juvenile idiopathic arthritis: functional outcome. Rheumatology 2002;41:1428–35.

[69] Lien G, Flato B, Haugen M, Vinje O, Sorskaar D, Dale K, et al. Frequency of osteopenia in adolescents with early-onset juvenile idiopathic arthritis: a long-term outcome study of one hundred five patients [see comment]. Arthritis Rheum 2003;48:2214–23.

[70] French AR, Mason T, Nelson AM, Crowson CS, O'Fallon WM, Khosla S, et al. Osteopenia in adults with a history of juvenile rheumatoid arthritis. A population based study. J Rheumatol 2002;29:1065–70.

[71] Kocak I, Yenisey C, Dundar M, Okyay P, Serter M. Relationship between seminal plasma interleukin-6 and tumor necrosis factor alpha levels with semen parameters in fertile and infertile men. Urol Res 2002;30:263–7.

[72] Naz RK, Butler A, Witt BR, Barad D, Menge AC. Levels of interferon-gamma and tumor necrosis factor-alpha in sera and cervical mucus of fertile and infertile women: implication in infertility. J Reprod Immunol 1995;29:105–17.

[73] Packham JC, Hall MA. Premature ovarian failure in women with juvenile idiopathic arthritis (JIA). Clin Exp Rheumatol 2003;21:347–50.

[74] Yokota S. Interleukin 6 as a therapeutic target in systemic-onset juvenile idiopathic arthritis. Curr Opin Rheumatol 2003;15:581–6.

[75] Frosch M, Vogl T, Seeliger S, Wulffraat N, Kuis W, Viemann D, et al. Expression of myeloid-related proteins 8 and 14 in systemic-onset juvenile rheumatoid arthritis. Arthritis Rheum 2003;48:2622–6.

[76] Savolainen HA, Isomaki HA. Decrease in the number of deaths from secondary amyloidosis in patients with juvenile rheumatoid arthritis. J Rheumatol 1993;20:1201–3.

[77] Grom AA. Macrophage activation syndrome and reactive hemophagocytic lymphohistiocytosis: the same entities? Curr Opin Rheumatol 2003;15:587–90.

[78] Henter JI. Biology and treatment of familial hemophagocytic lymphohistiocytosis: importance of perforin in lymphocyte-mediated cytotoxicity and triggering of apoptosis. Med Pediatr Oncol 2002;38:305–9.

[79] Aggarwal A, Misra R. Methotrexate inhibits interleukin-6 production in patients with juvenile rheumatoid arthritis. Rheumatol Int 2003;23:134–7.

[80] Quartier P, Taupin P, Bourdeaut F, Lemelle I, Pillet P, Bost M, et al. Efficacy of etanercept for the treatment of juvenile idiopathic arthritis according to the onset type. Arthritis Rheum 2003; 48:1093–101.

[81] Yokota S, Imagawa T, Miyamae T, Mori M, Nishimoto N, Kishimoto T. Long-term therapeutic experience of humanized anti-IL-6 monoclonal antibody in systemic onset juvenile idiopathic arthritis [abstract]. Arthritis Rheum 2004;50(Suppl):1100.

[82] Dekker L, Armbrust W, Rademaker CM, Prakken B, Kuis W, Wulffraat NM. Safety of anti-TNFalpha therapy in children with juvenile idiopathic arthritis. Clin Exp Rheumatol 2004;22: 252–8.

[83] Nielsen OH, Bukhave K, Elmgreen J, Ahnfelt-Ronne I. Inhibition of 5-lipoxygenase pathway of arachidonic acid metabolism in human neutrophils by sulfasalazine and 5-aminosalicylic acid. Dig Dis Sci 1987;32:577–82.

[84] Bissonnette EY, Enciso JA, Befus AD. Inhibitory effects of sulfasalazine and its metabolites on histamine release and TNF-alpha production by mast cells. J Immunol 1996;156:218–23.

[85] Lovell DJ, Giannini EH, Reiff A, Jones OY, Schneider R, Olson JC, et al. Long-term efficacy and safety of etanercept in children with polyarticular-course juvenile rheumatoid arthritis: interim results from an ongoing multicenter, open-label, extended-treatment trial. Arthritis Rheum 2003;48:218–26.

[86] Lovell DJ, Giannini EH, Reiff A, Cawkwell GD, Silverman ED, Nocton JJ, et al. Etanercept in children with polyarticular juvenile rheumatoid arthritis. Pediatric Rheumatology Collaborative Study Group. N Engl J Med 2000;342:763–9.

[87] Isomaki P, Panesar M, Annenkov A, Clark JM, Foxwell BM, Chernajovsky Y, et al. Prolonged exposure of T cells to TNF down-regulates TCRzeta and expression of the TCR/CD3 complex at the cell surface. J Immunol 2001;166:5495–507.

[88] Brown SL, Greene MH, Gershon SK, Edwards ET, Braun MM. Tumor necrosis factor antago-
     nist therapy and lymphoma development: twenty-six cases reported to the Food and Drug
     Administration. Arthritis Rheum 2002;46:3151–8.
[89] Gomez-Reino JJ, Carmona L, Valverde VR, Mola EM, Montero MD. Group B: treatment
     of rheumatoid arthritis with tumor necrosis factor inhibitors may predispose to significant
     increase in tuberculosis risk: a multicenter active-surveillance report. Arthritis Rheum 2003;
     48:2122–7.

ELSEVIER
SAUNDERS

PEDIATRIC CLINICS
OF NORTH AMERICA

Pediatr Clin N Am 52 (2005) 359–372

Measurement of Health Status, Functional Status, and Quality of Life in Children with Juvenile Idiopathic Arthritis: Clinical Science for the Pediatrician

Ciarán M. Duffy, MB, BCh, MSc, FRCPC[a,b,c,*]

[a]Division of Paediatric Rheumatology, Montreal Children's Hospital, 2300 Tupper Street,
Room C503, Montreal, Quebec, H3H 1P3 Canada
[b]McGill University Health Centre, 1650 Avenue Cedar, Montreal, Quebec, H3G 1A4, Canada
[c]McGill University, 845 Sherbrooke St. W. Montreal, Quebec, H3A 2T5 Canada

The historical focus in assessment of children with juvenile idiopathic arthritis (JIA) [1] has been on hard outcomes such as persistent disease activity, disease remission, joint damage, and organ system damage. A number of the measures of these outcomes have been grouped as a core set and used to define improvement in JIA [2]. These outcomes are important and need to be measured. JIA, however, like most other chronic diseases of childhood, influences virtually all aspects of the child's life, including physical, social, emotional, intellectual, and economic aspects, and affects the entire family with ultimate effects on the child's overall outcome [3,4]. Thus, there is also a need for a more all-encompassing picture of the health status, functional status, socioeconomic status, and quality of life (QoL) of these children.

Unfortunately, the terminology in this area can be confusing, because the terms health status, functional status, and QoL are frequently used interchangeably. Thus they merit definition. Health status is an overall point estimate of a person's well being in physical, psychologic, and social terms compared with some baseline assessment. Functional status is a broad summary statement

* Division of Rheumatology, Montreal Children's Hospital, 2300 Tupper Street, Room C503, Montreal, Quebec, H3H 1P3 Canada.
 E-mail address: ciaran.duffy@muhc.mcgill.ca

0031-3955/05/$ – see front matter © 2005 Elsevier Inc. All rights reserved.
doi:10.1016/j.pcl.2005.01.009

with respect to the effect of a disease on the patient's ability to carry out usual tasks, such as the activities of daily living. QoL includes both health status and functional status. Moreover, measurement of QoL should attempt to incorporate some aspect of the patient's own perception of which aspects of his/her life are significantly affected and the extent to which this perception is influenced by the disease [5]. QoL measures used in the clinical domain tend to focus on health-related quality of life (HRQoL).

All such measures may be divided into generic and disease-specific measures [6]. Generic measures have broad application across different types and severity of disease, across different treatments, and across cultural subgroups. Disease-specific measures are designed to assess specific diseases or patient populations and, as such, are usually more responsive to changes in the status of the individual subject. Considerable work has been conducted in JIA in the past 15 years to develop new measures, including functional status and HRQoL measures, in an effort to define better the overall outcomes for these children. Comprehensive reviews provide a more detailed discussion of these issues [7–9]. This article focuses on the general process of measure development, some of the specific measures developed for JIA, and their use in defining patient outcomes.

Process of outcome measure development

Although the processes of developing and validating outcome measures have been well established [10,11], a short discussion is necessary because the approach is unfamiliar to most pediatricians. In setting out to develop a measure, one must clearly understand the precise purpose of the measurement. There are many compendia of measures, and it is incumbent upon the investigator to review what measures are available before pursuing the laborious task of developing a new one. One may be surprised to find that such a measure already exists. When no such measure exists, the long process of development commences. This process entails a series of steps including item generation, item reduction, item presentation and scaling, and assessing reliability, validity, and responsiveness (Box 1). Each step, in essence, entails a different study. The initial phases aim to establish the content of the format of the measure. The later phases aim to establish the measurement properties of the instrument. The process of developing and validating disease-specific measures for children with JIA has been described thoroughly [12,13]. The approach is discussed here briefly.

Items for inclusion in the measure may be derived from a review of the literature, together with a series of interviews of patients, parents of patients, and experts in the field of pediatric rheumatology including pediatric rheumatologists, nurses, therapists, and other members of the extended health care team. Examples of potential items include using a scissors to cut paper, brushing teeth, school absences, feeling sad, and so forth. This process generates many items. The number of items must be reduced to a more manageable number by

---

Box 1. Steps involved and properties required for an ideal measure for juvenile idiopathic arthritis

Steps involved

    Item generation
    Item reduction
    Item presentation
    Item scaling

Required properties

    Reliability
    Validity
    Responsiveness (sensitivity to change)
    Discriminative ability
    Ease of use and scoring
    Applicability to a wide age range and heterogeneous population

---

identifying those that are most pertinent to the purpose of the measure, most important to the patient, and occur most frequently. This reduction is generally performed by a panel of experts in the field of pediatric rheumatology, patients, and parents of patients. The panel scores the items in some categorical fashion, and these scores are used to reduce the item number. Thereafter, items are presented, and a process of scaling is determined. Generally, this process entails ensuring that the components and their description make sense, are presented in an easily understood way, and are easy to complete within a short time frame. Clearly, the process is much more intricate than this simplified description.

Once the initial version is developed, it must be tested to ensure that it is reliable (it provides the same result on repeated testing in stable subjects), that it is valid (it measures what it purports to measure by demonstrating appropriate correlations with other measures, usually based on a priori predictions of the degree of such correlation, thereby demonstrating construct validity), and that it is responsive to change (its score changes in a meaningful way as the patient's condition changes). Changes are usually made to the measure after initial testing. With changes to the instrument, the same process of demonstration of measurement properties must be undertaken once more. Given the complexity associated with the development of measures for assessing children, the various age groups and thus various stages of physical and psychosocial development involved, information that is usually obtained from a third party (the parent), and the heterogeneity of JIA, developing an assessment tool is an onerous task.

Outcome measures in use in juvenile idiopathic arthritis

Over the past 15 years, a number of JIA-specific measures of functional status and HRQoL have been developed (Box 2).

Additionally, several generic measures have been modified for use in JIA. A complete description of these various measures can be found in the original publications. Here, examples of each type of measure are discussed, and the advantages and disadvantages of various measures are highlighted (Table 1).

The Childhood Health Assessment Questionnaire

The CHAQ [17] is a disease-specific measure of functional status that comprises two indices, disability and discomfort; both indices focus on physical function. The disability index assesses function in eight areas that include dressing, grooming, eating, and general physical activities distributed among a total of 30 items. Each question is rated on difficulty in performance and is scored from 0 to 3. The disability index is calculated as the mean of the eight

---

Box 2. Instruments developed/used to assess juvenile idiopathic arthritis

Measures of physical function

> Childhood Arthritis Impact Measurement Scales (CHAIMS) [14]
> Juvenile Arthritis Assessment Scale (JAFAS) and Report (JAFAR) [17]
> Childhood Health Assessment Questionnaire (CHAQ) [15,16]
> Juvenile Arthritis Self-Report Index (JASI) [12,18]

Measures of quality of life

Disease-specific

> Juvenile Arthritis Quality of Life Questionnaire (JAQQ) [13,19]
> Childhood Arthritis Health Profile (CAHP) [20]

Generic

> Childhood Health Questionnaire (CHQ) [21]
> Pediatric Quality of Life Inventory Scales (Peds QL) [22]
> Quality of My Life Questionnaire (QoMLQ) [23]

Table 1
Comparison of measures used to assess health-related quality of life in juvenile idiopathic arthritis

	CHAQ	JAQQ	CHQ	Peds QL	QoMLQ
Reliability	Very good	Good	Good	Moderately good	Moderately good
Validity	Very good	Very good	Very good	Good	Good
Responsiveness	Moderately good	Excellent because patients can select items	Excellent	Moderately good	NA
Discriminative ability	Excellent but has ceiling and floor effects	Moderately good; does not have ceiling and floor effects	Moderately good	NA	NA
Applicable to a heterogeneous population	Excellent	Excellent because patients can select items	Excellent	Very good	NA
Measures physical function comprehensively	Good	Very good	Very good	Very good	No
Measures quality of life comprehensively	No	Very good	Very good	Very good	Measures QoL but not comprehensively
Measures pain	Good	Good	Good	Good	No
Tested widely	Excellent, used most widely and available in many languages	Moderately good; available in several languages	Excellent, used very widely and available in many languages	No	No
East to use	Excellent	Very good	Very good	Very good	Excellent
Time to complete	5 minutes	15 minutes, initially; 5 subsequently	20 minutes	15 minutes	1 minute
Clinical application	Excellent	Very good	Moderately good	Very good	Excellent
Parent completion	Yes	Yes	Yes	Yes	Yes
Patient completion	Yes; > 9 years	Yes; > 7 years	No	Yes; various forms for different ages	Yes; age not clearly established

functional areas. Discomfort is determined by the presence of pain measured by a 100-mm visual analogue scale. In the original study, reliability was very good, and validity was also very good, with excellent correlations with functional class and measures of disease activity. The CHAQ was completed by the parents in all cases and also by children 8 years of age or older, in a mean time of 10 minutes.

The CHAQ has been shown to be a useful instrument for evaluating outcome in longitudinal studies [24–31]. It has also been used in a variety of settings and translated into a number of different languages [32–36]. It has been shown to have reasonable responsiveness in clinical drug trials [37,38] and in the evaluation of rehabilitative interventions [39–41]. Scores of 0.13, 0.63, and 1.75 seem to represent mild, mild to moderate, and moderate disability, respectively [42]. A change in score of 0.13 represents an important change in clinical status.

The CHAQ has excellent reliability and validity, and reasonable responsiveness. It also has good discriminative properties and can be administered to children of all ages and in several languages. Thus, it is of value for longitudinal studies as well as clinical trials and has become the preferred measure in both settings. Because it is short and easy to use, it is used with increasing frequency in the clinical setting.

The Juvenile Arthritis Quality of Life Questionnaire

The JAQQ [13] is a disease-specific measure of HRQoL in which children with JIA and their parents were interviewed to generate items, a process that showed a very high level of agreement between patients and parents over a wide array of perceived difficulties in both physical and psychosocial function [19]. Generated items were subsequently reduced and categorized into four dimensions (gross motor function, fine motor function, psychosocial function, and general symptoms), each with approximately 20 items. A seven-point scale was then applied (scored 1–7, with higher scores indicating worse function). The JAQQ score is computed as the mean of the four dimension scores. The JAQQ was completed in 15 minutes initially, and then 5 minutes subsequently in 30 patients, showing good construct validity, with moderate correlations with measures of disease activity and excellent correlations with pain. As predicted, correlations for the psychosocial dimension were less close; the best correlation was with pain. Responsiveness was demonstrated by correlations of changes in scores; correlations were moderate with measures of disease activity and were excellent with pain.

After this initial study, the number of items was reduced to 74, and a pain dimension was added. Face and content validity of this version were confirmed by 20 experts. Construct validity and responsiveness were also established [43]. Responsiveness was established before and after commencement of new drug therapy, with a mean of 8 weeks between assessments. In further studies, responsiveness of the JAQQ was at least as good as that for the CHAQ or CHQ [44]. English and French versions are available, and a Dutch translation has been validated [45].

The JAQQ was developed in a detailed fashion, resulting in excellent validity and responsiveness. It can be administered to children of all ages and disease-onset types in a reasonable period of time with minimal assistance and can also be scored quickly by hand. These features make it practical for use in the clinical setting.

The Child Health Questionnaire

The CHQ [21] is a generic instrument that comprises a number of different forms. The form used most commonly in children with JIA is the Parent Form 50 (PF 50) that contains 50 items distributed in several dimensions including general health, physical activities, pain, self-esteem, and family issues. These sections are complemented by general questions about the child and the caregiver. Two separate scores can be computed that estimate physical and psychosocial function; both are scored from 0 to 100, with the higher score indicating better function.

The CHQ has been validated, along with the CHAQ, for use in 32 languages [36] and was used in a study of short-term outcome in 116 children with JIA [46]. It has been used in combination with the CHAQ in a trial of methotrexate, in which it was shown to be highly responsive [38]. Because of its generalizability, it has become the preferred measure of HRQoL for JIA trials. Because of its length, however, it is of less use in the clinical setting.

The Pediatric Quality of Life Inventory

The Peds QL is a modular instrument designed to measure HRQoL in children and adolescents aged 2 to 18 years [22]. It contains a generic core integrated with a disease-specific core. The generic core has undergone various iterations, the most recent of which, the Peds QL 4.0 Generic Core Scales, contains 23 items distributed in four scales: physical, emotional, social, and school functioning. The Peds QL 3.0 rheumatology module contains 22 disease-specific items distributed in five scales (pain, daily activities, treatment, worry, and communication). It is completed by both patients and their parents and has developmentally appropriate forms for varying age groups. The parent–child concordance has been demonstrated to be good when the instrument is completed separately by parents and children,. It takes approximately 15 minutes to complete. Each item is scored on a five-point scale (0–4), with the higher score indicating worse function. Total scale scores are computed as the mean across all items scored in that scale.

This instrument was shown to have excellent reliability, validity, and responsiveness in a study of 271 children with various rheumatic diseases, 91 of whom had JIA, and their parents [47]. Reliability varied with the age of the child, being less good for younger children. Reliability was also not as good for the rheumatology module. Responsiveness has not been tested in a trial setting. Nonetheless, this instrument represents an important addition to the outcome measures available for use in JIA, and further studies will be followed with interest.

The Quality of My Life Questionnaire

The QoMLQ was developed in an attempt to distinguish between difficulties resulting from the disease itself and difficulties that are generic [23]. It comprises two separate 100-mm visual analogue scales, anchored with the descriptors "worst" or "best," that respondent uses to indicate quality of life in relation to the disease itself and to overall difficulties not necessarily directly caused by the disease. This approach demonstrated the importance of distinguishing between these factors, because respondents indicated clear differences between these two separate entities. The QoMLQ is a short and easy-to-use generic instrument that has been demonstrated to be highly reliable and valid. Thus, it is a practical measure and is of great use in the clinical setting. It needs further study, however.

In a recent study in children with JIA that compared a number of HRQoL measures, the Peds QL, JAQQ, and QoMLQ were moderately to highly correlated with one another [48]. Overall, children's HRQoL significantly decreases with increasing disability. This study also showed that parents are moderate to good proxy reporters of HRQoL, disability, and overall well being in children with JIA, confirming the results of a prior study [19].

Health outcomes in juvenile idiopathic arthritis

Remission rates

Prior studies of remission rates in JIA [24–28], which have recently been reviewed comprehensively [49,50], have used a variety of definitions of remission and disease flare, resulting in considerable variation in reported remission rates. This variation makes definitive interpretation of the studies difficult. Overall, these studies suggest that JIA is not a benign disease, that it frequently continues into adulthood, and that most remissions occur in the first 5 years after disease onset. The probability of remission 10 years after onset approximates 30% to 35% overall; thus 65% to 70% of children with JIA have a disease that remains active into adulthood. This persistence varies considerably with disease-onset type; the rate of disease remission is about 50% for oligoarticular arthritis but only approaches 5% polyarticular rheumatic-factor–positive (RF-positive) arthritis (the best and worst cases, respectively). The probability of remission decreases progressively after 10 years. If remission does not occur within 10 years of disease onset, it is unlikely to occur at all. Recently, new definitions of disease remission and disease flare in JIA have been proposed [51,52]. If these definitions are applied to new studies outcomes can be reported more accurately and thus provide with better prognostic data.

Disability, health-related quality of life, psychosocial and socioeconomic outcomes

Most early studies of disability used a basic measure of functional assessment and showed a progressive decrease in the numbers of JIA patients with poor functional outcomes, from as many as 40% in the 1970s to as few as 0% in the 1990s for some disease-onset types [49]. Trends in improvement overall seem impressive, but considerably less improvement is seen in patients systemic JIA or with RF-positive polyarticular JIA [24–28].

Of the newer measures, the CHAQ is the instrument used in most recent studies of outcome. The CHAQ places most patients in the category of no or mild functional disability, but up to 15% to 20% of patients with systemic JIA and polyarticular RF-positive JIA were classified as having severe disability [26]. In a study of adults with JIA, 36% had impaired physical functioning using the adult Health Assessment Questionnaire [28]. In a study that used the CHQ, poorer physical status but minimal psychologic impairment was noted in JIA patients relative to controls, although follow-up in this study was quite brief (mean of 2.5 years) [46].

Studies that have focused on high school and higher education and marital and employment status have shown varied results. A recent study showed a high rate of high school completion for JIA patients (>85%) relative to controls (>79%) [26]. The rate of postsecondary education completion, however, was considerably lower for females with JIA (55%) relative to controls (71%). Another study demonstrated that a significant proportion of patients had difficulty completing full days at school and needed some assistance [30]. Rates of unemployment seem to be higher for JIA patients relative to controls, and this decrement increases over time [26,29].

Taken together, these data suggest that there is overall improvement in these outcomes for all JIA patients, except for patients with systemic and polyarticular RF-positive JIA, who exhibit greater evidence of severe disabilities. Nonetheless, the lower rate of employment in JIA patients, overall, relative to controls, does suggest ongoing functional impairment for a significant proportion of JIA patients.

Joint damage and osteopenia

Radiographic damage has been found in all JIA subtypes, with erosions evident in 25% to 75% and joint space narrowing in 14% to 79%, being for worse patients with systemic and polyarticular RF-positive JIA, a mean of 8 years from disease onset [28,53]. Radiographic damage correlates strongly with disability as measured by the CHAQ. The requirement for arthroplasty was surprisingly high in one study, again being highest in patients with systemic and polyarticular RF-positive JIA, 23% of whom underwent this procedure, predominantly for hip and knee disease [26].

Decreased bone mineral density is a significant problem in children with JIA. If a sound foundation for peak bone mass is not established during the second decade of life, osteopenia and increased fracture risk occur [54]. In a recent Norwegian study of 103 adolescent JIA patients with mean disease duration of 14.2 years, 41% had low total-body bone mineral content, and 34% had low total-body bone mineral density [55].

Factors predictive of poor outcomes

The factors predictive of poor outcome have been reviewed comprehensively recently [56]. Some of the main findings are highlighted here. In an attempt to determine factors predictive of outcomes in JIA, Oen at al [31] conducted a series of multivariate analyses on their data from a three-center Canadian study. Male sex correlated with worse disability in systemic arthritis but with less disability in polyarticular RF-negative JIA. Positive antinuclear antibody titer correlated with longer duration of active disease in oligoarticular arthritis. Younger age of disease onset predicted longer duration of active disease in oligoarticular and polyarticular RF-negative JIA and a shorter duration of active disease in systemic arthritis. There were no clear predictors of outcome in polyarticular RF-positive JIA, which in general had a poor prognosis. Predictors of persistent disease activity and erosions, overall, were young age of onset, large number of affected joints, long duration of elevated sedimentation rate (ESR), and positive RH [28]. Predictors of physical disability were female sex, symmetric arthritis, hip joint involvement, long duration of elevated ESR, and RF positivity. Other studies have looked at the predictive value of joint patterns in oligoarticular JIA. One study showed that the early presence of ankle or wrist disease, symmetric joint involvement, and an elevated ESR in a child with oligoarticular JIA are predictive of disease progression [57]. Another study showed that small joint and wrist disease in a patient with oligoarthritis is associated with juvenile psoriatic arthritis [58].

Clearly, it is difficult to generalize from these studies, given the variations in study design and factors evaluated. Nonetheless, persistent disease activity seems to be the single most important determinant of poor outcomes, and all attempts to eradicate disease activity seem to be appropriate. Additionally, systemic arthritis and RF-positive polyarthritis have a poor prognosis, and early aggressive treatment is merited in these onset types.

Summary

There has been a tremendous emphasis on the development of measures of function and HRQoL for application in JIA over the past 15 years. Of the measures that are currently available, the CHAQ and the CHQ are the most widely used, although the use of others, including the JAQQ, the Peds QL, and the QoMLQ, is growing. As evidence emerges from better longitudinal studies with these measures, it will be possible to describe patient outcomes in JIA more accurately.

From the outcome studies that have been conducted to date, one can conclude that JIA is not a benign disease. It frequently continues into adulthood, and most remissions occur in the first 5 years after disease onset. The probability of remission 10 years after onset approximates 30% to 35%, overall, and decreases progressively thereafter. Thus, if remission does not occur within 10 years of disease onset, it is unlikely to occur at all. Although remission rates have not changed substantially, functional outcomes have improved tremendously, with fewer patients exhibiting severe outcomes. Nonetheless, the degree of impaired functional outcome is still unacceptable and needs to be improved. Significant joint damage is still a consequence of this disease, with relatively high rates of arthroplasty, and increasing data reveal significant problems of osteopenia and osteoporosis that are not being addressed adequately.

A large prospective study with strict application of the JIA classification, using the new definitions of remission and disease flare and coupled with the use of the newer functional and HRQoL measures will provide more accurate outcome data and better means of predicting good and poor outcomes. Such a study is under way in Canada. It will be interesting to see if there is a significant change in remission rates in this study, because the current approach to therapy, especially with the availability of biologic agents, is more aggressive than that used in most patients in the reported studies. Pediatricians need to be aware of this change in approach and should refer patients for evaluation to a pediatric rheumatologist early in the disease course to maximize ultimate patient outcomes.

Acknowledgments

Dr. Duffy is recipient of the Sessenwein Award for research, McGill University.

References

[1] Petty RE, Southwood TR, Manners P, et al. International League of Associations of Rheumatology classification of juvenile idiopathic arthritis: second revision, Edmonton, 2001. J Rheumatol 2004;31:390–2.

[2] Giannini EH, Ruperto R, Ravelli A, and the Paediatric Rheumatology International Trials Organization (PRINTO). Preliminary definition of improvement in juvenile arthritis. Arthritis Rheum 1997;40:1202–9.

[3] Miller JJ. Psychosocial factors related to rheumatic diseases in childhood. J Rheumatol 1993; 20:1–4.

[4] Allaire SH, DeNardo BS, Szer IS, et al. The economic impact of juvenile chronic arthritis. J Rheumatol 1992;19:952–5.

[5] Gill TM, Feinstein AR. A critical appraisal of the quality of quality of life measurements. JAMA 1994;272:619–26.

[6] Guyatt GH, Veldhuyzen Van Zanten SJO, et al. Measuring quality of life in clinical trials: a taxonomy and review. Can Med Assoc J 1989;140:1441–8.

[7] Duffy CM, Duffy KN. Health assessment in the rheumatic diseases of childhood. Curr Opin Rheumatol 1997;9:440–7.

[8] Duffy CM, Lovell DJ. Outcome assessment in paediatric rheumatic diseases. In: Cassidy JT, Petty RE, editors. Textbook of pediatric rheumatology. Toronto: W.B. Saunders; 2001. p. 189–99.

[9] Murray KJ, Passo MH. Functional measures in children with rheumatic diseases. Pediatr Clin North Am 1995;42:1127–53.

[10] Kirshner B, Guyatt G. A methodologic framework for assessing health indices. J Chron Dis 1985;38:27–36.

[11] Streiner DK, Norman GR. Health measurement scales: a practical guide to their development and use. Oxford (UK): Oxford University Press; 1989.

[12] Wright FV, Law M, Goldsmith CH, et al. Development of a self-report functional status index for juvenile rheumatoid arthritis. J Rheumatol 1994;21:536–44.

[13] Duffy CM, Arsenault L, Duffy KNW, et al. The juvenile arthritis quality of life questionnaire— development of a new responsive index for juvenile rheumatoid arthritis and juvenile spon- dyloarthritides. J Rheumatol 1997;24:738–46.

[14] Coulton CJ, Zborowsky E, Lipton J, et al. Assessment of the reliability and validity of the arthritis impact measurement scales for children with juvenile arthritis. Arthritis Rheum 1987;30:819–24.

[15] Lovell DJ, Howe S, Shear E, et al. Development of a disability measurement tool for juve- nile rheumatoid arthritis. The Juvenile Arthritis Functional Assessment Scale. Arthritis Rheum 1989;32:1390–5.

[16] Howe S, Levinson J, Shear E, et al. Development of a disability measurement tool for juvenile rheumatoid arthritis. The Juvenile Arthritis Functional Assessment Report for children and their parents. Arthritis Rheum 1991;34:873–80.

[17] Singh G, Athreya BH, Fries JF, et al. Measurement of health status in children with juvenile rheumatoid arthritis. Arthritis Rheum 1994;37:1761–9.

[18] Wright FV, Kimber JL, Law M, et al. The juvenile arthritis functional status index (JASI): a validation study. J Rheumatol 1996;23:1066–79.

[19] Duffy CM, Arsenault L, Duffy KNW, et al. Level of agreement between parents and chil- dren in rating dysfunction in juvenile rheumatoid arthritis and juvenile spondyloarthritides. J Rheumatol 1993;20:2134–9.

[20] Tucker LB, De Nardo BA, Schaller JG. The childhood arthritis health profile: correlation of JRA-specific scales with disease severity and activity. Arthritis Rheum 1996;39:S57.

[21] Landgraf JM, Abetz L, Ware JE. Child Health Questinnaire (CHQ): a user's manual. Boston: The Health Institute, New England Medical Center; 1996.

[22] Varni JW, Seid M, Rode CA. The Peds QL: measurement model for the Pediatric Quality of Life Inventory. Med Care 1999;37:126–39.

[23] Feldman BM, Grundland B, McCullough L, et al. Distinction of quality of life, health-related quality of life, and health status in children referred for rheumatology care. J Rheumatol 2000;27:226–33.

[24] Minden K, Kiessling U, Listing J, et al. Prognosis of patients with juvenile chronic arthritis and juvenile spondyloarthropathy. J Rheumatol 2000;27:2256–63.

[25] Spiegel LR, Schneider R, Lang BA, et al. Early predictors of poor functional outcome in systemic onset juvenile rheumatoid arthritis: a multicentre cohort study. Arthritis Rheum 2000;43:2402–9.

[26] Oen K, Malleson P, Cabral D, et al. Disease course and outcome of juvenile rheumatoid arthritis in a multicentre cohort. J Rheumatol 2002;29:1989–99.

[27] Fantini F, Gerloni V, Gattinara M, et al. Remission in juvenile chronic arthritis: a cohort study of 683 consecutive cases with a mean 10 year follow up. J Rheumatol 2003;30:579–84.

[28] Flato B, Lien G, Smerdel A, et al. Prognostic factors in juvenile rheumatoid arthritis: a case- control study revealing early predictors and outcome after 14.9 years. J Rheumatol 2003;30: 386–93.

[29] Foster HE, Marshall N, Myers A, et al. Outcome in adults with juvenile idiopathic arthritis. Arthritis Rheum 2003;48:767–75.

[30] Bowyer S, Roettcher PA, Higgins GC, et al. Health status of patients with juvenile rheumatoid arthritis at 1 and 5 years after diagnosis. J Rheumatol 2003;30:394–400.

[31] Oen K, Malleson P, Cabral D, et al. Early predictors of long-term outcome in patients with juvenile rheumatoid arthritis: subset-specific correlations. J Rheumatol 2003;30:585–93.

[32] Fantini F, Corvaglia G, Bergomi P, et al. Validation of the Italian version of the Stanford Childhood Health Assessment Questionnaire for measuring functional status for children with chronic arthritis. Clin Exp Rheumatol 1995;13:785–91.

[33] Goycochea-Robles MV, Garduno-Espinosa J, Vilchis-Guizar E, et al. Validation of a Spanish version of the Childhood Health Assessment Questionnaire. J Rheumatol 1997;24:2242–5.

[34] Arguedas O, Andersson-Gare B, Fasth A, et al. Development of a Costa Rican version of the Childhood Health Assessment Questionnaire. J Rheumatol 1997;24:2233–41.

[35] Flato B, Soskaar D, Vinje O, et al. Measuring disability in early juvenile arthritis: evaluation of a Norwegian version of the Childhood Health Assessment Questionnaire. J Rheumatol 1998;25:1851–8.

[36] Ruperto N, Ravelli A, Pistorio A, et al. Cross-cultural adaptation and psychometric evaluation of the Childhood Health Assessment Questionnaire (CHAQ) and the Child Health Questionnaire (CHQ) in 32 countries. Clin Exp Rheumatol 2001;19(Suppl 23):S1–9.

[37] Lovell DJ, Giannini EH, Reiff A, et al. Etanercept in children with polyarticular juvenile rheumatoid arthritis. Pediatric Rheumatology Collaborative Study Group. N Engl J Med 2000; 342:763–9.

[38] Ruperto N, Murray K, Gerloni V, et al. A randomized trial of parenteral methotrexate comparing an intermediate dose with a higher dose in children with juvenile idiopathic arthritis who failed to respond to standard doses of methotrexate. Arthritis Rheum 2004;50:2191–201.

[39] Fan JS, Wessel J, Ellsworth J. The relationship between strength and function in females with juvenile rheumatoid arthritis. J Rheumatol 1998;25:1399–405.

[40] Wessel J, Kaup C, Fan J, et al. Isometric strength in children with arthritis: reliability and relation to function. Arthritis Care Res 1999;12:238–46.

[41] Takken T, van der Net J, Helders PJ. Relationship between functional ability and physical fitness in juvenile idiopathic arthritis patients. Scand J Rheumatol 2003;32:174–8.

[42] Dempster H, Porepa M, Young N, et al. The clinical meaning of functional outcome scores in children with juvenile arthritis. Arthritis Rheum 2001;44:1768–74.

[43] Duffy CM, Arsenault L, Watanabe Duffy KN, et al. Validity and sensitivity to change of the Juvenile Arthritis Quality of Life Questionnaire (JAQQ) [abstract]. Arthritis Rheum 1993;36(Suppl):S144.

[44] Duffy CM, Watanabe Duffy KN, Gibbon M, et al. Accuracy of functional outcome measures in defining improvement in juvenile idiopathic arthritis [abstract]. Ann Rheum Dis 2000; 59:724.

[45] Takken T, van der Net J, Kuis W, et al. Aquatic fitness training for children with juvenile idiopathic arthritis. Rheumatology 2003;42:1408–14.

[46] Selvaag AE, Flato B, Lien G, et al. Measuring health status in early juvenile idiopathic arthritis: determinants and responsiveness of the Child Health Questionnaire. J Rheumatol 2003;30:1602–10.

[47] Varni JW, Seid M, Smith Knight T, et al. The Peds QL in pediatric rheumatology. Reliability, validity and responsiveness of the Pediatric Quality of Life Inventory Generic Core Scales and Rheumatology Module. Arthritis Rheum 2002;46:714–25.

[48] Brunner HI, Klein-Gitelman M, Miller MJ, et al. Health of children with chronic arthritis: relationship of different measures and the quality of parent proxy reporting. Arthritis Rheum 2004;51:763–73.

[49] Oen K. Long-term outcomes and predictors of outcomes for patients with juvenile idiopathic arthritis. Best Pract Res Clin Rheumatol 2002;16:347–60.

[50] Duffy CM. Health Outcomes in paediatric rheumatic diseases. Curr Opin Rheumatol 2004; 16(2):102–8.

[51] Wallace CA, Ruperto N, Giannini EH, for the Childhood Arthritis and Rheumatology Research Alliance (CARRA), The Pediatric Rheumatology International Trials Organizations (PRINTO), and The Pediatric Rheumatology Collaborative Study Group (PRCSG). Preliminary criteria for clinical remission for select categories of juvenile idiopathic arthritis. J Rheumatol 2004; 31:2290–4.

[52] Brunner HI, Lovell DJ, Finck BK, et al. Preliminary definition of disease flare in juvenile rheumatoid arthritis. J Rheumatol 2002;29:1058–64.

[53] Oen K, Reed M, Malleson P, et al. Radiologic outcome and its relationship to functional disability in juvenile rheumatoid arthritis. J Rheumatol 2003;30:832–40.

[54] Cassidy JT. Osteopenia and osteoporosis in children. Clin Exp Rheumatol 1999;17:245–50.

[55] Lien G, Flato B, Haugen M, et al. Frequency of osteopenia in adolescents with early-onset juvenile idiopathic arthritis. A long-term outcome study of one hundred five patients. Arthritis Rheum 2003;48:2214–23.

[56] Ravelli A, Martini A. Early predictors of outcome in juvenile idiopathic arthritis. Clin Exp Rheumatol 2003;21(Suppl 31):S89–93.

[57] Al-Matar MJ, Petty RE, Tucker LB, et al. The early pattern of joint involvement predicts disease progression in children with oligoarticular (pauciarticular) juvenile rheumatoid arthritis. Arthritis Rheum 2002;46:2708–15.

[58] Huemer C, Malleson PN, Cabral D, et al. Patterns of joint involvement at onset differentiate oligoarticular juvenile psoriatic arthritis from pauciarticular juvenile rheumatoid arthritis. J Rheumatol 2002;29:1531–5.

ELSEVIER
SAUNDERS

Pediatr Clin N Am 52 (2005) 373–411

PEDIATRIC CLINICS
OF NORTH AMERICA

Radiologic Investigation of Rheumatic Diseases

Paul Babyn, MDCM[a,b,*], Andrea S. Doria, MD, MSc, PhD[a,b]

[a]Department of Diagnostic Imaging, Hospital for Sick Children, 555 University Avenue,
Toronto, Ontario, M5G 1X8 Canada
[b]Department of Medical Imaging University of Toronto, Fitzgerald Building, 150 College Street,
Room 112, Toronto, Ontario, M5G 1X8 Canada

A variety of imaging techniques is now available to investigate the child with rheumatic disease. Sonography and MRI, for example, are playing an increasing role in the evaluation of joint, tendon, and soft tissue inflammation or other abnormalities in children with rheumatic diseases. Imaging modalities offer the potential for earlier visualization and diagnosis of inflammatory abnormalities such as synovitis or cartilage damage along with improved assessment of therapeutic response. Each imaging modality has advantages and disadvantages when applied to selected anatomic regions and in imaging of children (Boxes 1, 2). These advantages and disadvantages must be understood before an appropriate investigative can be selected.

To understand the imaging appearance of the growing joint, especially when using conventional radiography, one must recognize the significant postnatal development that occurs in the musculoskeletal system. In the newborn, there is extensive unossified epiphyseal cartilage that cannot be distinguished from adjacent soft tissues by conventional radiography. With increasing age, epiphyseal cartilage transforms to bone, narrowing the radiographic joint space to the thickness of the opposing layers of articular cartilage as seen in adolescence or adulthood. Normal articular soft tissue components are primarily of a similar radiographic density and cannot be clearly differentiated from each other or from adjacent muscles, fascia, tendons, ligaments, nerves, or vessels by conventional radiography. Displacement of fat deposits in fascial and intermuscular planes

---

* Corresponding author. Department of Diagnostic Imaging, Hospital for Sick Children, 555 University Avenue, Toronto, Ontario M5G 1X8.
  E-mail address: paul.babyn@sickkids.on.ca (P. Babyn).

0031-3955/05/$ – see front matter © 2005 Elsevier Inc. All rights reserved.
doi:10.1016/j.pcl.2005.02.002   *pediatric.theclinics.com*

Box 1. Utility of imaging modalities [1–4]

Conventional radiography

Traditional standard for assessment of established joint damage including bone erosions, joint space narrowing, joint subluxation, misalignment, or ankylosis
Advantages: Low cost, high availability, helpful in differential diagnosis, reasonable reproducibility, validated assessment methods
Disadvantages: Not sensitive in detecting early bone disease or soft tissue manifestations, projectional superimposition, use of ionizing radiation

Ultrasound

Ultrasound can assess effusion or synovitis by detecting thickening of synovial membrane of inflamed joints, bursas, or tendon sheaths by grey-scale and Doppler techniques. Follow-up studies have shown improvement in ultrasound measures of synovitis following treatment with glucocorticoids or tumor necrosis factor-alpha antagonists
Advantages: Noninvasive, relatively low cost, lack of ionizing radiation, ability to visualize both inflammatory and destructive disease manifestations, easy repeatability, possibility of examining several joint regions at one session, potential for guiding interventions
Disadvantages: Physical limitations, not all joint areas accessible, operator dependence

MRI

MRI directly visualizes both inflammatory and destructive aspects of arthritic disease. It has potential for accurate monitoring of treatment efficiency. Allows assessment of all structures in arthritic disease including synovial membrane, intra- and extra-articular fluid collections, cartilage, bone erosions and edema, ligaments, tendons, tendon sheaths
Advantages: Multiplanar tomographic imaging, marked soft tissue contrast, lack of ionizing radiation, more sensitive than clinical and radiographic examination for detection of inflammatory soft tissue changes and early bone changes. Safety, availability, acceptable costs, acceptable duration
Disadvantages: Potential allergic contrast reactions, higher cost/lower availability compared with radiography, longer examination times, and evaluation of only a few joints per session

---

Box 2. Clinical situations in which MRI and/or ultrasound may be of benefit [2]

MRI and/or ultrasound can be used in evaluation of suspected but not definite inflammatory joint disease to determine presence or absence of synovitis, tenosynovitis, enthesitis, or bone erosions. Demonstration or exclusion of joint-related signs of inflammation or destruction in patients without a clear clinical presentation may be helpful in excluding or verifying inflammatory disease and in choosing the appropriate follow-up therapeutic strategy.

MRI can be helpful in

Assisting in establishing the differential diagnosis process by detecting enthesitis in spondyloarthritides
Monitoring therapeutic response to determine whether a treatment satisfactorily suppresses joint inflammation
Assessing disease activity in clinically difficult cases or joints such as the temporomandibular joint
Potential prognostication of patients to different therapeutic regimens

Ultrasound can be used to guide punctures of joints, bursas, and tendon sheaths, improving the success rates of diagnostic or therapeutic aspirations and injections

---

may aid in determination of joint effusions in the elbow, knee, or ankle but not around the hip.

This article reviews the current use of the wide variety of imaging modalities now available, presenting the imaging features of common and important causes of acute and chronic rheumatic disorders including juvenile idiopathic arthritis (JIA), spondyloarthropathies/enthesitis-related arthritis, sepsis, autoimmune diseases, vasculitis, and osteoporosis.

Juvenile idiopathic arthritis

Clinically diagnosed, JIA is a chronic inflammatory arthritis that begins in patients younger than 16 years and that persists for longer than 6 weeks. All other diseases that can cause arthritis need to be considered and excluded before the diagnosis of JIA is made. JIA is the most important rheumatic disease affecting children and one of the most common chronic diseases of childhood.

Although JIA may be self-limited, with most patients having no active syno-vitis in adulthood, many children have significant joint complications [5]. JIA includes several subgroups, including systemic arthritis, oligoarthritis, polyar-thritis, enthesitis-related arthritis, and psoriatic arthritis, which are distinguished by clinical and laboratory features, including disease onset [6]. In JIA, the synovium is the target tissue for inflammation. Early in the disease course, the affected joints develop synovial proliferation and infiltration by inflammatory cells including polymorphonuclear leukocytes, lymphocytes, and plasma cells with subsequent increased secretion of synovial fluid and pannus formation. Inflammation of synovial coverings of tendons and bursas, which can also be affected, can lead to periostitis. With prolonged inflammation, destruction of cartilage, adjacent bone erosions, and even joint ankylosis may be seen.

Musculoskeletal system

In early arthritis, plain radiography is often nonspecific, reflecting the early response of the soft tissues and bones to inflammation with soft tissue swelling, osteopenia, joint effusions, and periosteal reaction [7]. The osteopenia is initially periarticular, becoming more diffuse over time. Rarely, one sees the bandlike pattern observed in leukemia. Periosteal reaction is commonly seen in the phalanges, metacarpals, and metatarsals but can occur in the long bones. Soft tissue nodules can be noted, as may periarticular calcification, although this manifestation usually is a consequence of prior intra-articular therapy. Joint space narrowing and erosions are usually later radiographic findings (Fig. 1). In rheumatoid factor–positive polyarthritis and in up to one third of patients with systemic arthritis early erosive disease can occur. Abnormalities in growth and maturation may lead to accelerated osseous growth, altered maturation, and enlarged epiphyses. Late sequelae of JIA are common and include epiphyseal deformity, abnormal angular carpal bones, and premature fusion of the growth plate with brachydactyly and cystlike, well-corticated erosions. At the hip, protrusio acetabuli, premature degenerative changes, coxa magna, and coxa valga can be seen [8]. Joint space loss can progress to ankylosis, particularly in the apophyseal joints of the cervical spine and wrist (Fig. 1). Subluxation of the joints, especially in the atlantoaxial location, may also occur. Growth disturbance of the temporomandibular joint may lead to micrognathia and abnormalities of the temporomandibular disk.

Although total joint assessment is often hindered by acoustic barriers [9], sonography can be used to assess articular cartilage thickness and to detect synovial thickening, joint effusions, and associated synovial cysts [1,9,10]. Sonography is sensitive in detecting joint effusion, particularly in the hips and shoulders where plain films are insensitive. Sonography can also be used to assess tendon sheath synovial proliferation and bursal hypertrophy [11] and to guide joint aspiration or injection. Power Doppler sonography shows promise in evaluating the amount and activity of pannus [1].

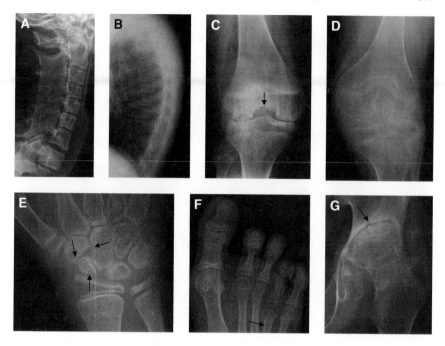

Fig. 1. Radiographic findings of advanced JIA. (*A*) Multilevel cervical apophyseal joint ankylosis. (*B*) Thoracic kyphosis with diffuse osteoporosis and slight decreased height of the vertebral bodies, probably the result of chronic steroid use. (*C*) Widening of the trochlear notch (*arrow*) and joint space narrowing of the knee. (*D*) Epiphyseal deformity and overgrowth. (*E*) Irregularity in contour and erosive changes in the carpal bones (*arrows*). (*F*) Brachydactyly with shortening of the fourth metatarsal (*arrow*). (*G*) Protrusio acetabuli (*arrow*).

With MRI, one can directly image synovial proliferation, joint fluid, popliteal cysts, meniscal hypoplasia or atrophy, pannus formation, and erosion of cartilage and bone (Fig. 2). MRI is suitable for assessing disease severity or progression and is playing an increasing role in diagnosis and outcome assessment [1]. It is more sensitive than plain films in detecting bone erosions [12]. Uncomplicated joint fluid usually has low signal on T1- and high signal on T2-weighted images [13]. MR enhancement of the synovium can be used for early detection of synovial proliferation, which precedes destructive changes. Normal synovium is thin and shows slight enhancement. Proliferating synovium on MRI without contrast appears as intermediate density soft tissue on T1- and T2-weighted sequences. It may have slightly higher signal than adjacent fluid on unenhanced T1 images [1,13]. Pannus appears as intermediate to low signal intensity on T2-weighted images, best seen when outlined by high signal intensity joint fluid. Its variable signal intensity reflects differing amounts of fibrous tissue and hemosiderin. Contrast enhancement improves visualization of the thickened synovium. In particular, the use of fat suppression allows the synovium proliferating in regions normally devoid of synovium to be seen as enhancing

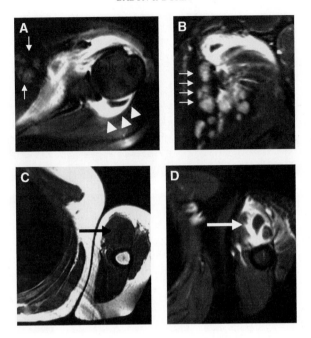

Fig. 2. Fat-suppressed T1-weighted MR images of the left shoulder of an 8-year-old boy with JIA presenting with an arm mass. (*A*) Contrast-enhanced axial and (*B*) coronal images show marked synovial enhancement within the glenohumeral joint, with enhancement seen extending medially subjacent to the scapula. Enlarged lymph nodes are seen medial to the joint (*small arrows*). (*C*) Unenhanced axial non–fat-suppressed and (*D*) contrast-enhanced fat-suppressed T1-weighted MR images of the proximal arm of this patient reveal biceps tenosynovitis (*long arrows*).

linear, villous, or nodular tissue (Fig. 3) [1,7]. Images should be obtained immediately after contrast injection because contrast medium diffuses over time from the synovium into the joint fluid. Hypervascular inflamed pannus enhances significantly, whereas fibrous inactive pannus shows much less enhancement [1]. Quantitative techniques may be used to determine synovial volume. Hemosiderin

Fig. 3. Important differential diagnostic considerations for synovial abnormalities of the pediatric knee. *Upper row*: (*A*) Multiplanar gradient-recalled echo (MPGR), (*B,C*) unenhanced non–fat-saturated, (*D*) contrast-enhanced non–fat-saturated, and (*E*) fat-saturated sagittal T1-weighted images of knees of different patients presenting with hemophilia, lipoma arborescens, nodular synovitis, synovial hemangioma, and soft tissue chondroma, respectively. MPGR MR images clearly demonstrate deposition of hemosiderin components resulting from previous bleeding episodes in hemophiliacs along the capsular and cartilage surface of the joint (*arrows, A*). *Lower row*: multiple knees imaged after administration of gadolinium present with diagnoses that are differentials for knee synovitis in children: (*F*) JIA, (*G*) pigmented villonodular synovitis, (*H*) foreign body, (*I*) septic arthritis with an associated epiphyseal abscess related to on-going osteomyelitis, and (*J*) Klippel-Trénaunnay. Arrows indicate abnormalities that mimic or result in synovial disorders in *B, C, D,* and *E*. The intravenous administration of gadolinium DTPA chelates better delineates the extent of synovial thickening and enhancement (*arrows, F,G,H,I*) representing different degrees of synovial inflammation.

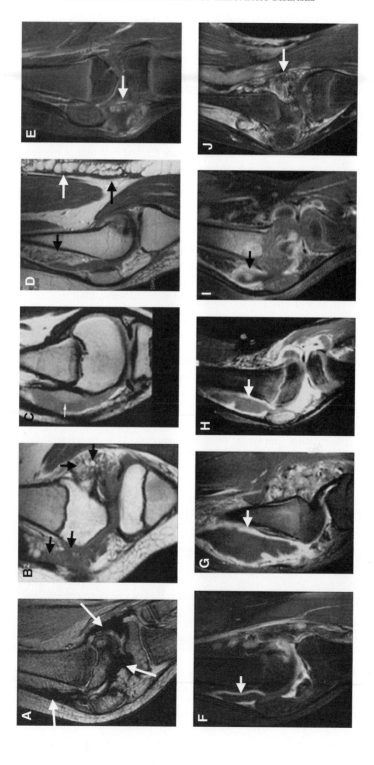

deposition can occur in JIA but is seen more often in disorders typically accompanied by hemarthrosis including pigmented villonodular synovitis, hemophilic arthropathy, synovial hemangioma, and posttraumatic synovitis. Gradient-echo sequences are most sensitive in detecting hemosiderin deposition within the synovium with signal loss resulting from increased magnetic susceptibility.

With prolonged synovial inflammation, as occurs in JIA or tuberculosis, well-defined intra-articular nodules arising from detached fragments of hypertrophied synovial villi can be noted. These nodules are termed rice bodies because of their characteristic macroscopic appearance [14].

Extra-articular manifestations

Sonography may also be used to identify extra-articular complications such as hepatosplenomegaly or serositis. Rarely, retroperitoneal fibrosis may be associated with autoimmune disorders or idiopathic arthritis [15]. Cross-sectional imaging with sonography, CT, or MRI may demonstrate directly the retroperitoneal fibrosis and associated vascular and ureteral narrowing.

Response to therapy

Assessment of disease activity is important for monitoring treatment efficacy and for predicting outcome. Histopathologic evidence of persistent synovitis and radiologic deterioration has been observed in patients assumed clinically and biochemically to have inactive disease. Radiography can be used to quantify joint destruction and to assess disease treatment, with absence of change and lack of progression implying treatment success [16]. Intra-articular corticosteroids can be used to suppress local joint inflammation temporarily (Fig. 4)

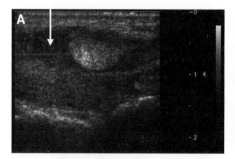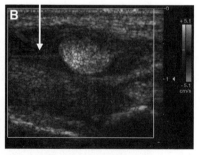

Fig. 4. Transverse gray-scale sonogram of the tendon sheath in a 15-year-old boy with polyarticular JIA and symptomatic tenosynovitis around his left ankle who underwent steroid injection under ultrasound guidance. (*A*) Hypoechoic synovial fluid surrounding the tendon. The injection needle appears as a sharply echoic band (*arrows*). The tip of the needle is noted just by the synovium. (*B*) No significant peritendineus soft tissue hyperemia is noted on color Doppler examination.

[17]. Following injection of intra-articular corticosteroids, periarticular calcification can be noted. Other changes related to intra-articular therapy seem to be uncommon even with repeated joint injections [18]. Sonography may be used to support a clinical suspicion of disease activity in clinically mild or silent joints and in deciding whether to discontinue therapy [9,19]. Increases in synovial thickening and synovial fluid accompany clinical worsening, but the significance of residual synovial thickening and effusion seen on ultrasound in asymptomatic patients remains unclear. It may represent silent active disease or inactive fibrous pannus in a quiescent phase. Following intra-articular therapy for JIA in the hips and knees, decreases in synovial effusion, synovial proliferation, and adenopathy were noted on ultrasound [6]. Several studies in adults [20–23] and children [24,25] have demonstrated the ability of color and power Doppler sonography, with or without intravenous injection of contrast agents, to estimate synovial activity in JIA (Fig. 5). Resistive indices and fraction of color pixels may be used as quantitative measurements of the blood flow.

Contrast-enhanced MRI can be used to monitor synovial membrane volumes, effusion volumes, and cartilage and bone erosion scores quantitatively. Synovial membrane volume may reflect the degree of edema, dilated vessels, and cellular infiltration in the synovial membrane and may be a measure of synovial inflammatory activity. Synovial volume, however, may also reflect the cumulated synovial proliferative disease activity and seems to correlate with duration of clinical remission [1,17]. A close relationship between the rate of contrast enhancement and inflammatory activity has been noted, with the enhancement rate apparently decreasing after intra-articular steroid administration, remaining low during clinical remissions, and increasing before the return of symptoms, indicating subclinical increase in synovial inflammatory activity [26].

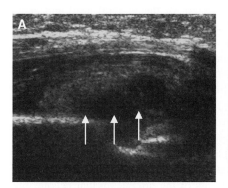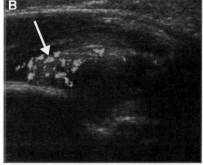

Fig. 5. (A) Gray-scale sonogram of the elbow of a young child with JIA shows joint effusion (*arrows*) displacing the articular capsule and anterior fat pad anterosuperiorly. (B) Corresponding color Doppler sonogram reveals synovial proliferation and hyperemia (*arrow*) from active synovitis.

Juvenile spondyloarthropathies/enthesitis-related arthritis

The juvenile spondyloarthropathies are a group of disorders that affect the axial and extra-axial joints and are associated with the HLA-B27 antigen [27]. They currently fall under the classification of JIA and the subclassification of enthesitis-related arthritis. The spondyloarthropathies, which include juvenile ankylosing spondylitis, reactive arthritis, and arthritis associated with inflammatory bowel disease, all with onset in persons younger than 16 years, constitute the second most common form of chronic arthritis in children [28], but joint findings are generally limited in this group of disorders. Some forms of juvenile psoriatic arthritis are also similar to the spondyloarthropathies, but, like enthesitis-related arthritis, form their own group within the rubric of JIA. Other entities related to the seronegative spondyloarthropathies include the arthritis associated with hyperostosis, acne, or palmar pustolosis, Whipple's disease, and Behcet's disease [29]. Synovitis and enthesitis (inflammation at the site of attachment of ligaments or tendons to bone) are major types of inflammation. Enthesitis is most commonly present at the insertions of the Achilles tendon, plantar fascia, and the patellar and quadriceps tendons.

Musculoskeletal system

Peripheral skeleton

Radiographic findings are common among all the spondyloarthropathies and similar to findings in JIA. Sacroiliitis and enthesitis are exceptions in which the findings are more specific for spondyloarthropathy. Plain films are usually normal initially but later may demonstrate soft tissue swelling, effusion, osteopenia, joint space narrowing, or erosion and, rarely, fusion. Erosions are typically associated with irregular bone apposition at joint margins referred to as "whiskering" (Fig. 6). Rapid joint destruction can be noted [27]. With hip involvement, these proliferative changes are noted at the junction of the femoral head and neck. Dactylitis may be seen with periosteal reaction along the shaft of metacarpals, metatarsals, or phalanges. Soft tissue edema and synovial proliferation resulting in sausagelike digits can best seen on contrast-enhanced T1-weighted MR images and are characteristic of juvenile psoriasis. In juvenile ankylosing spondylitis, extra-axial arthritis usually involves one or more large joints of the lower extremities (eg, hips, knees, and ankles) along with the sacroiliitis. In psoriatic arthritis, severe erosions can be seen, particularly in the digits [30].

Enthesitis may be revealed by soft tissue swelling, localized osteopenia, or by a bone erosion or spur formation (particularly at the site of insertion of the Achilles tendon into the calcaneus, plantar aponeurosis, or patella) (Fig. 6). Grayscale ultrasound of enthesitis may show loss of the normal fibrillar echotexture of tendon, absence of the homogeneous pattern, blurring of tendon margins, and irregular fusiform thickening [31]. The ability of color and power Doppler sonography to assess low-velocity blood flow in small vessels (eg, synovium) allows

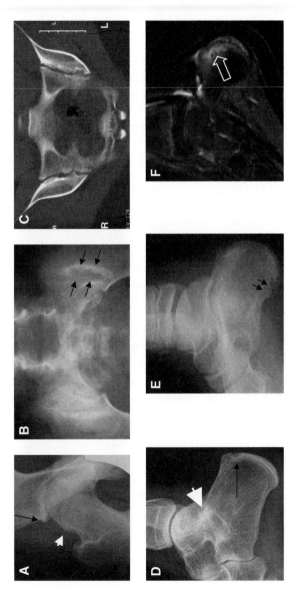

Fig. 6. Enthesitis-related arthritis. (*A*) Frontal radiograph of the right hip shows bone proliferation at the border of the right acetabular roof (*long arrow*) and along the lateral aspects of the femoral head (*short arrow*). (*B*) Diffuse sclerosis and irregularity of the sacroiliac joints with bilateral joint space widening (*arrows*) are characteristic features of sacroiliitis. (*C*) Corresponding CT scan of the sacroiliac joints confirms the radiographic findings seen in this patient with juvenile ankylosing spondylitis. (*D*) Right ankle radiograph of this 15-year-old boy shows loss of the posterior subtalar joint space consistent with partial fusion (*short arrow*). A small lucency is noted at the supero-posterior aspect of the calcaneus at the insertion of the Achilles tendon, which represents a small erosion (*long arrow*). (*E*) A 17-year-old male presents with small plantar calcaneal spurring seen radiographically (*short arrows*) suggestive of enthesitis. (*F*) Corresponding STIR MR image of the ankle shows a focal area of high signal intensity, probably representing bone edema, in the posterior aspect at the insertion of the Achilles tendon (*open arrow*).

a clear depiction of minimal increases of perfusion in spondyloarthropathy [32]. Recently, Tse et al [33] demonstrated the ability of color and power Doppler sonography to reflect the response of the joint to treatment with biologic agents in children with spondyloarthropathy, suggesting that this technique may add valuable information to gray-scale sonography [34–36]. With MRI one may see bone marrow edema, granulation tissue, or cortical erosion.

Axial skeleton

Sacroiliitis and vertebral involvement usually follow later on. Plain films may demonstrate unilateral or bilateral sacroiliitis with indistinct articular margins, pseudowidening, erosions, and reactive sclerosis particularly on the iliac side of the joint (Fig. 6). CT or MRI can be used if necessary to diagnose sacroiliitis earlier than is possible radiologically [30]. On CT, angled scans through the sacroiliac joint should be used to lower the radiation dose [30]. On MRI, inflammatory changes in bone marrow can be seen as periarticular low signal on T1-weighted images and as high signal on T2-weighted images (Fig. 6), whereas bone sclerosis will be seen as low signal. MRI may also demonstrate changes in articular cartilage with erosions. MRI evaluation, particularly with administration of gadolinium diethylenetriamine pentaacetic acid (DTPA) chelates, may allow earlier diagnosis of back pain caused by acute sacroiliitis than possible with conventional radiography [37]. Differentiating spondyloarthropathy from septic sacroiliitis can be difficult. Changes of sequestration and abscess formation do not typically occur in spondyloarthropathy-associated sacroiliitis. Late changes often encountered in the seronegative spondyloarthropathies, including sub-chondral sclerosis and transarticular bone bridges, are not typically found in septic sacroiliitis. Bone scintigraphy can overcome the difficulty in recognizing early sacroiliac abnormalities on plain radiography. There is normally a high concentration of physiologic activity in the sacroiliac joints, and mild to moderate increases in the radioisotope uptake may evade visual detection. In addition, because bilateral and symmetrically enhanced sacroiliac uptake can occur in juvenile ankylosing spondylitis, quantitative analysis of the sacroiliac joints is usually necessary. Asymmetric uptake is more common in other childhood spondyloarthropathies.

Vertebral involvement is not usually present, because it develops quite late. Occasionally there may be localized osteitis, erosions, and sclerosis, particularly at vertebral margins. Syndesmophytes, paraspinal calcification, and atlanto-axial subluxation are rarely seen in children [30,38,39].

Miscellaneous arthritis and joint disorders

Septic arthritis

Acute purulent infection of the joints is more common in infancy and early childhood [7] because of the greater blood flow to the joints during the active stages of growth. The usual cause is hematogenous dissemination related to upper respiratory infection or pyoderma. Infection may also spread from adjacent osteomyelitis, cellulitis, abscess, or traumatic joint invasion [7,40]. In children, septic arthritis develops commonly from osteomyelitis in metaphyses that are intra-articular, such as the hip [7,40,41]. The identification of the obvious septic joint is not much of a diagnostic challenge although time to diagnosis is critical to avoid a poor outcome such as destruction of the femoral head, degenerative arthritis, or permanent deformity.

Most septic arthritides are monoarticular, with the most commonly affected joints being the knee, hip, and ankle [40]. In septic arthritis, bacterial contamination causes hypertrophy and edema of the synovium. In infants with septic arthritis, distension of the joint capsule may result in pathologic dislocation, particularly in the hip or shoulder. Joint space narrowing results from cartilage destruction by proteolytic enzymes. There may be associated bone erosion and destruction or periosteal reaction [42]. Pus in the joint increases intra-articular pressure and may result in osteonecrosis of the epiphysis [40]. Other sequelae include angular deformities, leg length discrepancy, and ankylosis.

The classic radiographic findings of acute septic arthritis are rapid joint space loss and erosions with relative preservation of mineralization. These findings indicate advanced irreversible destruction of the joint but are not specific for infection. Early radiographic findings of joint effusion may be detected in the knee, ankle, or elbow, but radiographs are insensitive for detecting effusion in the shoulder, hip, or sacroiliac joints [43].

Radionuclide imaging is more sensitive than radiographs in diagnosis of septic arthritis and osteomyelitis and may be used to localize the site of infection. In septic arthritis, there is increased articular activity in the blood flow and blood pool phases, and there may be uptake in the juxta-articular bones on the delayed phase because of hyperemia [43]. Increased intra-articular pressure from joint effusion may result in reduced radionuclide uptake within the epiphysis because of ischemia.

Ultrasound, CT, and MRI are sensitive in demonstrating joint effusion but cannot distinguish infected from noninfected joint effusion, and aspiration is still necessary for diagnosis. Ultrasound or CT can be used for guiding diagnostic aspiration or drainage of the joint. CT may be the best modality for evaluating certain joints such as the sternoclavicular joint [43]. MRI may be used to demonstrate early bone erosions and cartilage destruction. In addition to joint effusions, associated findings include synovial thickening and enhancement, septations, and debris within the joint (see Fig. 3) [13,44]. Uncomplicated septic arthritis may cause abnormal signal within the bone marrow on both sides of the joint secondary to reactive edema that may be difficult to differentiate from osteomyelitis [7,41,44]. A secondary complication of septic arthritis includes soft tissue abscess, which demonstrates as a localized fluid collection with peripheral enhancement following gadolinium enhancement. Edema within periarticular structures or fluid collections in tendon sheaths also show increased signal on T2-weighted images [13]. MRI is also helpful for assessment of infection of the axial skeleton including pelvis and spine. Septic sacroiliitis in children is uncommon but can present with nonspecific clinical symptoms such as back pain and can mimic discitis, septic hip, intrapelvic and extrapelvic abscess, psoas abscess, osteomyelitis of the ileum, pyelonephritis, or appendicitis [45]. Plain radiographs will be normal early on, whereas skeletal scintigraphy using Technetium-99m-methylene diphosphonate (MDP) may reveal elevated tracer uptake within 2 to 6 days after the onset of clinical symptoms [45]. CT can demonstrate displacement or thinning of the periarticular fatty tissue layer, edema of adjacent muscles, and abscess formation. MRI provides better soft tissue contrast and has been shown to be more sensitive than CT or skeletal scintigraphy. MRI features of septic sacroiliitis include reduced signal intensity on T1-weighted images, elevated signal intensity on T2 weighted/short-tau inversion-recovery (STIR) images of the joint space and of the periarticular muscle tissue, and anterior or posterior subperiosteal infiltration [45,46]. Bone marrow edema and inflammatory changes of adjacent muscle tissue may be evident. Advanced stages of septic sacroiliitis may include demonstration of erosions, contrast enhancement, sequestration, and abscess formation. Subperiosteal infiltration is a specific sign not seen in other inflammatory causes of sacroiliitis. CT-guided puncture of the sacroiliac joint may be needed when blood culture fails to isolate the pathogen. MRI can also be used to assess progression or regression at follow-up, with the understanding that MRI findings will lag behind clinical improvement [45,46].

Transient synovitis

Transient synovitis is the most common cause of childhood hip pain and can be mimicked by a number of more serious hip disorders including Legg-Calve-Perthes' disease, slipped capital femoral epiphysis, JIA, septic arthritis, and malignancy [30]. It is an acute, self-limiting disorder of unknown origin [30]. Imaging is usually performed with conventional radiography or ultrasound. It has been proposed that radiography should not be used in the primary evaluation of most children with hip pain because the results are generally normal or show only subtle findings of joint effusion. Exceptions should be made in infants younger than 1 year of age and in children older than 8 years because of the lower incidence of transient synovitis in these age groups, with the higher risk of child abuse and septic arthritis in infancy, and the occurrence of slipped capital femoral epiphysis in the older age group [30]. Sonography is a sensitive and noninvasive method of detecting hip joint effusion in transient synovitis [47,48]. Sonography findings, however, led to changes in management in less than 1% of cases in large series. Aspiration is required if infection is a consideration [47]. Other modalities such as bone scans, CT, and MRI are not used initially in the evaluation of irritable hips because of their higher cost and limited benefit [44,49].

Hemophilia

Hemophilia is an X-linked recessive disorder characterized by abnormality of the coagulation mechanism. It may be secondary to a deficiency in factor VIII as in classic hemophilia (hemophilia A) or secondary to a deficiency of factor IX in Christmas disease (hemophilia B) [50]. Hemarthrosis occurs in approximately 75% to 90% of patients with hemophilia [51]. The most commonly affected joints are the knee, elbow, and ankle. Hemorrhage may be secondary to trauma or may occur spontaneously [52]. Recurrent hemarthrosis leads to synovial inflammation and proliferation associated with absorption of hemosiderin and red cell products (see Fig. 3) [53]. With synovial inflammation, cartilage destruction and subchondral bone damage lead to joint space narrowing. With hyperemia and prolonged inflammation epiphyseal overgrowth, early growth plate fusion and fibrosis of ligaments can be seen [54].

The radiographic changes may be identical to JIA, but clinical findings and typical joint involvement help distinguish these entities. Radiodense joint effusions and subchondral changes are more common in hemophilic arthropathy. In the knee, the classic radiographic findings include squaring of the femoral condyles, a widened intercondylar notch, and squaring of the patella [55].

MRI may be used to determine whether hemarthrosis has occurred so that therapy with factor VIII can be administered to prevent chronic joint damage [50,51]. Acute hemarthrosis and chronic joint effusion may be indistinguishable, with low signal intensity on T1-weighted and high signal intensity on T2-weighted images [53]. Subacute hemarthrosis has high signal intensity on both T1- and T2-weighted images because of the presence of extracellular methemoglobin [53]. The synovial thickening often has areas of low signal intensity on T1- and T2-weighted images because of fibrosis or hemosiderin deposition (see Fig. 3) [53]. Gadolinium better delineates the extent of synovial thickening in the hemophilic joint, which shows less enhancement than the JIA joint does. This lack of enhancement is probably secondary to hypovascular connective tissue and hemosiderin deposition within the synovium [56]. Gradient-echo MRI is helpful for evaluation of hemosiderin and cartilage abnormalities [51]. Subchondral cysts may result from intraosseous bleeding, and, rarely, pseudotumors may develop secondary to hemorrhage in bone or in the periarticular soft tissues. Signal characteristics are variable depending on the age of the soft tissue hematoma [57].

Intra-articular masses

A number of articular masses may arise from either the synovium or the joint capsule and lead to joint dysfunction mimicking chronic arthritis. These masses include vascular malformations and nodular synovitis (see Fig. 3). Imaging findings may be diagnostic. Vascular malformations are benign lesions most commonly involving the knee joint [58]. Radiographs are often normal but may demonstrate a soft tissue mass, joint effusion, phleboliths, erosions, and epiphyseal overgrowth [59–62]. MRI findings are usually diagnostic showing a lobulated mass of low or intermediate signal similar to muscle on T1-weighted images and high signal on T2-weighted images [60]. There may be fluid levels and extensive enhancement after contrast administration.

Nodular and pigmented villonodular synovitis are uncommon synovial proliferative disorders (see Fig. 3) [63]. Radiographic findings are usually normal but may show bone erosions or cysts [63,64]. MRI demonstrates multinodular synovial masses with variable amounts of hemosiderin, which causes marked signal dropout on gradient echo images [63,65,66]. The synovial masses may show prominent contrast enhancement after gadolinium administration [67]. If the typical features are present, the MRI appearance is diagnostic. In villonodular synovitis, a synovial mass is seen without hemosiderin deposition or the low MRI signal associated with hemosiderin. Lipoma arborescens is a rare, benign intra-articular lesion with villous lipomatous proliferation of the synovium [68]. Radiographs may demonstrate a joint effusion and mass, usually about the knee [69]. The MRI findings are pathognomonic, with frondlike synovial masses with signal characteristics paralleling fat on all pulse sequences (see Fig. 3) [70–72].

Foreign-body synovitis

Wood splinters, especially plant thorns such as palm or blackthorn, may produce a chronic synovitis or tendinitis. Foreign-body synovitis usually presents with a monoarticular synovitis and may be suggested by the presence of a puncture wound. Extraction of the foreign body is essential for recovery, and identification of the foreign body by imaging allows a localized synovectomy [73]. Plant thorns have slightly higher density than soft tissue and may be detected on CT. Non-radiopaque foreign bodies may also be identified with ultrasound or MRI (see Fig. 3).

Malignancies

Any of the childhood malignancies, especially the leukemias (Fig. 7) and neuroblastoma, can mimic rheumatic disease. Leukemic arthritis typically presents with transient arthralgias and joint pain, often involving the knees, shoulders, and ankles [74]. Although often normal, radiologic findings can include joint effusion, osteopenia, periostitis, lytic or sclerotic bone lesions, and metaphyseal radiolucent bands [75,76]. Diffuse abnormal signal intensity of bone marrow, low on T1- and high on T2-weighted sequences, can be seen on MRI.

Storage disorders, skeletal dysplasias, and syndromes

A variety of storage disorders, skeletal dysplasias, and syndromes may present with joint symptoms. In mucopolysaccharidosis IS (Scheie's syndrome), a

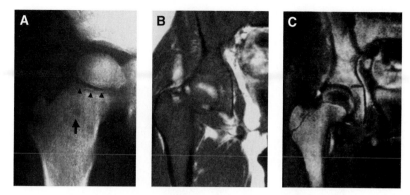

Fig. 7. (*A*) Frontal radiograph of the right hip of a leukemic child shows metaphyseal lucent band (*arrowheads*), and small lytic lesions (*arrow*) within the proximal femoral metaphysis. On the corresponding coronal (*B*) T1-weighted MR image and (*C*) inversion-recovery image, low signal intensity and high speed intensity, respectively, are seen within the bone marrow of the patient's pelvis and proximal femur representing leukemic bone marrow.

lysosomal storage disease, joint abnormalities include stiffness with claw hand deformity and cystic changes in the carpals, metacarpals, tarsals, metatarsals, and femoral heads [77]. Abnormal low signal around affected joints has been described in patients with mucolipidosis III on MRI [78].

In progressive pseudorheumatoid arthritis of childhood, initial symptoms include difficulty in walking that develops between 3 and 8 years of age [79]. There is generalized, progressive joint stiffness and swelling related to osseous enlargement, which is most marked in the hands [79]. Characteristic skeletal abnormalities, particularly in the spine, with platyspondy distinguish this disorder from JIA. Other skeletal dysplasias associated with joint symptoms include Kniest dysplasia, multiple epiphyseal dysplasia, and spondyloepiphyseal dysplasia tarda [77–80]. Rarely, mild synovitis including MR evidence of synovial enhancement and thickening may be present.

Camptodactyly-arthropathy-coxa vara-pericarditis syndrome is a rare disorder consisting of congenital camptodactyly, arthropathy, and pericarditis [81]. The lack of inflammation and absence of joint narrowing with chronic disease help differentiate this disorder from JIA [82]. Flexion deformities are symmetric involving the proximal interphalangeal joint of the hands. Arthropathy predominantly affects large joints, and radiographic findings are most marked in the hips with coxa vara and intraosseous cysts [81].

Chronic recurrent multifocal osteomyelitis

Chronic recurrent multifocal osteomyelitis is a well-established skeletal disorder of unknown origin mainly occurring in children and adolescents [83].

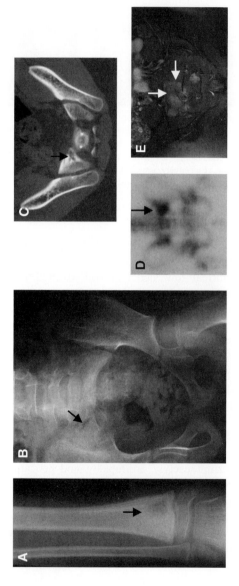

Fig. 8. (*A*) Anterior-posterior radiograph of the right ankle of a 17-year-old girl with chronic recurrent multifocal osteomyelitis shows an ill-defined lytic metaphyseal lesion adjacent to the tibial growth plate (*arrow*) and adjacent periosteal reaction. (*B*) The oblique radiograph of the patient's pelvis reveals a subtle radiolucency within the right sacral wing (*arrow*), which is more clearly demonstrated on (*C*) the corresponding CT (*arrow*), (*D*) posterior view bone scan (*arrow*), and (*E*) MRI. On the T2-weighted MRI, a focal area of high signal intensity is seen within the right sacral promontory extending laterally adjacent to the right sacroiliac joint (*arrows*).

This clinical entity is a diagnosis of exclusion, distinct from bacterial osteomyelitis, based on the following criteria:

1. Bone lesions with a radiographic picture suggesting subacute or chronic osteomyelitis (Fig. 8)
2. An unusual location of lesions when compared with infectious osteomyelitis and frequent multifocality
3. No abscess formation, fistula, or sequestra
4. Lack of a causative organism
5. Nonspecific histopathologic and laboratory findings compatible with subacute or chronic osteomyelitis
6. A characteristic prolonged, fluctuating course with recurrent episodes of pain
7. Occasional accompanying skin disease [83]

The lesions of chronic recurrent multifocal osteomyelitis are predominantly located on tubular bones followed by the clavicle, the spine, and pelvic bones [84,85].

Autoimmune diseases

Systemic lupus erythematosus

Systemic lupus erythematosus is an autoimmune disease characterized by a persistent nonspecific polyclonal B-cell activation that results in widespread tissue deposition of immune complexes that may cause organ damage [86]. Antiphospholipid antibodies, which are associated with a hypercoagulable state, have been associated with a variety of abnormalities including coronary artery and microvascular thrombotic occlusion, myocardial and cerebral infarction, and diffuse cardiomyopathy [87,88].

Musculoskeletal system

Arthropathy affects most children with systemic lupus erythematosus [89]. Although synovial proliferation may be present, erosive changes are rare [90]. The joint space is generally preserved. Conventional radiography may show soft tissue swelling, joint effusion, and periarticular osteopenia in addition to the characteristic digital hyperextension at the proximal interphalangeal joints ("swan neck" deformities) and proximal interphalangeal flexion associated with distal interphalangeal hyperextension ("boutonniere" deformity) The changes of deforming nonerosive arthropathy are usually reversible [91]. Contrast-enhanced T1-weighted MRI can demonstrate the extent and distribution of abnormal synovium, which appears as brightly enhancing, linear, villous, or nodular tissue lining the joint [7] as well as the presence of joint effusion. Fat-suppressed three-dimensional fast spoiled gradient-recalled echo (3-D SPGR) MR images may be useful for early depiction of osteochondral changes. Children with systemic lupus erythematosus are at risk of developing osteonecrosis in weight-bearing bones (femoral heads and tibial plateaus), especially if they have a previous history of longstanding corticotherapy [92,93]. Ultrasonography can detect fluid within the synovial sheath of the tendons, synovial thickening, and partial and complete tendon ruptures [94]. Typically, sonography is the first imaging modality used to evaluate children with clinical suspicion of tenosynovitis or bursitis. MRI is reserved for cases in which findings on ultrasonography were inconclusive [7].

Heart

Echocardiography and MRI may disclose the presence of pericardial effusion, fibrous pericardial disease, Libman-Sacks verrucae, calcified valvular leaflets, and abnormal ventricular function [95]. Thallium-201 scintigraphic studies may reveal segmental perfusion abnormalities that are either reversible (ischemia) or persistent (scar) or both [87,95]. Technetium-99m sestamibi (Tc99m-MIBI) offers several advantages over thallium-201 for myocardium perfusion imaging, including higher quality images, on-site availability, and the possibility of monitoring the state of mitochondrial energetics [96].

Lungs

Pulmonary involvement includes pleural effusion, alveolitis, pneumonia, obliterative bronchiolitis, pulmonary vasculitis and hemorrhage, pulmonary arterial hypertension, and thromboembolic disease [97,98]. High-resolution CT is a sensitive technique to detect interstitial lung disease, bronchiectasis, mediastinal or hilar lymphadenopathy, and pleural or pericardial effusion. It is especially useful in patients who present with normal chest plain radiographs and pulmonary function tests [99].

Urinary tract

Renal involvement produces abnormalities indistinguishable from those caused by other diseases that progress with glomerulonephritis and end-stage renal failure. Ultrasonography may show enlarged kidneys because of nephritis or secondary to renal vein thrombosis and signs of ureteric obstructions at the level of the vesicoureteric junction caused by interstitial cystitis [89,100,101].

Central nervous system

Imaging is useful in children who present with cerebral hemorrhages (CT or conventional MRI), focal ischemic brain lesions (diffusion-weighted MRI)

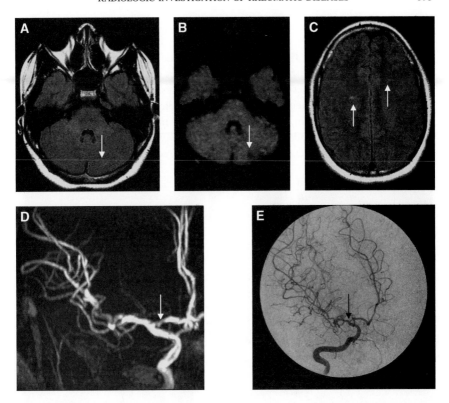

Fig. 9. Subtle high signal intensity abnormalities (*arrows*) are noted (*A,B*) in the left cerebellar hemisphere (FLAIR)/diffusion-weighted MRI images and (*C*) in the centrum semiovale bilaterally (FLAIR image) representing areas of previous stroke in a 14-year-old girl with systemic lupus erythematosus. (*D*) Her corresponding MR angiography and (*E*) conventional angiogram show focal narrowing at the origin of the right middle cerebral artery (*arrows*) resulting from her lupus vasculitis.

(Fig. 9), and venous sinus thrombosis (MR venogram) [102,103]. Single photon emission tomography scanning is a sensitive but poorly specific technique for assessing cerebral blood flow and for detecting subtle areas of decreased perfusion in systemic erythematosus lupus [104].

Juvenile dermatomyositis

Juvenile dermatomyositis (JDM) is an autoimmune inflammatory myopathy characterized by diffuse, nonsuppurative inflammation of muscle fibers and skin [105]. Clinical findings include severe proximal muscle weakness, fatigue, heliotrope rash, and underlying vasculitic pathology [106,107].

Musculoskeletal system

In the acute stage of JDM, incipient soft tissue swelling and subcutaneous edema represented by blurring of fatty tissue planes can be noted in the proximal appendicular skeleton in some cases. The muscles of the scapular and pelvic girdles are most frequently affected, and their involvement is typically symmetrical [108,109]. In chronic disease, plain radiographs demonstrate loss of soft tissue bulk secondary to muscle atrophy (Fig. 10). There also may be marked osteoporosis of the long bones and vertebral bodies. The most

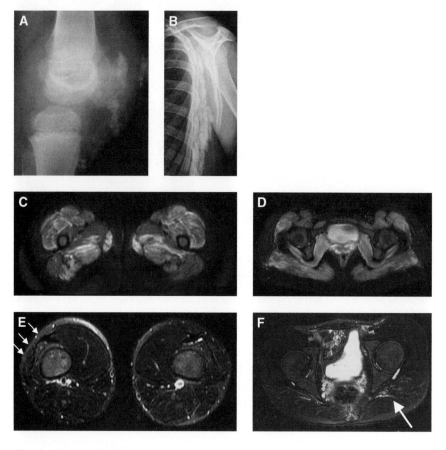

Fig. 10. (*A*) Lateral radiograph of the knee and (*B*) oblique radiograph of the chest wall reveal extensive soft tissue calcium deposits in patients with juvenile dermatomyositis. (*C–F*) Axial fast spin-echo inversion-recovery MR images of the pelvic girdle and thigh musculature of two other patients with dermatomyositis. (*C,D*) Diffuse increased signal intensity is seen in most muscles of an 18-year-old girl, sparing only some muscle groups such as the gluteus maximus, tensor of fascia lata, and vastus lateralis. (*E,F*) Focal areas of atrophy and fatty involution are noted along the rectus femoris and vastus lateralis muscles (*small arrows*, *E*). In a 16-year-old girl, only subtle, ill-defined areas of increased signal intensity are seen involving the gluteus maximus muscle (*long arrow*, *F*). This differing pattern is likely related to the inflammatory activity of the disease.

characteristic finding of chronic disease, however, which is identified in 25% to 50% of the cases, is the deposition of calcium in the soft tissues (Fig. 10) [110]. The calcium deposits may present as subcutaneous plaques, nodules, periarticular calcific foci, and large clumps or sheets of calcium within the musculature or subcutaneous tissue [111]. The arthritis associated with JDM is usually transient and nondeforming [111].

Sonographic scanning of the involved musculature shows diffusely increased echogenicity of the soft tissues and acoustic shadowing within the musculature regions that correspond to calcium deposits. Other sonographic findings that may be seen in JDM include atrophy, decreased muscular bulk, soft tissue fasciculation, tenosynovitis, and soft tissue nodularity [112].

MRI is more sensitive than sonography for the detection of edema, representing inflammation, in the acute phase of the disease. Although both MRI and sonography allow guided biopsy and aspiration of muscle pathology [113–116], ultrasonography has the advantage over MRI of not requiring sedation for younger children. MRI reveals increased water content (edema) within infarcted muscles resulting from the vasculitis process [117]. This intramuscular edema is depicted as increased signal intensity on T2-weighted and STIR images (Fig. 10). T2 relaxation time can be used as a quantitative measure of muscle inflammation and correlates well with other measures of disease activity [118]. In chronic disease, focal areas of low signal intensity, which represent calcific and fibrotic foci, are usually seen on all MRI sequences. Focal areas of increased signal intensity on T1-weighted images representing partial fatty replacement of muscles and tenosynovitis-related changes may also be identified on MRI [117,119].

Although CT is not indicated for detection of inflammatory changes in muscle tissue, it is the modality of choice for identifying calcifications in soft tissues, which are characteristically associated with JDM [120].

Phosphorus-31 MR spectroscopy is able to characterize metabolic abnormalities in vivo and to localize nonhomogeneous inflammation in JDM patients [107]. Biochemical abnormalities in JDM are probably related to decreased delivery of energy substrates and oxygen expressed by reduced levels of ATP and phosphocreatine within the muscle region-of-interest. An additional potential role of this technique is to monitor joints after the disappearance of inflammation and normalization of serum levels of muscle enzymes [107].

Scleroderma

Scleroderma is an autoimmune connective tissue disease that involves the microvascular system. Childhood onset is uncommon and accounts for only a small proportion of patients [121]. Two main categories of scleroderma have been described: systemic (also known as systemic sclerosis) and localized disease [122], the latter being the most common form of disease in children (rate of localized versus systemic scleroderma, 9:1). With increasing severity of the disease, the excessive production of collagen and its accumulation in the extracellular matrix leads to thickening of the skin and to interstitial fibrosis of the organs [122,123].

Musculoskeletal system

Radiologic findings of systemic sclerosis in children include resorption of the extremities of the distal phalanges (acro-osteolysis) (Fig. 11), resorption of

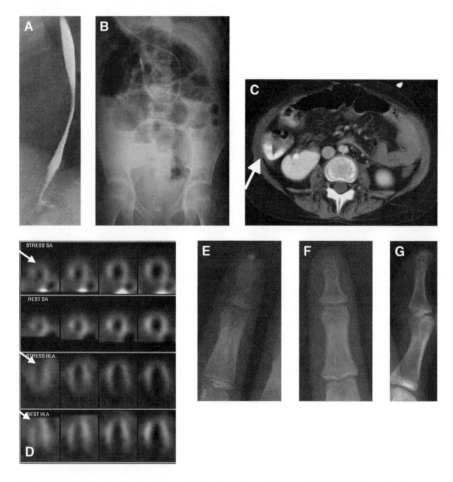

Fig. 11. Multisystemic manifestations of scleroderma in an 11-year-old girl. (*A*) The patient's upper barium meal showed poor motility of the distal esophagus with slow emptying into the stomach. (*B*) The frontal radiograph of the abdomen reveals moderate bowel dilatation with multiple air fluid levels suggestive of a partial small bowel obstruction. (*C*) A CT scan of the abdomen obtained 2 months after the abdominal radiograph shows a thickened bowel loop in the right lower quadrant (*arrow*), probably representing ileum. (*D*) The patient's MIBI study shows a large perfusion defect in the inferior cardiac wall near the apex (*arrows*) with minimal reversibility. (*E*) A small, rounded radiopaque density, (*F*) acro-osteolysis, and (*G*) stippled calcific foci are shown at the digital tips.

the distal ends of ribs, clavicles, radius, and ulna [124,125], polyarthritis, flexion contractures, subcutaneous and periarticular calcification, and thickening of the periodontal membrane [124,125].

Sonography may depict soft tissue calcifications and narrowing of the distance between phalanx apex and skin surface [126]. Recently, high-resolution ultrasonography has been shown to be valuable for evaluating the dermis and hypodermis of patients with localized scleroderma [127–130]. Sonograms may disclose undulations, disorganization, and loss of thickness of the dermis, and thickened hyperechoic bands in the hypodermis, as well as a characteristic flattened "yo-yo" image caused by retraction of the hypodermis [128].

Gastrointestinal tract

The esophagus is the most commonly affected organ in pediatric systemic sclerosis [124]. Barium- or water-soluble contrast radiographic studies may reveal decreased or absent peristalsis (Fig. 11), hiatal hernia, strictures in the distal esophagus, and bowel abnormalities. The degree of esophageal involvement can also be assessed by measuring the esophageal transit time with radioisotopes [131]. Bowel abnormalities are most commonly represented by focal dilatations of the second and third parts of the duodenum and proximal jejunum [131,132], loss of the colonic haustra, development of diverticula in the antimesenteric border [133], and intestinal pseudo-obstruction (see Fig. 10) [134].

Lungs

Basal interstitial shadowing may be identified on conventional radiography [135], but high-resolution CT scan is the method of choice for evaluation of the lungs [136]. In the initial stage of the disease, poorly defined subpleural

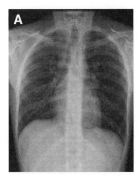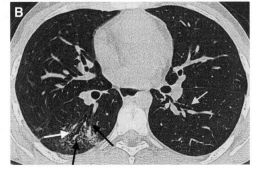

Fig. 12. (*A*) Frontal radiograph of the chest of a 17-year-old boy with scleroderma displays only subtle increased interstitial markings. (*B*) The corresponding high-resolution CT scan obtained within 2 days of the radiograph reveals the presence of traction bronchiectasis (*arrows*) in the superior segment of the right lower lobe and thickening and fibrosis of the interlobular septa.

densities are typically seen in the posterior segments of the lower lobes. Later on, subpleural reticulonodularities [137], ground-glass opacities, septal thickening, and honeycombing are identified (Fig. 12). Gallium and calcium trisodium DTPA also have been used to assess the degree of pulmonary inflammation in the initial stage of diffuse systemic sclerosis [122,136].

Vasculitis

Vasculitis is an inflammatory process that affects arteries, veins, and capillaries. The vessel wall is infiltrated by inflammatory cells that may or may not produce vascular destruction [138]. The vessels involved may be small, medium, or large. Most of the vasculitides affect vessels of varying sizes, although one particular size can be more commonly affected. Among the vasculitides described here, Kawasaki disease is the most common in the pediatric age group [138].

Kawasaki disease

Kawasaki disease is an acute vasculitis characterized by fever, rash, conjunctival injection, exanthem, redness and swelling of the hands and feet, and cervical adenitis [139]. This disease is seen almost exclusively in young children; approximately 80% of affected patients are under the age of 5 years [139]. The histopathogic features of vasculitis involving arterioles, capillaries, and venules appear in the earliest phase of the disease. Coronary aneurysms or ectasia develop in approximately 15% to 20% of untreated patients within 4 to 6 weeks of disease onset [140]. The long-term clinical issue in Kawasaki disease concerns the coronary artery lesions, which involve aneurysm formation, thrombotic occlusion, progression to ischemic heart disease, and premature atherosclerosis [141]. Various peripheral and central arterial segments may also develop aneurysms in patients with Kawasaki disease (Fig. 13).

Heart

Two-dimensional echocardiography and selective coronary angiography are standard methods to evaluate coronary artery lesions [140]. Intravascular ultrasonography may show intimal thickening with calcification at the site of the resolved coronary aneurysm years after the onset of the disease. Although transthoracic echocardiography is often sufficient for evaluation of the distribution and size of coronary artery aneurysms, visualization of the coronary arteries becomes progressively more difficult as the children grow. 3-D coronary MR angiography provides a noninvasive alternative imaging tool when echo-

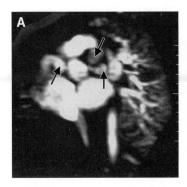
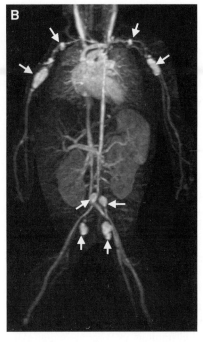

Fig. 13. Reformatted contrast-enhanced 3-D SPGR MR angiography images of a 4-month-old infant with Kawasaki's disease display multiple irregular aneurysms (*arrows*) involving (*A*) both coronary arteries and (*B*) brachial and subclavian arteries, and both common and internal iliac arteries.

cardiography image quality is insufficient and reduces the need for serial X-ray coronary angiography in the pediatric population (Fig. 13) [142].

Polyarteritis nodosa

Polyarteritis nodosa is characterized clinically by a necrotizing vasculitis caused by immune complex deposition in vessel walls that predominantly involve medium-sized arteries of kidneys, central nervous system, muscles, and viscera [143]. The inflammation may skip areas along the course of the involved vessel [138].

Central nervous system

Aneurysms often form at the branching points of small- and medium-sized arteries. Their rupture may result in spontaneous hemorrhage in approximately 6% of cases [144]. Cerebral angiography demonstrates alternating segments of narrowed and widened arteries, occlusion of small arteries, or, less frequently, intracranial aneurysms [145]. Aneurysms in children differ from those in adults: a greater propotion of aneurysms seen in children are infections and peripheral, or involve the posterior cerebral circulation [146]. T2-weighted MRI may show high signal intensity abnormalities, consistent with infarcts, in cortical and white matter [147].

Wegener's granulomatosis

Wegener's granulomatosis is a multisystemic disorder characterized by necrotizing granulomas in the upper or lower respiratory tract, with or without focal necrotizing glomerulonephritis and a systemic vasculitis [148]. This vasculitis predominantly affects medium and small blood vessels [138].

Upper respiratory tract

Erosion of nasal septum, bleeding material from mucosal ulcers of nose, granulomatous masses filling nasal cavities, destruction of the nasal cartilage, and thickening of the membranes of the paranasal sinuses are common radiographic findings in Wegener's granulomatosis (Fig. 14) [149].

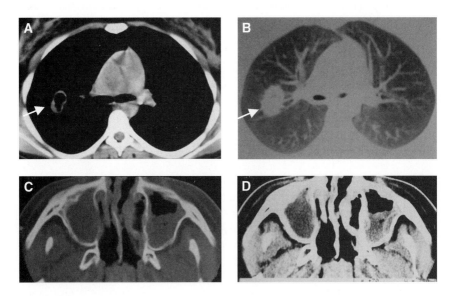

Fig. 14. (*A*) Mediastinal and (*B*) lung windows of enhanced helical CT scans of a child with Wegener's granulomatosis reveal a large, thick-walled cavity with irregular inner lining (*arrows*) within the right upper lobe. This cavitated nodular lesion represents a noncaseous granuloma. This patient also presented with bilateral thickening of the mucous membranes of the maxillary sinus, most notably on the right (*C,D*) and nasal septal deviation as shown on bone and soft tissue windows.

Lungs

Radiographs and CT scans may show pulmonary infiltrates (granulomata), which can be discrete and solitary or multiple and bilateral, having a predilection for the lower lobes of the lungs [150]. Cavitation of the pulmonary granulomatous lesions (Fig. 14), pneumothorax, and pleural effusions may also develop.

Urinary tract

Although the appearances of the renal parenchyma may be nonspecific on ultrasonography, an abnormally reflective renal cortex suggests active interstitial renal disease. In the acute stages of glomerulonephritis the kidney may be enlarged with a smooth outline, eventually becoming smaller in the later stage with generalized cortical atrophy. These findings can be demonstrated by gray-scale ultrasonography or CT [151].

Central nervous system

Cerebral angiography can be negative in suspected cases of cerebral vasculitis related to Wegener's granulomatosis because of the involvement of small vessels (50–300 μm) [152]. On MRI, granulomatous lesions in the brain parenchyma can appear as homogeneously enhancing or ring-enhancing masses on T1-weighted images and as regions of hyperintense signal intensity on T2-weighted images, typically in the white matter [153].

Takayasu's arteritis

Takayasu's arteritis is a chronic, progressive, and obliterative arteritis of large vessels that has a predilection for the aorta and its major branches but may also involve the coronary and pulmonary arteries [138]. It is characterized by a granulomatous inflammation of the arterial wall with marked intimal proliferation and fibrosis of the media and adventitia. This may lead to stenosis, occlusion, poststenotic dilatations, and aneurysm formation [154]. This arteritis is uncommon in children, but its mortality rate in this age group is as high as 40% [155].

Arterial involvement in Takayasu's arteritis can be detected by sonography when there is an acoustic window for the vessel section involved [156]. Otherwise, MR or CT angiography should be considered [157,158]. Sonography can demonstrate segmental or diffuse circumferential thickening of the arterial wall, whereas angiography provides information solely about the vascular lumen. Contrast-enhanced T1-weighted spin-echo MRI may show more enhancement in the thickened aorta wall (usually >3 mm) than in the myocardium, thus suggesting active disease (Fig. 15) [157]. During the early phase of Takayasu's arteritis, only mild luminal changes of the arteries may be present without sig-

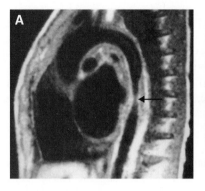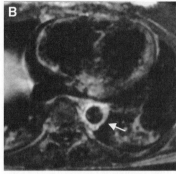

Fig. 15. Contrast-enhanced fat-suppressed (*A*) sagittal and (*B*) axial T1-weighted spin-echo MR images of the aorta of a child with Takayasu's arteritis show markedly enhanced wall thickening and luminal narrowing at the level of the proximal descending thoracic aorta (*arrows*). No significant involvement of the innominate, common carotid, or subclavian arteries was noted.

nificant stenosis. These may not be detectable by conventional or digital subtraction angiography [157]. In this phase of the disease, when luminal stenosis has not yet occurred, cross-sectional imaging techniques (helical CT or MR angiography) are better suited for the evaluation of subtle vascular changes [154,159].

Osteoporosis

Osteoporosis is a skeletal disease characterized by low bone mass and microarchitectural deterioration of bone tissue, which leads to increased bone fragility and fracture [160]. In JIA, multiple risk factors are associated with decreased bone mass including severity of inflammatory disease, decreased mobility, and use of glucocorticoids. Fractures may occur with low or minimal trauma, particularly in skeletal sites rich in trabecular bone (wrist, femoral neck, and spine) [161]. In adults, osteoporosis is defined as a loss of measured bone mineral density compared with the expected peak bone mass of young adults (T-score), measured with dual energy X-ray absorptiometry (DEXA) at any skeletal site. In children, there are currently no generally accepted definitions for osteoporosis and osteopenia, and a Z-score (obtained with comparison to age- and sex-matched controls) is used. Increasingly, it is recognized that osteopenia and osteoporosis are common in pediatric rheumatic diseases. Normal peak bone mass may not be achieved in children and adolescents with chronic rheumatic disease, predisposing them to risk of premature osteoporosis and fracture. Periodic measurement of bone mineral density with DEXA has been suggested for high-risk patients. Studies on drug treatment of osteoporosis in pediatric rheumatic disease are limited but suggest that bone mass can be enhanced with growth hormone and biphosphonates.

Several imaging methods are currently available for diagnosis of osteoporosis in children and adolescents [162]. DEXA has several advantages, such as fast scanning, low cost, low radiation dose, and applicability to clinically relevant sites of osteoporotic fracture. However, DEXA provides two-dimensional imaging of 3-D objects, does not distinguish between trabecular and cortical bone [163], and is size dependent (a potential problem in growing children). A further drawback is that in vivo bone strength is related to bone quality as well as to bone density [164–166]. Radiographs are generally unhelpful, but a new radiographic scoring system that uses lateral radiographs to assess vertebral morphology and to measure vertebral body dimensions in spinal radiographs of pediatric patients with suspected osteoporosis seems useful [167]. Quantitative CT can assess both bone volume and bone density in the axial and appendicular skeletons independent of skeletal size and can provide separate measures of cortical and trabecular bone. The need for more irradiation for examination often precludes its use for assessment of normal persons in research studies, limiting normal comparative data. Quantitative ultrasound is a recently introduced modality that is inexpensive, easy to use, and does not require radiation. Ultrasound values, however, are dependent on many structural bone properties not yet fully understood, which limits its use.

Future developments

A number of novel imaging techniques are under evaluation for better or earlier assessment of synovial, cartilaginous, or osseous abnormalities. These techniques include MR techniques such as diffusion-weighted and perfusion imaging, delayed gadolinium-enhanced cartilage imaging, and T2 quantification. Diffusion-weighted imaging demonstrates the normal translational movement (Brownian motion) of water molecules that occurs in all tissues [76,77]. Alteration of normal diffusion can occur in pathologic events with a loss of tissue integrity. This technique is promising for evaluating ischemic tissues [78] and functional changes associated with osteoporosis [79]. Perfusion imaging assesses blood flow using intravenously administered paramagnetic contrast agents and may be helpful in characterizing ischemic or hyperemic areas [81,82]. Potential uses of this technique include recognition of epiphyseal ischemia [8], quantification and monitoring of synovial inflammation [8], and directing therapeutic scheduling for rheumatoid arthritis according to enhancement patterns [83].

Delayed gadolinium-enhanced MR cartilage imaging (dGEMRIC) is a sensitive technique for assessing cartilage proteoglycan content using the negative charge of the paramagnetic MR contrast agent. The contrast agent distributes into the cartilage inversely to the fixed charge density of negatively charged glycosaminoglycans (GAG) [84]. Thus, T1 relaxation time in presence of this contrast agent is approximately linearly related to the glycosaminoglycan content. dGEMRIC may be used to assess early cartilage injury with depletion of glycosaminoglycans. Other cartilage assessment can be provided by mapping T2 relaxation time [92,93]. T2 measurements may characterize the structural integrity of the cartilaginous tissue and quantitatively assess the degree of cartilaginous degeneration, as previously shown in the pediatric population [95].

Summary

Extensive evidence now supports the increasing role of all the cross-sectional imaging modalities, but especially MRI and sonography, in investigating rheumatic disease. CT plays a more limited role because of its need for radiation and its relatively poorer soft tissue contrast. MRI provides exquisite detail of all joint and periarticular soft tissues, which can be used to provide earlier and more accurate diagnosis and follow-up of inflammatory arthritides. The application of these techniques should enable better-targeted therapy and evaluation of potential complications.

References

[1] Lamer S, Sebag GH. MRI and ultrasound in children with juvenile chronic arthritis. Eur J Radiol 2000;33(2):85–93.
[2] Ostergaard M, Ejbjerg B, Szkudlarek M. Imaging in early rheumatoid arthritis: roles of magnetic resonance imaging, ultrasonography, conventional radiography and computed tomography. Best Pract Res Clin Rheumatol 2005;19(1):91–116.
[3] Ostergaard M, Duer A, Moller U, et al. Magnetic resonance imaging of peripheral joints in rheumatic diseases. Best Pract Res Clin Rheumatol 2004;18(6):861–79.
[4] Grassi W, Filippucci E, Busilacchi P. Musculoskeletal ultrasound. Best Pract Res Clin Rheumatol 2004;18(6):813–26.
[5] Schanberg LE, Sandstrom MJ. Causes of pain in children with arthritis. Rheum Dis Clin North Am 1999;25(1):31–53.
[6] Johnson K, Gardner-Medwin J. Childhood arthritis: classification and radiology. Clin Radiol 2002;57(1):47–58.
[7] Gylys-Morin VM. MR imaging of pediatric musculoskeletal inflammatory and infectious disorders. Magn Reson Imaging Clin N Am 1998;6(3):537–59.
[8] Patriquin HB, Camerlain M, Trias A. Late sequelae of juvenile rheumatoid arthritis of the hip: a follow-up study into adulthood. Pediatr Radiol 1984;14(3):151–7.
[9] Cellerini M, Salti S, Trapani S, et al. Correlation between clinical and ultrasound assessment of the knee in children with mono-articular or pauci-articular juvenile rheumatoid arthritis. Pediatr Radiol 1999;29(2):117–23.
[10] Eich GF, Halle F, Hodler J, et al. Juvenile chronic arthritis: imaging of the knees and hips before and after intraarticular steroid injection. Pediatr Radiol 1994;24(8):558–63.
[11] Ruhoy MK, Tucker L, McCauley RG. Hypertrophic bursopathy of the subacromial-subdeltoid bursa in juvenile rheumatoid arthritis: sonographic appearance. Pediatr Radiol 1996;26(5): 353–5.
[12] Graham TB, Blebea JS, Gylys-Morin V, et al. Magnetic resonance imaging in juvenile rheumatoid arthritis. Semin Arthritis Rheum 1997;27(3):161–8.
[13] White EM. Magnetic resonance imaging in synovial disorders and arthropathy of the knee. Magn Reson Imaging Clin N Am 1994;2(3):451–61.
[14] Chung C, Coley BD, Martin LC. Rice bodies in juvenile rheumatoid arthritis. AJR Am J Roentgenol 1998;170(3):698–700.

[15] Tsai TC, Chang PY, Chen BF, et al. Retroperitoneal fibrosis and juvenile rheumatoid arthritis. Pediatr Nephrol 1996;10(2):208–9.

[16] Pettersson H, Rydholm U. Radiologic classification of knee joint destruction in juvenile chronic arthritis. Pediatr Radiol 1984;14(6):419–21.

[17] Ostergaard M, Stoltenberg M, Gideon P, et al. Changes in synovial membrane and joint effusion volumes after intraarticular methylprednisolone. Quantitative assessment of inflammatory and destructive changes in arthritis by MRI. J Rheumatol 1996;23(7):1151–61.

[18] Sparling M, Malleson P, Wood B, et al. Radiographic followup of joints injected with triamcinolone hexacetonide for the management of childhood arthritis. Arthritis Rheum 1990;33(6):821–6.

[19] Sureda D, Quiroga S, Arnal C, et al. Juvenile rheumatoid arthritis of the knee: evaluation with US. Radiology 1994;190(2):403–6.

[20] Klauser A, Frauscher F, Schirmer M, et al. The value of contrast-enhanced color Doppler ultrasound in the detection of vascularization of finger joints in patients with rheumatoid arthritis. Arthritis Rheum 2002;46(3):647–53.

[21] Stone M, Bergin D, Whelan B, et al. Power Doppler ultrasound assessment of rheumatoid hand synovitis. J Rheumatol 2001;28(9):1979–82.

[22] Terslev L, Torp-Pedersen S, Savnik A, et al. Doppler ultrasound and magnetic resonance imaging of synovial inflammation of the hand in rheumatoid arthritis: a comparative study. Arthritis Rheum 2003;48(9):2434–41.

[23] Terslev L, Torp-Pedersen S, Qvistgaard E, et al. Estimation of inflammation by Doppler ultrasound: quantitative changes after intra-articular treatment in rheumatoid arthritis. Ann Rheum Dis 2003;62(11):1049–53.

[24] Doria AS, Kiss MH, Lotito AP, et al. Juvenile rheumatoid arthritis of the knee: evaluation with contrast-enhanced color Doppler ultrasound. Pediatr Radiol 2001;31(7):524–31.

[25] Shahin AA, el Mofty SA, el Sheikh EA, et al. Power Doppler sonography in the evaluation and follow-up of knee involvement in patients with juvenile idiopathic arthritis. Z Rheumatol 2001;60(3):148–55.

[26] Smith HJ. Contrast-enhanced MRI of rheumatic joint disease. Br J Rheumatol 1996; 35(Suppl 3):45–7.

[27] Jacobs JC, Berdon WE, Johnston AD. HLA-B27-associated spondyloarthritis and enthesopathy in childhood: clinical, pathologic, and radiographic observations in 58 patients. J Pediatr 1982;100(4):521–8.

[28] Bollow M, Braun J, Kannenberg J, et al. Normal morphology of sacroiliac joints in children: magnetic resonance studies related to age and sex. Skeletal Radiol 1997;26(12):697–704.

[29] Azouz EM, Duffy CM. Juvenile spondyloarthropathies: clinical manifestations and medical imaging. Skeletal Radiol 1995;24(6):399–408.

[30] Azouz EM, Babyn P, Chlem RK. MRI of the pediatric knee. In: Munk PL, Helms CA, editors. MRI of the knee. Philadelphia: Lippincott-Raven; 1995. p. 281–314.

[31] Kamel M, Eid H, Mansour R. Ultrasound detection of heel enthesitis: a comparison with magnetic resonance imaging. J Rheumatol 2003;30(4):774–8.

[32] D'Agostino MA, Said-Nahal R, Hacquard-Bouder C, et al. Assessment of peripheral enthesitis in the spondylarthropathies by ultrasonography combined with power Doppler: a cross-sectional study. Arthritis Rheum 2003;48(2):523–33.

[33] Tse SML, Doria AS, Babyn PS, et al. Anti-tumor necrosis factor alpha therapy leads to improvement of both enthesitis and synovitis in children with enthesitis-related arthritis. In: Programs and Abstracts of Park City and Beyond IX: 2003. p. 1.

[34] Balint PV, Kane D, Wilson H, et al. Ultrasonography of entheseal insertions in the lower limb in spondyloarthropathy. Ann Rheum Dis 2002;61(10):905–10.

[35] Lehtinen A, Taavitsainen M, Leirisalo-Repo M. Sonographic analysis of enthesopathy in the lower extremities of patients with spondylarthropathy. Clin Exp Rheumatol 1994;12(2):143–8.

[36] Lehtinen A, Leirisalo-Repo M, Taavitsainen M. Persistence of enthesopathic changes in patients with spondylarthropathy during a 6-month follow-up. Clin Exp Rheumatol 1995; 13(6):733–6.

[37] Bollow M, Braun J, Biedermann T, et al. Use of contrast-enhanced MR imaging to detect sacroiliitis in children. Skeletal Radiol 1998;27(11):606–16.

[38] Foster HE, Cairns RA, Burnell RH, et al. Atlantoaxial subluxation in children with seronegative enthesopathy and arthropathy syndrome: 2 case reports and a review of the literature. J Rheumatol 1995;22(3):548–51.

[39] Prieur AM. Spondyloarthropathies in childhood. Baillieres Clin Rheumatol 1998;12(2): 287–307.

[40] Jaramillo D, Treves ST, Kasser JR, et al. Osteomyelitis and septic arthritis in children: appropriate use of imaging to guide treatment. AJR Am J Roentgenol 1995;165(2):399–403.

[41] Brower AC. Septic arthritis. Radiol Clin North Am 1996;34(2):293–309.

[42] Mitchell CS, Parisi MT. Pediatric acetabuloplasty procedures: radiologic evaluation. AJR Am J Roentgenol 1998;170(1):49–54.

[43] Forrester DM, Feske WI. Imaging of infectious arthritis. Semin Roentgenol 1996;31(3): 239–49.

[44] Lee SK, Suh KJ, Kim YW, et al. Septic arthritis versus transient synovitis at MR imaging: preliminary assessment with signal intensity alterations in bone marrow. Radiology 1999; 211(2):459–65.

[45] Sandrasegaran K, Saifuddin A, Coral A, et al. Magnetic resonance imaging of septic sacroiliitis. Skeletal Radiol 1994;23(4):289–92.

[46] Sturzenbecher A, Braun J, Paris S, et al. MR imaging of septic sacroiliitis. Skeletal Radiol 2000;29(8):439–46.

[47] Marchal GJ, Van Holsbeeck MT, Raes M, et al. Transient synovitis of the hip in children: role of US. Radiology 1987;162(3):825–8.

[48] Robben SG, Lequin MH, Diepstraten AF, et al. Anterior joint capsule of the normal hip and in children with transient synovitis: US study with anatomic and histologic correlation. Radiology 1999;210(2):499–507.

[49] Ranner G, Ebner F, Fotter R, et al. Magnetic resonance imaging in children with acute hip pain. Pediatr Radiol 1989;20(1–2):67–71.

[50] Yulish BS, Lieberman JM, Strandjord SE, et al. Hemophilic arthropathy: assessment with MR imaging. Radiology 1987;164(3):759–62.

[51] Rand T, Trattnig S, Male C, Heinz-Peer G, et al. Magnetic resonance imaging in hemophilic children: value of gradient echo and contrast-enhanced imaging. Magn Reson Imaging 1999;17(2):199–205.

[52] Rodriguez-Merchan EC. Effects of hemophilia on articulations of children and adults. Clin Orthop 1996;328:7–13.

[53] Baunin C, Railhac JJ, Younes I, et al. MR imaging in hemophilic arthropathy. Eur J Pediatr Surg 1991;1(6):358–63.

[54] Nuss R, Kilcoyne RF, Geraghty S, et al. Utility of magnetic resonance imaging for management of hemophilic arthropathy in children. J Pediatr 1993;123(3):388–92.

[55] Kottamasu SR. Bone changes in diseases of the blood and blood-forming organs. In: Kuhn JP, Slovis TL, Haller JO, editors. Caffey's pediatric diagnostic imaging. Philadelphia: Elsevier; 2004. p. 2417–35.

[56] Nagele M, Kunze V, Hamann M, et al. [Hemophiliac arthropathy of the knee joint. Gd-DTPA-enhanced MRI; clinical and roentgenological correlation]. Rofo 1994;160(2):154–8 [in German].

[57] Hermann G, Gilbert MS, Abdelwahab IF. Hemophilia: evaluation of musculoskeletal involvement with CT, sonography, and MR imaging. AJR Am J Roentgenol 1992;158(1): 119–23.

[58] Llauger J, Monill JM, Palmer J, et al. Synovial hemangioma of the knee: MRI findings in two cases. Skeletal Radiol 1995;24(8):579–81.

[59] Resnick D, Oliphant M. Hemophilia-like arthropathy of the knee associated with cutaneous and synovial hemangiomas. Report of 3 cases and review of the literature. Radiology 1975; 114(2):323–36.

[60] Cotten A, Flipo RM, Herbaux B, et al. Synovial haemangioma of the knee: a frequently misdiagnosed lesion. Skeletal Radiol 1995;24(4):257–61.

[61] Greenspan A, Azouz EM, Matthews J, et al. Synovial hemangioma: imaging features in eight histologically proven cases, review of the literature, and differential diagnosis. Skeletal Radiol 1995;24(8):583–90.

[62] Wong K, Sallomi D, Janzen DL, et al. Monoarticular synovial lesions: radiologic pictorial essay with pathologic illustration. Clin Radiol 1999;54(5):273–84.

[63] Goldman AB, DiCarlo EF. Pigmented villonodular synovitis. Diagnosis and differential diagnosis. Radiol Clin North Am 1988;26(6):1327–47.

[64] Lin J, Jacobson JA, Jamadar DA, et al. Pigmented villonodular synovitis and related lesions: the spectrum of imaging findings. AJR Am J Roentgenol 1999;172(1):191–7.

[65] Eustace S, Harrison M, Srinivasen U, et al. Magnetic resonance imaging in pigmented villonodular synovitis. Can Assoc Radiol J 1994;45(4):283–6.

[66] Hughes TH, Sartoris DJ, Schweitzer ME, et al. Pigmented villonodular synovitis: MRI characteristics. Skeletal Radiol 1995;24(1):7–12.

[67] Bravo SM, Winalski CS, Weissman BN. Pigmented villonodular synovitis. Radiol Clin North Am 1996;34(2):311–3.

[68] Hallel T, Lew S, Bansal M. Villous lipomatous proliferation of the synovial membrane (lipoma arborescens). J Bone Joint Surg [Am] 1988;70(2):264–70.

[69] Cardinal E, Dussault RG, Kaplan PA. Imaging and differential diagnosis of masses within a joint. Can Assoc Radiol J 1994;45(5):363–72.

[70] Donnelly LF, Bisset III GS, Passo MH. MRI findings of lipoma arborescens of the knee in a child: case report. Pediatr Radiol 1994;24(4):258–9.

[71] Grieten M, Buckwalter KA, Cardinal E, et al. Case report 873: Lipoma arborescens (villous lipomatous proliferation of the synovial membrane). Skeletal Radiol 1994;23(8):652–5.

[72] Feller JF, Rishi M, Hughes EC. Lipoma arborescens of the knee: MR demonstration. AJR Am J Roentgenol 1994;163(1):162–4.

[73] Maillot F, Goupille P, Valat JP. Plant thorn synovitis diagnosed by magnetic resonance imaging. Scand J Rheumatol 1994;23(3):154–5.

[74] Spilberg I, Meyer GJ. The arthritis of leukemia. Arthritis Rheum 1972;15(6):630–5.

[75] Evans TI, Nercessian BM, Sanders KM. Leukemic arthritis. Semin Arthritis Rheum 1994;24(1):48–56.

[76] Gallagher D, Heinrich SD, Craver R, et al. Skeletal manifestations of acute leukemia in childhood. Orthopedics 1991;14(4):485–92.

[77] Taybi H, Lachman RS. Radiology of syndromes, metabolic disorders and skeletal dysplasias. St Louis (MO): Mosby-Year Book; 1996.

[78] Wihlborg CE, Babyn PS, Schneider R. The association between Turner's syndrome and juvenile rheumatoid arthritis. Pediatr Radiol 1999;29(9):676–81.

[79] Spranger J, Albert C, Schilling F, et al. Progressive pseudorheumatoid arthritis of childhood (PPAC). A hereditary disorder simulating rheumatoid arthritis. Eur J Pediatr 1983;140(1): 34–40.

[80] Poznanski AK. Radiological approaches to pediatric joint disease. J Rheumatol Suppl 1992; 33:78–93.

[81] Hugosson C, Bahabri S, McDonald P, et al. Radiological features in congenital camptodactyly, familial arthropathy and coxa vara syndrome. Pediatr Radiol 1994;24(7):523–6.

[82] Laxer RM, Cameron BJ, Chaisson D, et al. The camptodactyly-arthropathy-pericarditis syndrome: case report and literature review. Arthritis Rheum 1986;29(3):439–44.

[83] Jurik AG. Chronic recurrent multifocal osteomyelitis. Semin Musculoskelet Radiol 2004; 8(3):243–53.

[84] Huber AM, Lam PY, Duffy CM, et al. Chronic recurrent multifocal osteomyelitis: clinical outcomes after more than five years of follow-up. J Pediatr 2002;141(2):198–203.

[85] Job-Deslandre C, Krebs S, Kahan A. Chronic recurrent multifocal osteomyelitis: five-year outcomes in 14 pediatric cases. Joint Bone Spine 2001;68(3):245–51.

[86] Lehman TJ. A practical guide to systemic lupus erythematosus. Pediatr Clin North Am 1995; 42(5):1223–38.

[87] Gazarian M, Feldman BM, Benson LN, et al. Assessment of myocardial perfusion and function in childhood systemic lupus erythematosus. J Pediatr 1998;132(1):109–16.

[88] Miller DJ, Maisch SA, Perez MD, et al. Fatal myocardial infarction in an 8-year-old girl with systemic lupus erythematosus, Raynaud's phenomenon, and secondary antiphospholipid antibody syndrome. J Rheumatol 1995;22(4):768–73.

[89] Cassidy JT, Petty RE. Systemic lupus erythematosus. In: Cassidy JT, Petty RE, editors. Textbook of pediatric rheumatology. Philadelphia: W.B. Saunders; 1995. p. 260–322.

[90] Reilly PA, Evison G, McHugh NJ, et al. Arthropathy of hands and feet in systemic lupus erythematosus. J Rheumatol 1990;17(6):777–84.

[91] Resnick D. Lupus Erythematosus. In: Resnick D, editor. Bone and joint imaging. Philadelphia: W.B. Saunders; 1989. p. 347–52.

[92] Abeles M, Urman JD, Rothfield NF. Aseptic necrosis of bone in systemic lupus erythematosus. Relationship to corticosteroid therapy. Arch Intern Med 1978;138(5):750–4.

[93] Griffiths ID, Maini RN, Scott JT. Clinical and radiological features of osteonecrosis in systemic lupus erythematosus. Ann Rheum Dis 1979;38(5):413–22.

[94] van Holsbeeck M, Introcaso JH. Musculoskeletal ultrasonography. Radiol Clin North Am 1992;30(5):907–25.

[95] Roberts WC, High ST. The heart in systemic lupus erythematosus. Curr Probl Cardiol 1999; 24(1):1–56.

[96] Lagana B, Schillaci O, Tubani L, et al. Lupus carditis: evaluation with technetium-99m MIBI myocardial SPECT and heart rate variability. Angiology 1999;50(2):143–8.

[97] Gammon RB, Bridges TA, al Nezir H, et al. Bronchiolitis obliterans organizing pneumonia associated with systemic lupus erythematosus. Chest 1992;102(4):1171–4.

[98] Weinrib L, Sharma OP, Quismorio Jr FP. A long-term study of interstitial lung disease in systemic lupus erythematosus. Semin Arthritis Rheum 1990;20(1):48–56.

[99] Fenlon HM, Doran M, Sant SM, et al. High-resolution chest CT in systemic lupus erythematosus. AJR Am J Roentgenol 1996;166(2):301–7.

[100] Eberhard A, Shore A, Silverman E, et al. Bowel perforation and interstitial cystitis in childhood systemic lupus erythematosus. J Rheumatol 1991;18(5):746–7.

[101] Si-Hoe CK, Thng CH, Chee SG, et al. Abdominal computed tomography in systemic lupus erythematosus. Clin Radiol 1997;52(4):284–9.

[102] Graham JW, Jan W. MRI and the brain in systemic lupus erythematosus. Lupus 2003; 12(12):891–6.

[103] Steinlin MI, Blaser SI, Gilday DL, et al. Neurologic manifestations of pediatric systemic lupus erythematosus. Pediatr Neurol 1995;13(3):191–7.

[104] Russo R, Gilday D, Laxer RM, et al. Single photon emission computed tomography scanning in childhood systemic lupus erythematosus. J Rheumatol 1998;25(3):576–82.

[105] Pachman LM. Juvenile dermatomyositis. Pathophysiology and disease expression. Pediatr Clin North Am 1995;42(5):1071–98.

[106] Chan WP, Liu GC. MR imaging of primary skeletal muscle diseases in children. AJR Am J Roentgenol 2002;179(4):989–97.

[107] Park JH, Niermann KJ, Ryder NM, et al. Muscle abnormalities in juvenile dermatomyositis patients: P-31 magnetic resonance spectroscopy studies. Arthritis Rheum 2000;43(10): 2359–67.

[108] Ozonoff MB, Flynn Jr FJ. Roentgenologic features of dermatomyositis of childhood. Am J Roentgenol Radium Ther Nucl Med 1973;118(1):206–12.

[109] Steiner RM, Glassman L, Schwartz MW, et al. The radiological findings in dermatomyositis of childhood. Radiology 1974;111(2):385–93.

[110] Sullivan DB, Cassidy JT, Petty RE. Dermatomyositis in the pediatric patient. Arthritis Rheum 1977;20(2 Suppl):327–31.

[111] Cassidy JT, Petty RE. Juvenile dermatomyositis. In: Cassidy JT, Petty RE, editors. Textbook of pediatric rheumatology. Philadelphia: W.B. Saunders; 1995. p. 323–64.

[112] Rose AL. Childhood polymyositis. A follow-up study with special reference to treatment with corticosteroids. Am J Dis Child 1974;127(4):518–22.

[113] Bureau NJ, Cardinal E, Chhem RK. Ultrasound of soft tissue masses. Semin Musculoskelet Radiol 1998;2(3):283–98.

[114] Reimers CD, Finkenstaedt M. Muscle imaging in inflammatory myopathies. Curr Opin Rheumatol 1997;9(6):475–85.

[115] Fornage BD. The case for ultrasound of muscles and tendons. Semin Musculoskelet Radiol 2000;4(4):375–91.

[116] Yosipovitch G, Beniaminov O, Rousso I, et al. STIR magnetic resonance imaging: a noninvasive method for detection and follow-up of dermatomyositis. Arch Dermatol 1999; 135(6):721–3.

[117] Hernandez RJ, Keim DR, Sullivan DB, et al. Magnetic resonance imaging appearance of the muscles in childhood dermatomyositis. J Pediatr 1990;117(4):546–50.

[118] Maillard SM, Jones R, Owens C, et al. Quantitative assessment of MRI T2 relaxation time of thigh muscles in juvenile dermatomyositis. Rheumatology (Oxford) 2004;43(5): 603–8.

[119] Huppertz HI, Kaiser WA. Serial magnetic resonance imaging in juvenile dermatomyositis–delayed normalization. Rheumatol Int 1994;14(3):127–9.

[120] Reimers CD, Fleckenstein JL, Witt TN, et al. Muscular ultrasound in idiopathic inflammatory myopathies of adults. J Neurol Sci 1993;116(1):82–92.

[121] Cassidy JT, Petty RE. The sclerodermas and related disorders. In: Cassidy JT, Petty RE, editors. Textbook of pediatric rheumatology. Philadelphia: W.B. Saunders; 1995. p. 423–65.

[122] Uziel Y, Miller ML, Laxer RM. Scleroderma in children. Pediatr Clin North Am 1995;42(5): 1171–203.

[123] LeRoy EC, Black C, Fleischmajer R, et al. Scleroderma (systemic sclerosis): classification, subsets and pathogenesis. J Rheumatol 1988;15(2):202–5.

[124] Cassidy JT, Sullivan DB, Dabich L, et al. Scleroderma in children. Arthritis Rheum 1977; 20(2 Suppl):351–4.

[125] Resnick D. Scleroderma. In: Resnick D, editor. Bone and joint imaging. Philadelphia: WB Saunders; 1996. p. 298–304.

[126] Grassi W, Filippucci E, Farina A, et al. Sonographic imaging of the distal phalanx. Semin Arthritis Rheum 2000;29(6):379–84.

[127] Akesson A, Hesselstrand R, Scheja A, et al. Longitudinal development of skin involvement and reliability of high frequency ultrasound in systemic sclerosis. Ann Rheum Dis 2004; 63(7):791–6.

[128] Cosnes A, Anglade MC, Revuz J, et al. Thirteen-megahertz ultrasound probe: its role in diagnosing localized scleroderma. Br J Dermatol 2003;148(4):724–9.

[129] Kane D, Grassi W, Sturrock R, et al. Musculoskeletal ultrasound–a state of the art review in rheumatology. Part 2: clinical indications for musculoskeletal ultrasound in rheumatology. Rheumatology (Oxford) 2004;43(7):829–38.

[130] Szymanska E, Nowicki A, Mlosek K, et al. Skin imaging with high frequency ultrasound - preliminary results. Eur J Ultrasound 2000;12(1):9–16.

[131] Carette S, Lacourciere Y, Lavoie S, et al. Radionuclide esophageal transit in progressive systemic sclerosis. J Rheumatol 1985;12(3):478–81.

[132] Queloz JM, Woloshin HJ. Sacculation of the small intestine in scleroderma. Radiology 1972; 105(3):513–5.

[133] Martel W, Chang SF, Abell MR. Loss of colonic haustration in progressive systemic sclerosis. AJR Am J Roentgenol 1976;126(4):704–13.

[134] Ortiz-Alvarez O, Cabral D, Prendiville JS, et al. Intestinal pseudo-obstruction as an initial presentation of systemic sclerosis in two children. Br J Rheumatol 1997;36(2):280–4.

[135] Hanlon R, King S. Overview of the radiology of connective tissue disorders in children. Eur J Radiol 2000;33(2):74–84.

[136] Seely JM, Jones LT, Wallace C, et al. Systemic sclerosis: using high-resolution CT to detect lung disease in children. AJR Am J Roentgenol 1998;170(3):691–7.

[137] Remy-Jardin M, Remy J, et al. Pulmonary involvement in progressive systemic sclerosis: sequential evaluation with CT, pulmonary function tests, and bronchoalveolar lavage. Radiology 1993;188(2):499–506.

[138] Athreya BH. Vasculitis in children. Pediatr Clin North Am 1995;42(5):1239–61.

[139] Shulman ST, De Inocencio J, Hirsch R. Kawasaki disease. Pediatr Clin North Am 1995; 42(5):1205–22.

[140] Newburger JW, Takahashi M, Beiser AS, et al. A single intravenous infusion of gamma globulin as compared with four infusions in the treatment of acute Kawasaki syndrome. N Engl J Med 1991;324(23):1633–9.

[141] Hauser M, Bengel F, Kuehn A, et al. Myocardial blood flow and coronary flow reserve in children with "normal" epicardial coronary arteries after the onset of Kawasaki disease assessed by positron emission tomography. Pediatr Cardiol 2004;25(2):108–12.

[142] Greil GF, Stuber M, Botnar RM, et al. Coronary magnetic resonance angiography in adolescents and young adults with Kawasaki disease. Circulation 2002;105(8):908–11.

[143] Gallien S, Mahr A, Rety F, et al. Magnetic resonance imaging of skeletal muscle involvement in limb restricted vasculitis. Ann Rheum Dis 2002;61(12):1107–9.

[144] Lhote F, Guillevin L. Polyarteritis nodosa, microscopic polyangiitis, and Churg-Strauss syndrome. Clinical aspects and treatment. Rheum Dis Clin North Am 1995;21(4):911–47.

[145] Oran I, Memis A, Parildar M, et al. Multiple intracranial aneurysms in polyarteritis nodosa: MRI and angiography. Neuroradiology 1999;41(6):436–9.

[146] Kanaan I, Lasjaunias P, Coates R. The spectrum of intracranial aneurysms in pediatrics. Minim Invasive Neurosurg 1995;38(1):1–9.

[147] Provenzale JM, Allen NB. Neuroradiologic findings in polyarteritis nodosa. AJNR Am J Neuroradiol 1996;17(6):1119–26.

[148] Hoffman GS, Kerr GS, Leavitt RY, et al. Wegener granulomatosis: an analysis of 158 patients. Ann Intern Med 1992;116(6):488–98.

[149] Dahnert W. Radiology review manual. 3rd edition. Baltimore: Williams & Wilkins; 2005.

[150] Rottem M, Fauci AS, Hallahan CW, et al. Wegener granulomatosis in children and adolescents: clinical presentation and outcome. J Pediatr 1993;122(1):26–31.

[151] Rickards D, Jones S. The kidneys. In: Sutton D, editor. A textbook of radiology and imaging. Edinburgh (UK): Churchill Livingstone; 1993. p. 1099–125.

[152] Mentzel HJ, Neumann T, Fitzek C, et al. MR Imaging in Wegener granulomatosis of the spinal cord. AJNR Am J Neuroradiol 2003;24(1):18–21.

[153] Miller KS, Miller JM. Wegener's granulomatosis presenting as a primary seizure disorder with brain lesions demonstrated by magnetic resonance imaging. Chest 1993;103(1):316–8.

[154] Nastri MV, Baptista LP, Baroni RH, et al. Gadolinium-enhanced three-dimensional MR angiography of Takayasu arteritis. Radiographics 2004;24(3):773–86.

[155] Aluquin VP, Albano SA, Chan F, et al. Magnetic resonance imaging in the diagnosis and follow up of Takayasu's arteritis in children. Ann Rheum Dis 2002;61(6):526–9.

[156] Schmidt WA, Nerenheim A, Seipelt E, et al. Diagnosis of early Takayasu arteritis with sonography. Rheumatology (Oxford) 2002;41(5):496–502.

[157] Choe YH, Han BK, Koh EM, et al. Takayasu's arteritis: assessment of disease activity with contrast-enhanced MR imaging. AJR Am J Roentgenol 2000;175(2):505–11.

[158] Scatarige JC, Urban BA, Hellmann DB, et al. Three-dimensional volume-rendering CT angiography in vasculitis: spectrum of disease and clinical utility. J Comput Assist Tomogr 2001;25(4):598–603.

[159] Park JH, Chung JW, Im JG, et al. Takayasu arteritis: evaluation of mural changes in the aorta and pulmonary artery with CT angiography. Radiology 1995;196(1):89–93.

[160] Heaney RP. The natural history of vertebral osteoporosis. Is low bone mass an epiphenomenon? Bone 1992;13(Suppl 2):S23–6.

[161] Borah B, Gross GJ, Dufresne TE, et al. Three-dimensional microimaging (microMRI and microCT), finite element modeling, and rapid prototyping provide unique insights into bone architecture in osteoporosis. Anat Rec 2001;265(2):101–10.

[162] Gilsanz V. Bone density in children: a review of the available techniques and indications. Eur J Radiol 1998;26(2):177–82.

[163] Gomberg BR, Saha PK, Song HK, et al. Topological analysis of trabecular bone MR images. IEEE Trans Med Imaging 2000;19(3):166–74.

[164] Cody DD, Goldstein SA, Flynn MJ, et al. Correlations between vertebral regional bone mineral density (rBMD) and whole bone fracture load. Spine 1991;16(2):146–54.

[165] Lang SM, Moyle DD, Berg EW, et al. Correlation of mechanical properties of vertebral trabecular bone with equivalent mineral density as measured by computed tomography. J Bone Joint Surg [Am] 1988;70(10):1531–8.

[166] Mosekilde L, Bentzen SM, Ortoft G, et al. The predictive value of quantitative computed tomography for vertebral body compressive strength and ash density. Bone 1989;10(6): 465–70.

[167] Makitie O, Doria AS, Henriques F. Radiographic vertebral morphology. A diagnostic tool in pediatric osteoporosis. J Pediatr 2004.

ELSEVIER
SAUNDERS

PEDIATRIC CLINICS
OF NORTH AMERICA

Pediatr Clin N Am 52 (2005) 413–442

Juvenile Idiopathic Arthritis

Jennifer E. Weiss, MD[a], Norman T. Ilowite, MD[a,b,*]

[a]Division of Pediatric Rheumatology, Schneider Children's Hospital, 269-01 76th Avenue,
New Hyde Park, NY 11040, USA
[b]Albert Einstein College of Medicine, New York, NY, USA

Juvenile idiopathic arthritis (JIA) is an umbrella term referring to a group of disorders characterized by chronic arthritis. JIA is the most common chronic rheumatic illness in children and is a significant cause of short- and long-term disability. It is a clinical diagnosis made in a child less than 16 years of age with arthritis (defined as swelling or limitation of motion of the joint accompanied by heat, pain, or tenderness) for at least 6 weeks' duration with other identifiable causes of arthritis excluded. The incidence of JIA ranges from 1 to 22 per 100,000 with a prevalence of 8 to 150 per 100,000 [1–3].

Three separate systems are used currently to classify patients under 16 years of age with chronic arthritis: the American College of Rheumatology (ACR) [4], the European League Against Rheumatism (EULAR) [5], and the International League of Associations for Rheumatology (ILAR) systems [6] classification systems. Duffy et al [7] have written an excellent review of the history and relative advantages, disadvantages, and controversies surrounding the classification of chronic arthritis in children. None of the classification systems is perfect: some patients fulfill criteria for more than one subtype, whereas others are difficult to classify into any specific subgroup. (In the ILAR system, these patients are classified as "other.") Additionally, there is difficulty in characterizing juvenile spondyloarthropathies including juvenile ankylosing spondylitis and

* Corresponding author. Division of Pediatric Rheumatology, Schneider Children's Hospital, 269-01 76th Avenue, New Hyde Park, NY 11040.
  E-mail address: Ilowite@LIJ.edu (N.T. Ilowite).

0031-3955/05/$ – see front matter © 2005 Elsevier Inc. All rights reserved.
doi:10.1016/j.pcl.2005.01.007

pediatric.theclinics.com

Table 1
Summary of classification of chronic arthritis in children

ACR (1977) JRA	EULAR (1978) JCA	ILAR (1997) JIA
Systemic	Systemic	Systemic
Polyarticular	Polyarticular	Polyarticular RF-negative
	JRA	Polyarticular RF-positive
Pauciarticular	Pauciarticular	Oligoarticular
		persistent
		extended
	Juvenile psoriatric	Psoriatic
		Enthesitis-related
		Other

juvenile psoriatic arthritis (JPsA). All three schemata are shown in Tables 1 and 2. This article uses the ILAR system when applicable.

Etiology and pathophysiology

Although the causes of JIA remain unclear, JIA seems to be a complex genetic trait involving the effects of multiple genes related to immunity and inflammation. Some hypothesize that arthritis may be triggered in a genetically predisposed individual by psychologic stress, abnormal hormone levels, trauma to a joint, or bacterial or viral infection. Several studies have implicated rubella and parvovirus B19 as possible causes of JIA because rubella virus persists in lymphocytes and establishes a focus of persistent infection in the synovium resulting in chronic inflammation [8]. These data have been difficult to replicate in other laboratories, however. Highly conserved bacterial heat shock proteins may be potential disease triggers [9]. Results of studies investigating whether breastfeeding decreases the risk of developing JIA are inconclusive.

Table 2
Summary of the differences among the schemata

	ACR	EULAR	ILAR
Onset types	3	6	7
Age of onset	<16 years	<16 years	<16 years
Duration of arthritis	>6 weeks	>3 months	>6 weeks
Includes JAS, JpsA	No	Yes	Yes
Includes IBD	No	Yes	Yes
Includes course	No	No	Yes

Abbreviations: IBD, inflammatory bowel disease; JAS, juvenile ankyslosing spondylitis; JpsA, juvenile psoriatic arthritis.

Certain HLA class I and class II alleles are associated with an increased risk of JIA. The class I antigen HLA-A2 is associated with early-onset oligoarticular arthritis in girls [10]. The class II antigens HLA-DRB1*08 and *11, DQA1*04 and *05, and DQB1*04 are associated with persistent oligoarticular and extended oligoarticular JIA. HLA-DRB1*08 confers an increased risk of rheumatoid factor (RF)–negative polyarthritis, and HLA-DRB1*11 confers an increased risk of systemic-onset JIA (SOJIA). HLAB1*04, which is associated with adult rheumatoid arthritis, is associated with an increased risk of RF-positive polyarticular arthritis. The class I antigen HLA-B27 and class II antigens HLA-DRB1*01 and DQA1*0101are associated with enthesitis-related arthritis (ERA) and JPsA [11]. Other genes conferring risk include cytokine production–regulating genes [12–14]. Data using genome-wide scanning techniques in affected sib-pair families provide further evidence that multiple genes influence susceptibility to JIA [15].

There is evidence of immunodysregulation in JIA. Complement activation and consumption promote inflammation, and increasing serum levels of circulating immune complexes are found with active disease. Anti-nuclear antibodies (ANA) are found in approximately 40% of patient's with JIA, especially in young girls with pauciarticular disease [16]. Approximately 5% to10% of patients with JIA are RF positive [8].

The T-lymphocyte–mediated immune response is involved in chronic inflammation, and T cells are the predominant mononuclear cells in synovial fluid [17]. Patients with JIA have elevated serum levels of interleukin (IL)-1, -2, -6, and IL-2 receptor (R) and elevated synovial fluid levels of IL-1β, IL-6, and IL-2R, suggesting a Th1 profile [18]. Elevated serum levels of IL-6, IL2R, and soluble tumor necrosis factor (TNF) receptor correlate with inflammatory parameters, such as C-reactive protein, in JIA patients with active disease. Serum levels of IL-6 are increased in SOJIA and rise before each fever spike, correlating with active disease and elevation of acute-phase reactants. [19].

Classification of JIA

The ILAR classification of JIA includes seven subtypes: SOJIA, oligoarticular, polyarticular RF-positive and RF-negative, ERA, JpsA, and "other." This classification system was developed to identify clinically homogenous JIA subtypes to facilitate communication regarding epidemiology, therapeutics, and outcomes among physicians globally [6].

In order of frequency, the disease subtypes are oligoarticular JIA (50%–60%), polyarticular JIA (30%–35%), SOJIA (10%–20%), JPsA (2%–15%), and ERA (1%–7%). The subtypes are recognized based on the clinical features during the first 6 months of disease. Important clinical features that assist in classifying patients include the presence of enthesitis (inflammation at the sites of attachment of ligament, tendon, or fascia to bone), dactylitis, inflammatory lumbosacral pain, nail pitting, sacroiliitis, psoriasis, fever, rash, and serositis.

Oligoarticular JIA

Oligoarticular JIA is diagnosed in patients with arthritis in fewer than five joints during the first 6 months of disease. These patients tend to have involvement of the large joints of the lower extremities such as knees and ankles. Monoarticular onset affecting only the knee (Fig. 1) is common, seen in half of all patients [20,21]. These patients tend to function remarkably well and often do not complain of pain. Oligoarticular patients, especially ANA-positive girls, are at high risk for developing uveitis, usually their most serious clinical problem. Arthritis that remains confined to four or fewer joints is designated persistent oligoarticular JIA.

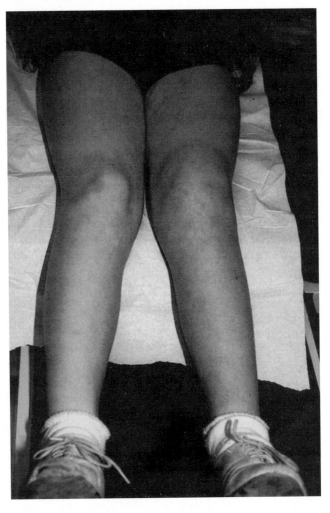

Fig. 1. Swollen left knee in a patient with oligoarticular JIA. Note the quadriceps atrophy.

A child who develops active arthritis of five or more joints after the first 6 months of disease is considered to have extended oligoarticular JIA. Up to 50% of oligoarticular patients may develop extended disease, and 30% will do so in the first 2 years after diagnosis. Risk factors for extended disease include ankle or wrist arthritis, hand disease, symmetric arthritis, arthritis of two to four joints, and an elevated erythrocyte sedimentation rate (ESR) and ANA titer [22]. Extended disease confers a worse prognosis. One study retrospectively evaluated JIA patients into adulthood with a median of 16.5 years of follow-up and found an overall remission rate of 12% in patients with extended oligoarticular JIA, compared with 75% in patients with persistent oligoarticular JIA [23].

Polyarticular JIA

Patients with arthritis in five or more joints within the first 6 months of disease are diagnosed as having polyarticular JIA. This subtype includes children with RF-negative disease (20% to 30% of JIA patients) and RF-positive disease (5% to 10% of JIA patients) [8]. Both types affect girls more frequently than boys.

RF-seronegative patients often develop polyarthritis in early childhood, in contrast to RF-seropositive patients, who develop arthritis during late childhood and adolescence. The seronegative patients have a variable prognosis. This subtype has no strong HLA association and may represent a group of disorders that can be further subtyped.

The seropositive patients are primarily adolescent girls with symmetric small joint involvement, and severe erosive disease. They may develop subcutaneous nodules (nontender, firm lesions over pressure points and tendon sheaths). The HLA associations in these patients are the same as in adult seropositive rheumatoid arthritis patients and probably represent the early expression of adult rheumatoid arthritis. The arthritis usually involves the large and small joints of the hands and feet, although the axial skeleton, including cervical spine and temporomandibular joints, may be affected. Boutonnière deformities (proximal interphalangeal joint flexion and distal interphalangeal joint hyperextension) and swan-neck deformities (proximal interphalangeal joint hyperextension and distal interphalangeal joint flexion) are common. Chronic uveitis develops less frequently than in oligoarticular disease.

Systemic onset juvenile idiopathic arthritis

SOJIA is the only subtype of JIA without a strong age, gender, or HLA association. At onset, extra-articular manifestations including rash, fever, lymphadenopathy, hepatosplenomegaly, and serositis predominate. Ten percent of patients may present with extra-articular manifestations only and may not develop arthritis for many months. In the right clinical setting, with characteristic fever and classic rash, the diagnosis of probable systemic onset disease may be made, with confirmation of the diagnosis when persistent arthritis develops [24].

Children with SOJIA typically have 2 weeks of high-spiking fever, classically with two peaks daily (double quotidian). During episodes of fever, chills are common, and the child appears ill, but when the fever breaks, the child appears well [25].

The classic rash is evanescent (usually coming and going with the fever spikes) and consists of discrete, circumscribed, salmon-pink macules 2 to 10 mm in size that may be surrounded by a ring of pallor or may develop central clearing. Lesions are more common on the trunk and proximal extremities, including the axilla and inguinal areas. Stress or a warm bath may exacerbate the rash. A linear streak on the skin, known as the Koebner phenomenon, may be elicited by scratching the skin. The rash is rarely pruritic and is never purpuric [25].

The arthritis associated with SOJIA is usually polyarticular and usually manifests within 6 months of systemic features. Both large and small joints are affected [24]. Asymmetric, oligoarticular arthritis is less common.

Laboratory findings in a patient with active SO JIA include anemia (which may be severe), leukocytosis, thrombocytosis, elevated liver enzymes, and elevated acute-phase reactants. The ANA titer is rarely positive [24].

SOJIA patients have a variable course, with 60% to 85% of patients going into remission or quiescence and up to 37% developing a chronic, destructive polyarthritis. It is usual for systemic systems to resolve over months to years; the mean period of disease activity is approximately 6 years [26]. Predictors of a poor prognosis include an age less than 6 years at diagnosis, disease duration longer than 5 years, IgA levels, and persistent systemic symptoms (defined by prolonged fever or sustained treatment with corticosteroids) or the presence of thrombocytosis (platelet count $\geq 600 \times 109/L$) 6 months into the disease course [27–29]. Radiographic changes consistent with disease progression are associated with a poor prognosis but not necessarily with poor functional status [26]. Patients with severe SOJIA who are inadequately treated have an increased incidence of amyloidosis (1.4%–9%) [23,26]. The mortality rate of patients with JIA is less than 0.3% in North America, where most deaths in SOJIA patients are secondary to macrophage activation syndrome, infection resulting from immunosuppression, or cardiac complications [30].

Macrophage activation syndrome is a rare but life-threatening complication of SOJIA characterized by increased activation and demonstration of histiophagocytosis in bone marrow. This complication is sometimes referred to as secondary or acquired hemophagocytic syndrome or hemophagocytic lymphohistiocytosis. Triggers include a preceding viral illness and the addition of or a change in medications, especially nonsteroidal anti-inflammatory drugs (NSAIDs), intramuscular gold injections, sulfasalazine, and more recently, etanercept [31]. Patients are acutely ill with hepatosplenomegaly, lymphadenopathy, purpura, and mucosal bleeding and may develop multiorgan failure. Pancytopenia, prolongation of the prothrombin time and partial thromboplastin time, elevated fibrin split products, hyperferritinemia, and hypertriglyceridemia are common. The sedimentation rate is often low (a clue to the diagnosis of macrophage activation syndrome versus exacerbation of SOJIA) because of hypofibrinogenemia secondary to consumptive coagulopathy and hepatic dysfunction [32–34]. Impaired cytotoxic activity of nuclear killer and CD8-positive T lymphocytes, low perforin levels, and endothelial activation may be involved in the pathogenesis [35]. Treatment includes pulse methylprednisolone (30 mg/kg with a maximum of 1 g), to which some patients do not respond, and cyclosporine A (2–5 mg/kg/day) [33]. Refractory patients may respond to dexamethasone and etoposide [36,37].

Enthesitis-related arthritis

Patients with juvenile ankylosing spondylitis and arthritis associated with inflammatory bowel disease are included in the ERA subtype (Table 2). ERA has a prevalence of 12 to 33 per 100,000 [38] and is most common in boys older than 8 years of age. It has a strong genetic predisposition as evidenced by a positive family history and the high frequency of the presence of HLA-B27 in affected patients. The hallmarks of the disease are pain, stiffness, and eventual loss of mobility of the back. ERA should be suspected in any child with chronic arthritis of the axial and peripheral skeleton, enthesitis (inflammation at points where tendons insert to bone), and RF and ANA seronegativity. Peripheral arthritis, usually affecting few joints of the lower extremity, precedes axial involvement, and arthritis of the sacroiliac joints may take years to develop. Radiographic changes of the sacroiliac joint include joint space narrowing, erosions, sclerosis, osteoporosis of the pelvis, and fusion (a late finding) [39].

The arthropathy of inflammatory bowel disease may present a diagnostic dilemma, because the arthritis may be the first manifestation of the disease. Clues to the diagnosis include gastrointestinal symptoms, weight loss or growth failure, and mucocutaneous abnormalities such as erythema nodosum, aphthous stomatitis, and pyoderma gangrenosum. There are two distinct forms of inflammatory disease–related arthritis. The first, an acute polyarticular form, generally mirrors the activity of the bowel disease; as a rule, the arthritis improves when the gastrointestinal disease is quiescent. In the second form, which is much more typical of ERA, the course of arthritis is independent of the course of the bowel disease.

Extra-articular manifestations include anterior uveitis, aortic insufficiency, aortitis, muscle weakness, and low-grade fever. Acute uveitis (distinguished from the chronic form common in oligo- and polyarticular disease) may develop in up to 27% of patients, is often unilateral and recurrent, and presents as a red, painful, photophobic eye, often without sequelae [40]. Laboratory data may show mild anemia, a normal to moderately elevated white blood cell count, and a thrombocytosis and elevated sedimentation rate [38,39].

Psoriatic arthritis

JPsA is chronic inflammatory arthritis with a peak age of onset in mid-childhood. JPsA is a difficult diagnosis to make, because the arthritis may

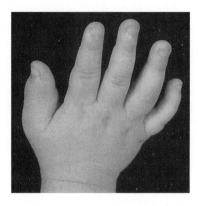

Fig. 2. Dactylitis involving the right thumb and fourth right finger.

develop many years before the rash. JPsA is an asymmetric arthritis that often affects the knees and ankles and the small joints of the hands and feet. Proximal interphalangeal joints, distal interphalangeal joints, and the tendon sheath are often inflamed, resulting in the diffuse swelling of the digit known as "sausage digit" (Fig. 2) [41].

Extra-articular manifestations include rash, nail changes (including pitting, onycholysis, oil-drop sign) and uveitis. One third of patients with JPsA develop the rash by 15 years of age [42]. All children with JPsA should have a slit-lamp examination every 6 months, because asymptomatic anterior uveitis may be found in up to 17% of patients [43].

Laboratory data show elevated acute-phase reactants, anemia of chronic disease, and thrombocytosis. ANA may be positive.

Extra-articular manifestations

Uveitis

Chronic, anterior, nongranulomatous uveitis (iridocyclitis) develops in up to 21% of patients with oligoarticular JIA and 10% of patients with polyarticular JIA [44]. Uveitis is most common in young girls with oligoarticular disease and a positive ANA titer [16]. The uveitis is usually asymptomatic, although patients may present with conjunctivitis, unequal pupils, eye pain, and headache. The uveitis may be present at diagnosis, develop during the course of JIA, or be an initial manifestation of the JIA. Patients with JIA should be screened routinely (Table 3) to prevent delay in diagnosis of uveitis. Complications of uveitis include posterior synechiae, cataracts, band keratopathy, glaucoma, and visual impairment (in up to 30%) (Fig. 3) [45]. A study of 703 JIA patients, followed for a period of 1 to 5 years, found that of the 13% of oligoarticular patients with

Table 3
Frequency of ophthalmologic examinations in patients with JIA

Sub-type at onset	Age at onset	
	< 7 years	≥ 7 years
Oligoarticular		
+ ANA	H	M
− ANA	M	M
Polyarticular		
+ ANA	H	M
− ANA	M	M
Systemic	L	L

Abbreviations: H, high risk (indicates ophthalmologic exam every 3–4 months); L, low risk (indicates ophthalmologic exam every 12 months); M, medium risk (indicates ophthalmologic exam every 6 months).
Data from Anonymous. Guidelines for ophthalmologic examinations in children with juvenile rheumatoid arthritis. Pediatrics 1993;92(2):295–6; with permission.

uveitis, 4% had loss of vision in 1 eye, and 17% had some loss of vision in both eyes. Of the 5% of polyarticular patients with uveitis, 17% had vision loss. None of the SOJIA patients was diagnosed as having uveitis [46].

Treatment of uveitis includes topical steroids and mydriatics to decrease inflammation and prevent posterior synechiae. Glucocorticoid ophthalmic drops may need to be given as often as hourly while the child is awake. Oral corticosteroids at a dose of 2 to 4 mg/kg/day with a maximum of 1 gram may be needed in patients who do not respond to topical therapy, and in some instances pulse intravenous methylprednisolone (30 mg/kg) has been used with benefit. Methotrexate, cyclosporine A, and a sub-tenon injection of steroids may benefit patients unresponsive to glucocorticoids. Preliminary case reports have shown infliximab and etanercept to be beneficial in treating refractory uveitis in children and adults [47,48].

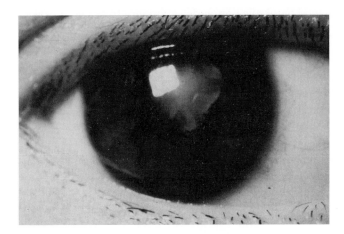

Fig. 3. Posterior synechiae and cataract formation in a JIA patient with iritis.

Nutrition

Nutritional impairment is common in children with rheumatic disease. The daily caloric requirement for a healthy child is approximately 80 to 120 kcal/kg/day for the first year of life with a decrease of approximately10 kcal/kg for each succeeding 3-year period [49]. In a random sample of 33 JIA patients, all had a total caloric intake of less than 50% of their estimated needs [50].

Children with JIA have a decrease in lean muscle mass and an increase in fat mass [51,52]. Increased resting energy expenditure was also found, especially in SOJIA patients, who had significantly elevated resting energy expenditure when compared with healthy controls [53]. These effects may be attributed to elevated levels of IL-1 and TNF-α [54].

It is important that the pediatrician use dietary guidelines on for healthy children based on sex and age instead of actual weight [53] and that a dietician or nutritionist be part of the treatment team, especially when significant malnutrition exists.

Growth disturbance

Generalized growth retardation and delayed puberty are common in patients with JIA. The causes are multifactorial (Box 1) [55–57].

Children with SOJIA and polyarticular disease of long duration are at greatest risk for diminished linear growth. It is important that diminished linear growth

---

Box 1. Causes of generalized growth delay

Metabolic

  Increased catabolic demands secondary to active disease [51,52]

Endocrinologic

  Decreased levels of insulin-like growth factor 1 (ILGF-1) in children secondary to elevated levels of IL-6 [53] and corticosteroids [52]
  Suppressive effect of corticosteroids on osteoblasts [52]

Malnutrition

  Cachexia secondary to increased levels of TNF-α and IL-1
  Mechanical (temporomandibular joint dysfunction, retrognathia)
  Anorexia secondary to nausea/vomiting and oral ulcers (methotrexate) and gastritis (corticosteroids and NSAIDs)

be recognized, because it is an undesirable and permanent disease outcome [52,53,55]. During periods of remission, patients may catch up if epiphyses have not closed prematurely. Alternate-day corticosteroid treatment or a daily dose of less than 0.5 mg/m^2 may lessen the adverse effects of corticosteroids on growth [58].

Growth hormone has been shown to be effective for severe growth retardation in select patients [59]. One study of prepubertal systemic and nonsystemic JIA patients treated with growth hormone found that patients had a net height gain of 1 SD over a period of 4 years, greater than the 0.7 SD height loss of the control group. This net gain of 1.7 SD may result in a greater final height [55].

Localized growth disturbance can result from destruction of a growth center, as in micrognathia (Fig. 4), accelerated bone maturation (Fig. 5), or premature

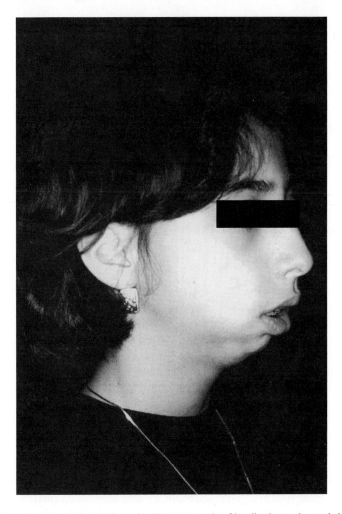

Fig. 4. Micrognathia in a patient with JIA, an example of localized growth retardation.

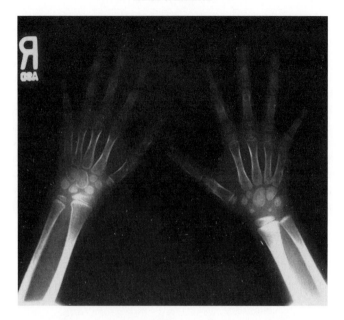

Fig. 5. Accelerated maturation of the right carpal bones in a patient with oligoarticular JIA secondary to active right wrist arthritis.

closure of the physis, as in brachydactyly of the digits. Overgrowth of a lower limb may develop in a patient with chronic inflammation of the knee secondary to hyperemia of inflammation [21]. Intra-articular steroid injections in the knee are helpful, because they control local inflammation and thereby reduce the incidence of leg-length discrepancy [60].

Osteopenia/osteoporosis

As a consequence of the disease and of corticosteroid treatment, children with JIA are at increased risk for osteopenia and osteoporosis, putting them at increased risk of fracture. Osteoporosis is defined as the parallel loss of bone mineral and matrix, resulting in a bone mineral density (BMD) more than 2.5 SD below the mean for age and sex. Osteopenia is a low bone mass for age with a BMD between 1 and 2.5 SD below the mean for age and sex. In interpreting results of dual energy X-ray photon absorptiometry scans, it is important to use pediatric, not adult, controls as normative data.

Low BMD in children with JIA has been associated with severe disease, younger age, lower body mass index, lower lean body mass, decreased intake of calcium and vitamin D, and decreased physical activity. Reduced levels of physical activity have been shown to correlate with osteopenia [61], and up to 5.6% of postpubertal female JIA patients have been found to be osteopenic based on lumbar spine BMD [62]. It is uncertain whether diminished BMD is secondary to increased bone resorption or decreased formation. Il-1, which is elevated during periods of active disease, stimulates osteoclast activity [63], and one study concluded that the insufficient skeletal growth results from depressed formation rather than increased bone resorption [52]. Roth et al [64] concluded that an important musculoskeletal abnormality in JIA is diminished muscle mass and force, resulting in abnormal bone geometry that may predispose a patient to fractures.

In most children with JIA, BMD and bone mineral content are below the norms for pre- and postpubertal children [52,62,64]. Total BMD and regional measurements, especially in postpubertal females with JIA, were significantly different from controls [52,65]. Patients with active JIA are at increased risk during their pubertal growth spurt because they may fail to achieve the normal increase in bone mass [66,67].

The best way to prevent these complications is to control disease activity, encourage appropriate caloric and calcium intake, and promote physical activity. Supplementation for any patient receiving oral corticosteroid treatment should start at 1200 to 1500 mg of calcium and 400 units of vitamin D [66,67]. The use of bisphosphonates should be considered in patients who develop osteoporosis, although there are concerns regarding the safety of these agents in children.

Special considerations

Psychosocial considerations/pain

Huygen et al [68] found children with JIA do not differ from healthy controls in regard to self-esteem, motivation for achievement and fear of failure, and physical appearance. Almost none of the JIA patients showed signs of depression. This finding is contrary to a study by Schanberg et al [69], which found depression in approximately 5% of JIA patients. Schanberg et al also found psychosocial anxiety, correlated with increased frequency and intensity of pain and fatigue, in approximately 10% of patients.

Pain is a major factor affecting the ability of JIA patients to perform activities of daily living, attend school, and participate in recreational activities. Children with polyarticular JIA report mild to moderate pain on most days, and pain and stiffness result in increased school absenteeism and less participation in social activities [68]. Up to 27% of polyarticular patients had limitation of school function, primarily in physical education [46]. A more recent study by Sällfors et al [70] confirmed that children with JIA missed an average of 3.7 days of school over a 2-month period, and more than half of the patients reported never or only sometimes attending physical education class. Seventy-four percent of patients had either 1 or no days free of pain during the 2-month study period, and they scored their pain at a level that interfered with their ability to concentrate and limited their activities. Reduced pain and attending physical education classes were found to be predictors of well being in patients with JIA [70].

Compared with healthy controls, mild to moderately active prepubertal JIA patients had significantly less physical activity and significantly more sleep [62,71]. These findings are in contrast to a study by Malleson et al [72], who found no association between physical fitness, functional ability, and joint pain. One study found mild to moderate pain in JIA patients, but their findings did not show that disease status, social support, or hopelessness and depressed mood account for the differences in patients' pain [73]. Because the degree of pain does not necessarily correspond with the degree of inflammation, treatment of the two should be separated. Cognitive behavioral pain management has been shown to be effective treatment for pain [74,75].

Disability

The Childhood Health Assessment Questionnaire (CHAQ) has been shown to be a reliable, valid, and sensitive tool for measuring functional status in JIA [76]. Median cut-off values corresponding to no, mild to moderate, and moderate disability and changes in CHAQ scores corresponding to a minimal clinically important improvement and deterioration have been quantified [77]. Based on the CHAQ score, polyarticular JIA patients have been shown to have mild to moderate functional limitations, and increased functional disability correlates with increased daily pain and stiffness [69]. Another study demonstrated that JIA patients had the most difficulty with gripping, activity, and getting up [70].

The Steinbrocker [78] classification has been used to assess functional outcome in JIA. Girls have a 2.5 times greater risk (95% confidence interval [CI], 1.1–5.4) and polyarticular JIA patients have a 5.5 times greater risk (95% CI, 1.6–9.8) of being classified as Steinbrocker class II–IV [79]. Based on this classification, no oligoarticular JIA patient had significant functional limitation outside of school. Twelve percent of the polyarticular patients and 30% of the SOJIA patients were in class III or class IV [46].

Outcome of adults with JIA

Studies have shown that 9% to 83% of JIA patients followed for up to 37 years have disease that persists into adulthood, and 14% to 48% of patients (31% overall) have a poor functional outcome as evidenced by a Steinbrocker class III or class IV [30,80–84]. Disease duration, polyarticular disease, and systemic corticosteroid treatment are important factors in determining disease outcome [80]. RF-positive polyarticular patients fared worst. They were predominantly females with onset in adolescence. They required significant assistance with hygiene, dressing, and domestic duties [81]. Foster et al [85] found that of 82 adult patients who had been diagnosed with JIA, 39% continued to have active disease. Compared with controls, JIA patients had a lower Medical Outcomes Study 36-item Short Form score indicating worse general health and quality of life.

In a study of JIA patients with a disease duration greater than 10 years, 28% of patients had depression (7% mild, 21% moderate-severe). Depression correlates with disability and persistently active disease [81]. Concerning education, 30% of patients did not graduate from high school, and 21% went on for higher education. Thirty percent of patients were unemployed, and they believed their unemployment was a result of their illness [81]. Foster [85] also reported that academic achievement in adults with a history of JIA was comparable to that of local controls, but the unemployment rate was threefold greater.

Up to 72% of patients, primarily extended oligoarticular, polyarticular, or SOJIA patients, had JIA-related surgery [80,81]. RF-positive patients had the greatest number of joint replacement surgeries and revisions [81].

The mortality rate, based on reports from the United States and Canada, is reported at 0.29/100 patients. Most deaths were patients with SOJIA [30].

Differential diagnosis

The diagnosis of JIA is a clinical one made after other identifiable causes of arthritis have been excluded by a careful history and examination in conjunction with appropriate radiographs and laboratory tests. Important clinical signs such as systemic illness, preceding infection, duration of fever, rash, and character of the arthritis help differentiate JIA from other causes of arthritis. The differential diagnosis of acute arthritis includes entities in the broad categories of reactive arthritis, inflammatory disease, infection, systemic disease, malignancy, and trauma (Box 2).

It may be difficult to differentiate SOJIA and polyarticular JIA from other causes of systemic disease with polyarthritis, such as acute rheumatic fever and other vasculitic and systemic rheumatic diseases. Acute rheumatic fever classically causes migratory arthritis, unlike the additive arthritis in JIA. The fever of SOJIA is more spiking in character and longer in duration. JIA patients never have overlying erythema, which is quite common in acute rheumatic fever. Endocardial disease strongly suggests acute rheumatic fever, but pericarditis can occur in both.

Sarcoidosis is a chronic noncaseating granulomatous disease, uncommon in children, manifesting as fever, arthritis, uveitis, rash, and pulmonary disease. The arthritis is characterized by substantial synovial hypertrophy and associated synovial cysts, especially in the ankles and wrists. The uveitis, either anterior or posterior, is granulomatous and nodular with formation of coarse keratic precipitates. The fixed macular eruption is unlike the evanescent rash of SOJIA [86].

Other multisystem rheumatic diseases can be distinguished from JIA by diagnostic clinical features and supporting laboratory data. Systemic lupus erythematosus (SLE) commonly presents in adolescence with fever and a painful, nonerosive polyarthritis affecting large and small joints [87]. The ANA titer can be positive in SLE and in polyarticular and oligoarticular JIA, and both SLE and SOJIA can manifest as polyserositis with fever, but hepatosplenomegaly and

Box 2. Differential diagnosis of arthritis

Reactive

    Postenteric
    Reiter's syndrome
    Rheumatic fever
    Poststreptococcal

Inflammatory

    Juvenile idiopathic arthritis
    Inflammatory bowel disease
    Sarcoidosis

Infection

    Septic
    Osteomyelitis
    Lyme disease
    Viral
    Bacterial sacroiliitis
    Discitis

Systemic

    Kawasaki disease
    Behcet's disease
    Henoch-Schönlein purpura
    Serum sickness
    Systemic lupus erythematosus
    Dermatomyositis
    Progressive systemic sclerosis

Malignancy

    Leukemia
    Neuroblastoma
    Malignant bone tumors:
        Osteosarcoma
        Ewing's sarcoma
        Rhabdosarcoma

Benign bone tumors:
    Osteoid osteoma
    Osteoblastoma

Trauma

    Accidental
    Nonaccidental

lymphadenopathy; malar erythema, nephritis, autoimmune pancytopenia, hypo-complementemia, and the presence of anti-double-stranded DNA and other autoantibodies are unique to SLE. Patients with systemic sclerosis and derma-tomyositis may have a mild, symmetric polyarthritis early on, but the proper diagnosis becomes apparent as symptoms progress. Patients with systemic scle-rosis may have limited range of motion secondary to sclerotic changes of the skin that should be distinguished from inflammatory arthritis.

Numerous causes of oligoarthritis need to be excluded before the diagnosis of oligoarticular JIA is made. In most cases, the distinction can be made based on the history of an antecedent infection and arthritis less than 6 weeks' duration. Septic arthritis must be excluded in any patient with acute onset of fever, severe joint pain, and an erythematous, hot, swollen joint with elevated acute-phase reactants. Synovial fluid should be examined and cultured, and treatment with antibiotics should be started immediately, because septic arthritis can rapidly lead to joint destruction. Bacterial sacroiliitis and discitis are more indolent in nature. Patients with gonococcal arthritis may present with systemic manifestations (fever, chills) and rash in addition to arthritis and tenosynovitis, especially of the wrist and ankles. It is important that the physician obtain a thorough sexual history, preferably without the parents present.

Reactive arthritis is an acute, sterile autoinflammatory arthritis that may be caused by T-cell– or B-cell–mediated cross-reactivity to similar antigens (molecular mimicry). Postenteric reactive arthritis (ReA) should be considered in any child with gastroenteritis and arthritis of the large joints of the lower extremity. The term Reiter's syndrome refers to the clinical syndrome of ReA that presents with the extra-articular manifestations of conjunctivitis and urethritis completing the classic triad. (It has been proposed that Reiter's name be removed from the medical lexicon because he was declared a Nazi war criminal [88].) HLA-B27 is strongly associated with ReA and with this syndrome [42]. Patients with sustained fever, arthritis, and a preceding streptococcal infection who do not fulfill Jones' criteria of acute rheumatic fever may be diagnosed as having poststreptococcal ReA.

Lyme disease, caused by *Borrelia burgdorferi*, is a major health problem in endemic areas [89]. Arthritis is a late manifestation of the disease but may be the presenting complaint, because the tick bite and initial rash may go unnoticed. The arthritis is episodic, with each episode being relatively short lived. The diagnosis should be confirmed with Lyme serology (ELISA and immunoblot assays). There are numerous viruses that cause arthritis including parvovirus B19, hepatitis B virus, rubella, varicella, herpesvirus, smallpox, and HIV. Identifiable infections should always be considered.

Arthritis of Kawasaki disease usually presents during the subacute phase of the illness and is commonly found in the knees and ankles, although the small joints of the hands may be involved. The arthritis of Kawasaki disease may be accompanied by desquamation and subcutaneous edema of the hands and feet, distinguishing it from SOJIA. Occasionally these distinctions are blurred. Behçet's disease (although rare) should be suspected in patients with recurrent oral and genital mucosal ulceration. When the arthritis of Henoch-Schönlein purpura precedes purpura, nephritis, or abdominal involvement, the diagnosis may be difficult. In Henoch-Schönlein purpura, arthritis rarely manifests with synovial effusions, and the inflammation is more likely to be periarticular.

Numerous conditions characterized by arthralgia or myalgia may be misdiagnosed as JIA. The presence of bone pain and bone tenderness should heighten suspicion for an underlying malignancy. A discrepancy between the blood counts and sedimentation rate (eg, relative thrombocytopenia) may be a clue to the diagnosis [90]. Night pain and low-grade fever should also lead to the suspicion of malignancy. Young children with generalized hypermobility complain predominantly of joint pain that occurs in the evening, often waking them from sleep, without associated swelling or morning stiffness, contrary to JIA. Overuse syndromes such as patellofemoral syndrome and Osgood–Schlatter's disease, are common in adolescents complaining of knee pain exacerbated by exercise. Fibromyalgia and reflex sympathetic dystrophy are chronic pain syndromes with onset in late childhood and adolescence. Musculoskeletal pain, without arthritis, is the predominant feature. These disorders are not inflammatory, and the diagnosis is suspect if the patient has evidence of synovitis.

Treatment

Objectives of the treatment of JIA include controlling pain and inflammation, preserving function, and promoting normal growth, overall development, and well being. During the past few years, remarkable advances in the treatment of JIA have been made with the advent of new disease-modifying antirheumatic agents (DMARDS), and biologic therapy.

Therapeutic modalities

Physical and occupational therapy are important adjuncts to medication because they help maintain and improve range of motion, muscle strength, and skills for activities of daily living. Splints may be used to prevent contractures or work to improve range of motion. Arthroplasty may be needed for patients with severe deformities.

Nonsteroidal anti-inflammatory medications

Initial treatment for most patients with JIA includes intra-articular long-acting corticosteroid injections and NSAIDs (Fig. 6). NSAIDs control pain and inflammation and are usually given for 4 to 8 weeks before starting treatment with a second-line agent. Naproxen (15–20 mg/kg divided into twice-daily doses; maximum dose of 500 mg BID), tolmentin (20–30 mg/kg divided into thrice-daily doses; maximum dose of 600 mg TID), diclofenac (2–3 mg/kg divided into thrice-daily doses; maximum dose; maximum dose of 50 mg TID), and ibuprofen (40 mg/kg/divided into thrice-daily doses; maximum dose of 800 mg TID) are commonly used and are usually well tolerated with little gastrointestinal discomfort. The choice of NSAID may be based on the taste of the medication and the convenience of the dosing regimen. Naproxen is prescribed most frequently but should be used with caution in fair-skinned children, because they may develop pseudoporphyria cutanea tarda, a scarring photosensitive rash [91]. Indomethacin (1–2 mg/kg/day; maximum dose of 200 mg/day) is a potent anti-inflammatory medication commonly used to treat ERA and SOJIA. When indomethacin is prescribed, patients should be warned about the possibility of headaches, difficulty in concentrating, and gastrointestinal upset [92].

The cyclo-oxygenase (COX)-2 inhibitors (ie, celecoxib) selectively inhibit the COX-2 enzyme allowing continued production of COX-1 and resulting in a decreased incidence of gastrointestinal side effects in adults. Although serious gastrointestinal complications are rare in children treated with conventional

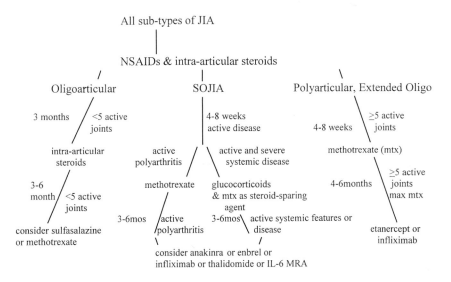

Fig. 6. Suggested treatment algorithm for JIA.

NSAIDS, COX-2 inhibitors may be useful in selected populations, especially children who have developed significant gastrointestinal symptoms [93–95]. Studies are now ongoing to assess the efficacy and pharmacokinetics of COX-2 inhibitors in children. An increased incidence of cardiovascular events, especially congestive heart failure, has been found in patients taking rofecoxib, more recently, celecoxib [96]. The mechanism by which COX-2 inhibitors increase cardiovascular risk may be, in part, the absence of inhibition of prostaglandin production in platelets, which would otherwise inhibit their function and thus promote thrombosis. The increased risk also may be related to sodium and water retention and blood pressure elevation [97]. These findings resulted in rofecoxib's being removed from the market shortly after being approved for use in children by the Food and Drug Administration. There is some evidence that naproxen sodium and celecoxib may be relatively cardioprotective [97,98], but some recent data suggest that in certain populations naproxen may actually demonstrate cardiovascular toxicity. Further studies are needed to determine whether cardiovascular toxicity is a class effect of all COX-2 inhibitors or all NSAIDs.

Glucocorticoids

Glucocorticoids are potent anti-inflammatory medications that should be used judiciously in patients with arthritis because the side-effect profile includes cushingoid appearance, hyperglycemia, immunosuppression, cataracts and glaucoma, adrenal suppression, peptic ulcer, dyslipoproteinemia, hypertension, avascular necrosis of bone, and central nervous system disturbance. Although glucocorticoids are the mainstay of treatment for controlling serious systemic manifestations of SOJIA, use in polyarticular patients should be limited to patients with extreme pain and functional limitation while waiting for a second-line agent to show some effect [99]. In rare instances pulse methylprednisolone (30 mg/kg; maximum of 1 gm) has been used to treat SOJIA patients who have not responded to oral glucocorticoids. Once disease improvement is noted, steroids should be tapered as quickly as possible (or used at the lowest dose that controls symptoms).

Treatment of a few joints with intra-articular long-acting corticosteroid injections is an effective method to treat arthritis while minimizing systemic side effects from oral medications. Triamcinolone hexacetonide (10–40 mg/joint or 1–2 mg/kg/joint) is commonly used and has been shown to result in improvement of signs and symptoms of arthritis, growth abnormalities, and gait disturbances that may last for many months [100–102]. Side effects may include infection, atrophic skin changes at the injection site, and asymptomatic calcifications on radiographs [99]. Injections can be given safely as often as every 3 months, but the same joint should not be injected more than three times in any year.

Disease-modifying antirheumatic agents

DMARDs that have been shown to be effective in JIA include sulfasalazine, methotrexate, and etanercept. Other DMARDs such as hydroxychloroquine, D-penicillamine, and auranofin have failed to show efficacy in double-blind, placebo-controlled trials [99]. Intramuscular or oral gold is rarely used for JIA currently because of poorer response rates and higher incidence of toxicity when compared with methotrexate and other DMARDs. SOJIA patients have shown improvement with monthly treatment with intravenous cyclophosphamide and intravenous immunoglobulin.

Sulfasalazine

Sulfasalazine was more effective than placebo in controlling arthritis and improving laboratory parameters in a double-blind, placebo-controlled trial [103]. Sulfasalazine is used commonly to treat oligoarticular JIA and HLA-B27 spondyloarthropathies, although a recent trial did not document efficacy [104]. Its use, however, is limited by side effects such as headache, rash, gastrointestinal toxicity, myelosuppression, and hypoimmunoglobulinemia. A complete blood count and liver transaminases must be obtained before the beginning of treatment and monitored every other week for the first 3 months, monthly for the next 3 months, and every 3 months thereafter [99].

Methotrexate

Methotrexate, a folate antagonist, is the most frequently used second-line agent for patients with JIA [105], particularly polyarticular and SOJIA. Up to 80% of JIA patients have some clinical response on methotrexate, and studies suggest it retards radiographic progression. Extended oligoarticular patients respond best to methotrexate; SOJIA patients may not do as well on this agent [92]. Methotrexate is also helpful in controlling the rash and arthritis of JPsA.

Methotrexate is tolerated quite well in children with doses starting at 0.3 mg/kg/week and increased to a maximum of 1 mg/kg/dose (no more than 25 mg/wk orally or 15 mg/m^2 subcutaneously to a maximum of 50). Subcutaneous methotrexate may be more effective than oral administration, but there seems to be a plateau in efficacy at about 15 mg/m^2 [106,107]. Gastrointestinal toxicity is the most common adverse event, occurring in 13% of the patients. Additional side effects include hepatotoxicity, oral mucosal ulcerations, teratogenicity, immunosuppression, pulmonary disease, pancytopenia, and an increased risk of lymphoproliferative malignancies [108]. Pulmonary disease is rare in the pediatric population, and there have not been convincing reports of lymphoma caused by methotrexate in JIA patients. These risks, therefore, may be theoretical in pediatric patients. Supplementation with folic acid has been shown to lessen the gastrointestinal and mucocutaneous side effects without altering the therapeutic effect of methotrexate [109]. Liver enzymes and a complete blood cell count should be monitored every 1 to 2 months, although serious, irreversible liver disease is rare in children [110]. The medication should be withheld if liver enzymes approach three times normal. Patients are advised not receive live virus vaccines because of the possible immunosuppressive effects of the medication.

It is the practice of some physicians, before the start of treatment to check varicella titers and to vaccinate patients if they are susceptible to varicella. Patients in remission for 1 year can gradually discontinue methotrexate to reduce potential long-term toxicity [92].

Leflunomide

Leflunomide, an immunosuppressive agent that reversibly inhibits de novo pyrimidine synthesis, is approved for the treatment of adult rheumatoid arthritis and is currently being studied for use in JIA. Preliminary results published in abstract form show efficacy similar to that of methotrexate [111]. Side effects include diarrhea, elevated liver enzymes, mucocutaneous abnormalities, and teratogenicity [92].

Biologic agents

The biologic agents, including the TNF inhibitors etanercept, infliximab, adalimumab, the IL-1 inhibitor anakinra, and the B-cell depleter rituximab, have improved the armamentarium for the treatment of patients with rheumatoid arthritis and JIA. All carry a risk of immunosuppression, and live virus vaccines are relatively contraindicated. Cases of reactivated tuberculosis have been reported in patients using the TNF inhibitors; tuberculin (PPD) nonreactivity should be demonstrated at the start of therapy. If the PPD is positive, the patient should be treated with isoniazid for at least 1 month before starting the biologic agent.

Etanercept

Elevated levels of TNF-α and soluble TNF receptor are found in serum of JIA patients. In addition, these patients also have elevated levels of TNF-α in the synovial fluid [112]. Etanercept, a soluble TNF receptor, is a fusion protein made up of two recombinant p75-soluble receptors fused with the Fc fragment from human IgG. It binds and inhibits TNF-α and lymphotoxin-α (TNF-β). In a double-blind, placebo-controlled study of polyarticular-course JRA patients who had not responded to or were intolerant of methotrexate, etanercept was proven effective in controlling pain and swelling and in improving laboratory parameters [113]. There is also evidence that it retards radiographic progression of disease. Approximately three fourths of patients who do not respond adequately to methotrexate will have a good response to etanercept. After 2 years of follow-up, patients in the initial clinical trial continue to have an excellent response [114]. Preliminary findings on etanercept in combination with a DMARD have shown it to be well tolerated [115].

Etanercept, 0.4 mg/kg (maximum 25 mg) given subcutaneously twice weekly has a dramatic response and is highly recommended for patients with extended oligoarticular and polyarticular JIA who have not responded to NSAIDs and methotrexate. The parents and possibly the adolescent patient are trained in reconstitution of the etanercept and administration of the injection using aseptic technique.

In placebo-controlled clinical trials, etanercept was well tolerated, and no increased incidence of infection was found. The most common adverse events were injection-site reactions (39%) and upper respiratory tract infection (35%). Less frequently, patients experienced headache, rhinitis, gastrointestinal symptoms, and rash [113]. Three cases of varicella zoster infection were reported, one resulting in aseptic meningitis [114]. It is recommended that varicella-susceptible children be immunized 3 months before the start of the drug, if possible. Any susceptible patient exposed to varicella should be treated with varicella-zoster immune globulin and acyclovir at the first sign of infection [114]. Pediatric patients with significant exposure to varicella should temporarily discontinue the etanercept [92].

Although etanercept is not currently approved for JPsA, a double-blind, placebo-controlled study of etanercept (25 mg subcutaneously two times per week) in adults with PsA showed remarkable improvement of arthritis and skin manifestations [116]. Etanercept has also shown promise in adults with spondyloarthropathy.

Infliximab

Infliximab is a chimeric monoclonal anti-TNF-α antibody. The variable region of a mouse monoclonal anti-TNF-α antibody is coupled to the constant region of human IgG1. Adult patients with rheumatoid arthritis are treated with infliximab, 3 to 10 mg/kg, at time 0, 2 weeks, 6 weeks, and then every 6 to 8 weeks. There are preliminary data on dosing, efficacy, and pharmacokinetics in pediatric patients. In a recent small, nonrandomized, open-label study, etanercept and infliximab (in combination with a DMARD) were found to be equally efficacious in treating patients with JPsA, polyarticular arthritis, and SOJIA. The incidence of adverse effects was higher and more serious in the infliximab group than in the etanercept group [117]. Results from a double-blind, placebo-controlled trial have recently been presented, demonstrating efficacy at a 3-mg/kg dose and a 6-mg/kg dose, with improved safety at the 6-mg/kg dose. Further studies are needed to evaluate the benefits and risks of infliximab in patients with JIA and JPsA [118].

Adalimumab

Adalimumab is a completely humanized monoclonal antibody to TNF given by subcutaneous injection every 2 weeks. The results of a recent open-label phase of a planned double-blind, placebo-controlled, randomized withdrawal study have recently been presented and suggest efficacy in polyarticular JRA [119].

Anakinra

Anakinra, a recombinant IL-1 receptor antagonist, has been studied in a manner similar to the seminal etanercept study in JIA in a randomized, placebo-controlled withdrawal design, but only the first, open-label portion of the study has been presented. Response was documented in 58% of subjects after 4 months of therapy but was highest (79%) in the systemic-onset patients. There have been a few reports of either isolated cases or small series of recalcitrant systemic-onset JIA patients responding dramatically in both rapidity of response and degree of response [120–123]. This agent may prove to be very effective in this subtype of JIA.

Humanized anti-interleukin-6 receptor antibody

There is evidence that SOJIA is in part an IL-6–mediated disease. In a dose-escalation study, SOJIA patients treated with humanized anti-interleukin-6 receptor antibody (MRA) at a dose of 8 mg/kg had significant improvement in the ACR improvement criteria and disease activity indices, in addition to a decrease in acute-phase reactants. No child withdrew from the trial because of disease flare or adverse effects [124]. MRA may be useful in patients with intractable disease who are receiving high-dose corticosteroids [125,126], but further randomized, placebo-controlled efficacy and long-term safety studies are needed.

Autologous stem cell transplantation

Autologous stem cell transplantation has been considered in recalcitrant cases of SOJIA. Drug-free remissions of disease have been reported, but the procedure carries a significant mortality risk, usually from macrophage activation syndrome [127]. Stem cell transplantation should be performed only in experienced centers after all other treatment options have failed [92].

In summary, all patients diagnosed with JIA should be given a trial of NSAIDs, and intra-articular corticosteroid injections should be considered. Patients with persistent oligoarticular JIA usually have a good response and need no further intervention. Patients with polyarticular disease benefit from aggressive therapy with methotrexate to improve function and prevent permanent damage. Intra-articular corticosteroids are a good adjunct to treatment. Extended oligoarticular JIA patients and JPsA patients who do not respond to first-line treatment should be treated like polyarticular patients. SOJIA patients with active systemic disease may require oral glucocorticoids for rapid relief of serious systemic manifestations including pericarditis, progressive anemia, malnutrition, and persistent fever. Methotrexate should be considered for articular disease treatment as well as a steroid-sparing agent. Sulfasalazine may be particularly effective in patients with ERA and extended oligoarticular patients who do not respond to NSAIDs. Presently, the only biologic agent that has been proved to be effective in JIA is etanercept, which should be used in patients with polyarticular disease who do not respond to methotrexate.

References

[1] Gare BA. Juvenile arthritis—who gets it, where and when? A review of current data on incidence and prevalence. Clin Exp Rheumatol 1999;17:367–74.

[2] Prieur AM, Le Gall E, Karman F, et al. Epidemiologic survey of juvenile chronic arthritis in France: comparison of data obtained from two different regions. Clin Exper Rheumatol 1987;5(3):217–23.

[3] Moe N, Rygg M. Epidemiology of juvenile chronic arthritis in northern Norway: a ten-year retrospective study. Clin Exp Rheumatol 1998;16(1):99–101.

[4] Brewer Jr EJ, Bass J, Baum J, et al. Current proposed revision of JRA criteria. Arthritis Rheum 1977;20:195–9.

[5] European League Against Rheumatism. EULAR Bulletin No. 4: nomenclature and classification of arthritis in children. Basel (Switzerland): National Zeitung AG; 1977.

[6] Petty RE, Southwood TR, Baum J, et al. Revision of the proposed classification criteria for juvenile idiopathic arthritis: Durban 1997. J Rheumatol 1998;25:1991–4.

[7] Duffy CM, Colbert RA, Laxer RM, et al for the Executive Committee, Pediatric Section, American College of Rheumatology. Nomenclature and classification in chronic childhood arthritis: time for a change? Arthritis Rheum, in press.

[8] Lang BA, Shore A. A review of current concepts on the pathogenesis of juvenile rheumatoid arthritis. J Rheumatol 1990;17(Suppl 21):1–15.

[9] Tucker LB. Juvenile rheumatoid arthritis. Curr Opin Rheumatol 1993;5:619–28.

[10] Murray KJ, Grom AA, Thompson SD, et al. Contrasting cytokine profiles in the synovium of different forms of juvenile rheumatoid arthritis and juvenile spondyloarthropathy: prominence of interleukin 4 in restricted disease. J Rheumatol 1998;25:1388–98.

[11] Thomson W, Barrett JH, Donn R, et al. Juvenile idiopathic arthritis classified by the ILAR criteria: HLA associations in UK patients. Rheumatology 2002;41:1183–9.

[12] Fishman D, Fauld G, Jeffrey R, et al. The effect of novel polymorphisms in the interleukin-6 (IL-6) gene on IL-6 transcription and plasma IL-6 levels and an association with systemic onset juvenile chronic arthritis. J Clin Invest 1998;102:1369–76.

[13] Woo P. Cytokines and juvenile idiopathic arthritis. Curr Rheumatol Rep 2002;4(6):452–7.

[14] Rosen P, Thompson S, Glass D. Non-HLA gene polymorphisms in juvenile rheumatoid arthritis. Clin Exp Rheumatol 2003;21(5):650–6.

[15] Donn R, Alourfi Z, Zeggini E, et al, British Paediatric Rheumatology Study Group. A functional promoter haplotype of macrophage migration inhibitory factor is linked and associated with juvenile idiopathic arthritis. Arthritis Rheum 2004;50(5):1604–10.

[16] Petty RE, Cassidy JT, Sullivan DB. Clinical correlates of antinuclear antibodies in juvenile rheumatoid arthritis. J Pediatr 1973;83(3):386–9.

[17] Mangee H, Schauenstein K. Cytokines in juvenile rheumatoid arthritis (JRA). Cytokine 1998; 10(6):471–80.

[18] Moore TL. Immunopathogenesis of juvenile rheumatoid arthritis. Curr Opin Rheumatol 1999; 11(5):377–87.

[19] Mangee H, Kenzian H, Gallistl S, et al. Serum cytokines in juvenile rheumatoid arthritis. Arthritis Rheum 1995;2:211–20.

[20] Cassidy JT, Levinson JE, Bass JL, et al. A study of classification criteria for a diagnosis of juvenile rheumatoid arthritis. Arthritis Rheum 1986;29(2):274–81.

[21] Calabro JJ. Juvenile rheumatoid arthritis. GP 1969;40(1):78–88.

[22] Al-Matar MJ, Petty RE, Tucker LB, et al. The early pattern of joint involvement predicts

disease progression in children with oligoarticular (pauciarticular) juvenile rheumatoid arthritis. Arthritis Rheum 2002;46(10):2708–15.

[23] Minden K, Niewerth M, Listing J, et al. Long-term outcome in patients with juvenile idiopathic arthritis. Arthritis Rheum 2002;46(9):2392–401.

[24] Schaller JG. Juvenile rheumatoid arthritis. Pediatr Rev 1980;2(6):163–74.

[25] Isdale IC, Bywaters EGL. The rash of rheumatoid arthritis and Still's disease. Q J Med 1956; 99:377–87.

[26] Svantesson H, Akesson A, Eberhardt K, et al. Prognosis in juvenile rheumatoid arthritis with systemic onset. A follow-up study. Scand J Rheumatol 1983;12(2):139–44.

[27] Spiegel LR, Schneider R, Lang BA, et al. Early predictors of poor functional outcome in systemic-onset juvenile rheumatoid arthritis: a multicenter cohort study. Arthritis Rheum 2000;43(11):2402–9.

[28] Calabro JJ, Holgerson WB, Sonpal GM, et al. Juvenile rheumatoid arthritis: a general review and report of 100 patients observed for 15 years. Semin Arthritis Rheum 1976;5:257–98.

[29] Cassidy JT. Abnormality in the distribution of serum immunoglobulin concentration in juvenile rheumatoid arthritis. J Clin Invest 1973;52:1931–6.

[30] Wallace CA, Levinson JE. Juvenile rheumatoid arthritis: outcome and treatment for the 1990's. Rheum Dis Clin North Am 1991;17(4):891–904.

[31] Ramanan AV, Schneider R. Macrophage activation syndrome following initiation of etanercept in a child with systemic onset juvenile rheumatoid arthritis. J Rheumatol 2003;30:401–3.

[32] Silverman ED, Miller III JJ, Bernstein B, et al. Consumption coagulopathy associated with systemic juvenile rheumatoid arthritis. J Pediatr 1983;103(6):872–6.

[33] Sawhney S, Woo P, Murray KJ. Macrophage activation syndrome: a potentially fatal complication of rheumatic disorders. Arch Dis Child 2001;85(5):421–6.

[34] Grom AA, Passo MD. Macrophage activation syndrome in systemic juvenile rheumatoid arthritis. J Pediatr 1996;129(5):630–2.

[35] Grom AA. Natural killer cell dysfunction: a common pathway in systemic-onset juvenile rheumatoid arthritis, macrophage activation syndrome, and hemophagocytic lymphohistiocytosis? Arthritis Rheum 2004;50(3):689–98.

[36] Henter JI, Arico M, Egeler RM, et al. HLH-94: a treatment protocol for hemophagocytic lymphohistiocytosis. HLH Study Group of the Histiocyte Society. Med Pediatr Oncol 1997; 28(5):342–7.

[37] Henter JI, Samuelsson-Horne A, Aricò M, et al for the Histiocyte Society. Treatment of hemophagocytic lymphohistiocytosis with HLH-94 immunochemotherapy and bone marrow transplantation. Blood 2002;100(7):2367–73.

[38] Burgos-Vargas R, Petty RE. Juvenile ankylosing spondylitis. Rheum Dis Clin North Am 1992; 18(1):123–42.

[39] Schaller J, Bitnum S, Wedgwood RJ. Ankylosing spondylitis with childhood onset. J Pediatr 1969;74(4):505–16.

[40] Ansell BM. Juvenile spondylitis and related disorders. In: Moll JMH, editor. Ankylosing spondylitis. Edinburgh (UK): Churchill Livingstone; 1980. p. 120.

[41] Shore A, Ansell BM. Juvenile psoriatic arthritis-an analysis of 60 cases. J Pediatr 1982; 100(4):529–35.

[42] Petty RE, Malleson P. Spondyloarthropathies of childhood. Pediatr Clin North Am 1986; 33(5):1079–96.

[43] Southwood TR, Petty RE, Malleson PN, et al. Psoriatic arthritis in children. Arthritis Rheum 1989;32:1007–13.

[44] Schneider R, Passo MH. Juvenile rheumatoid arthritis. Rheum Dis Clin North Am 2002; 28(3):503–30.

[45] Anonymous. Guidelines for ophthalmologic examinations in children with juvenile rheumatoid arthritis. Section on rheumatology and section on ophthalmology. Pediatrics 1993; 92(2):295–6.

[46] Bowyer SL, Roettcher PA, Higgins GC, et al. Health status of patients with juvenile rheumatoid arthritis at 1 and 5 years after diagnosis. J Rheumatol 2003;30:394–400.

[47] Schwartzman S, Flynn T, Barinstein L, et al. Infliximab therapy for resistant uveitis. Arthritis Rheum 2002;46(9):S326.

[48] Reiff A, Syuji T, Sadeghi S, et al. Etanercept therapy in children with treatment-resistant uveitis. Arthritis Rheum 2001;44(6):1411–5.

[49] Barness LA. Nutrition and nutritional disorders. In: Behrman RE, Kliegman RM, editors. Nelson textbook of pediatrics. Philadelphia: W.B. Saunders; 1992. p. 105–47.

[50] Henderson CJ, Lovell DJ. Nutritional aspects of juvenile rheumatoid arthritis. Rheum Dis Clin North Am 1991;17:403–13.

[51] Simon D, Lucidarme N, Prieur AM, et al. Effects on growth and body composition of growth hormone treatment ion children with juvenile idiopathic arthritis requiring steroid therapy. J Rheumatol 2003;30:2492–9.

[52] Pepmueller PH, Cassidy JT, Allen SH, et al. Bone mineralization and bone metabolism in children with juvenile rheumatoid arthritis. Arthritis Rheum 1996;39(5):746–57.

[53] Knops N, Wulffraat N, Lodder S, et al. Resting energy expenditure and nutritional status in children with rheumatoid arthritis. J Rheumatol 1999;26:2039–43.

[54] Ostrov BE. Nutrition and pediatric rheumatic diseases. Hypothesis: cytokines modulate nutritional abnormalities in rheumatic diseases. J Rheumatol 1992;19(Suppl 33):49–53.

[55] Bechtold S, Ripperger P, Hafner R, et al. Growth hormone improves height in patients with juvenile idiopathic arthritis: 4-year data on a controlled study. J Pediatr 2003;143:512–9.

[56] Davies UM, Jones J, Reeve J, et al. Juvenile rheumatoid arthritis: effects of disease activity and recombinant human growth hormone on insulin-like growth factor 1, insulin-like growth factor binding proteins 1 and 3. Arthritis Rheum 1997;40(2):332–40.

[57] De Benedetti F, Massa M, Robbioni P, et al. Correlation of IL-6 levels with joint involvement and thrombocytosis in systemic JCA. Arthritis Rheum 1991;34:1158–63.

[58] Ansell BM, Bywaters EGL. Alternate-day corticosteroids therapy in juvenile chronic polyarthritis. J Rheumatol 1974;1:176–86.

[59] Saha MT, Haapasaari J, Hannula S, et al. Growth hormone is effective in the treatment of severe growth retardation in children with juvenile chronic arthritis. Double blind placebo-controlled followup study. J Rheumatol 2004;31(7):1413–7.

[60] Sherry DD, Stein LD, Reed AM, et al. Prevention of leg length discrepancy in young children with pauciarticular juvenile rheumatoid arthritis by treatment with intraarticular steroids. Arthritis Rheum 1999;42(11):2330–4.

[61] Lovell DJ, Henderson CJ, Cawkwell G, et al. Bone mineral content in juvenile rheumatoid arthritis and healthy controls [abstract]. Arthritis Rheum 1993;36(Suppl 9):S171.

[62] Henderson CJ, Specker BL, Sierra RI, et al. Total-body bone mineral content in non-corticosteroid-treated postpubertal females with juvenile rheumatoid arthritis. Frequency of osteopenia and contributing factors. Arthritis Rheum 2000;43(3):531–40.

[63] Lipnick RN, Vieira NE, Stuff JE, et al. Calcium absorption and metabolism in children with juvenile rheumatoid arthritis assessed using stable isotopes. J Rheumatol 1993;20(7):1196–200.

[64] Roth J, Palm C, Scheunemann E, et al. Musculoskeletal abnormalities of the forearm in patients with juvenile idiopathic arthritis relate mainly to bone geometry. Arthritis Rheum 2004;50(4):1277–85.

[65] Hop RJ, Degan JA, Galllagher JC, et al. Estimation of bone mineral density in children with juvenile rheumatoid arthritis. J Rheumatol 1991;18:1235–9.

[66] Rabinovich CE. Bone metabolism in childhood rheumatic disease. Rheum Dis Clin North Am 2002;28(3):655–67.

[67] Cassidy JT. Osteopenia and osteoporosis in children. Clin Exp Rheumatol 1999;17(2):245–50.

[68] Huygen ACJ, Kuis W, Sinnema G. Psychological, behavioral, and social adjustment in children and adolescents with juvenile chronic arthritis. Ann Rheum Dis 2000;59:276–82.

[69] Schanberg LE, Anthony KK, Gil KM, et al. Daily pain and symptoms in children with polyarticular arthritis. Arthritis Rheum 2003;48(5):1390–7.

[70] Sällfors C, Hallberg LRM, Fasth A. Well-being in children with juvenile chronic arthritis. Clin Exp Rheumatol 1993;2:569–76.

[71] Henderson CJ, Lovell DJ, Specker BL, et al. Physical activity in children with juvenile rheumatoid arthritis: quantification and evaluation. Arthritis Care Res 1995;8(2):114–9.

[72] Malleson PN, Bennett SM, MacKinnon M, et al. Physical fitness and its relationship to other indices of health status in children with chronic arthritis. J Rheumatol 1996;23:1059–65.

[73] Hagglund KJ, Schopp LM, Alberts KR, et al. Predicting pain among children with juvenile rheumatoid arthritis. Arthritis Care Res 1995;8(1):36–42.

[74] Walco GA, Varni JW, Ilowite NT. Cognitive-behavioral pain management in children with juvenile rheumatoid arthritis. Pediatrics 1992;89:1075–9.

[75] Ilowite NT, Walco GA, Pochazchevsky R. Pain assessment in juvenile rheumatoid arthritis. The relationship between pain intensity and degree of joint inflammation. Ann Rheum Dis 1992;51:343–4.

[76] Singh G, Athreya BH, Fries JF, et al. Measurement of health status in children with juvenile rheumatoid arthritis. Arthritis Rheum 1994;37:1761–9.

[77] Dempster H, Porepa M, Young N, et al. The clinical meaning of functional outcome scores in children with juvenile arthritis. Arthritis Rheum 2001;44(8):1768–74.

[78] Steinbrocker O, Traeger CH, Batterman RC. Criteria for determination of progression of rheumatoid arthritis and functional capacity of patients with the disease. JAMA 1949;140:209.

[79] Andersson Gare B, Fasth A. The natural history of juvenile chronic arthritis: a population based cohort study. II. Outcome. J Rheumatol 1995;22:308–19.

[80] Zak M, Pederson FK. Juvenile chronic arthritis into adulthood: a long-term follow-up study. Rheumatology 2000;39:198–204.

[81] David J, Cooper C, Hickey L, Lloyd J, et al. The functional and psychological outcomes of juvenile chronic arthritis in young adulthood. Br J Rheumatol 1994;33:876–81.

[82] Laaksonen AL. A prognostic study of juvenile rheumatoid arthritis. Analysis of 544 cases. Acta Paediatr Scand 1966;(Suppl 166):1–163.

[83] Calabro JJ, Burnstein SL, Stanley HL. Prognosis in JRA: a fifteen year follow-up of 100 patients. Arthritis Rheum 1977;20(Suppl):285–90.

[84] Narayanan K, Rajendran CP, Porkodi R, et al. A follow-up study of juvenile rheumatoid arthritis into adulthood. J Assoc Physicians India 2002;50:1039–41.

[85] Foster HE, Marshall N, Myers A, et al. Outcome in adults with juvenile rheumatoid arthritis. A quality of life study. Arthritis Rheum 2003;48(3):767–75.

[86] Cimaz R, Ansell BM. Sarcoidosis in the pediatric age. Clin Exp Rheum 2002;20:231–7.

[87] Klein-Gittelman M, Reiff A, Silverman ED. Systemic lupus erythematosus in childhood. Rheum Dis Clin North Am 2002;28(3):561–77.

[88] Panush RS, Paraschiv D, Dorff RE. The tainted legacy of Hans Reiter. Semin Arthritis Rheum 2003;32(4):231–6.

[89] Szer IS, Taylor E, Steere AC. The long-term course of Lyme arthritis in children. N Engl J Med 1991;325(3):159–63.

[90] Cabral DA, Tucker LB. Malignancies in children who initially present with rheumatic complaints. J Pediatr 1999;134(1):53–7.

[91] Lang BA, Finlayson LA. Naproxen-induced pseudoporphyria in patients with juvenile rheumatoid arthritis. J Pediatr 1994;124:639–42.

[92] Ilowite NT. Current treatment of juvenile rheumatoid arthritis. Pediatrics 2002;109:109–15.

[93] Keenan GF, Giannini EH, Athreya BH. Clinically significant gastropathy associated with nonsteroidal antiinflammatory drug use in children with juvenile rheumatoid arthritis. J Rheumatol 1995;22(6):1149–51.

[94] Len C, Hilario MO, Kawakami E, et al. Gastroduodenal lesions in children with juvenile rheumatoid arthritis. Hepatogastroenterology 1999;46(26):991–6.

[95] Mulberg AE, Verhave M. Identification and treatment of nonsteroidal anti-inflammatory drug-induced gastroduodenal injury in children. Am J Dis Child 1993;147(12):1280–1.

[96] Mamdani M, Juurlink DN, Lee DS, et al. Cyclo-oxygenase-2 inhibitors versus non-selective non-steroidal anti-inflammatory drugs and congestive heart failure outcomes in elderly patients: a population based cohort study. Lancet 2004;363(9423):1751–6.

[97] Krum H, Liew D, Aw J, et al. Cardiovascular effects of selective cyclooxygenase-2 inhibitors. Expert Rev Cardiovasc Ther 2004;2(2):265–70.

[98] Weir MR, Sperling RS, Reicin A, et al. Selective COX-2 inhibition and cardiovascular effects: a review of the rofecoxib development program. Am Heart J 2003;146(4):591–604.

[99] Milojevic DS, Ilowite NT. Treatment of rheumatic diseases in children: special considerations. Rheum Dis Clin North Am 2002;28:461–82.

[100] Eberhard BA, Sison MC, Gottlieb BS, et al. A comparison of the intra-articular effectiveness of triamcinolone hexacetonide and triamcinolone acetonide in the treatment of children with juvenile rheumatoid arthritis. J Rheumatol 2004;31(12):2507–12.

[101] Brostrom E, Hagelberg S, Haglund-Akerlind Y. Effect of joint injections in children with JIA: evaluation by 3D-gait analysis. Acta Pediatr 2004;93(7):906–10.

[102] Zulian F, Martini G, Gobber D, et al. Triamcinolone acetonide and hexacetonide intra-articular treatment of symmetrical joints in juvenile idiopathic arthritis: a double blind trial. Rheumatology 2004;43:1288–91.

[103] van Rossum MAJ, Fiselier TJW, Franssen MJAM, et al. Sulfasalazine in the treatment of juvenile chronic arthritis: a randomized, double-blind, placebo-controlled, multi-center study. Dutch Juvenile Chronic Arthritis Study Group. Arthritis Rheum 1998;41:808–16.

[104] Burgos-Vargas R, Vazquez-Mellado J, Pacheco-Tena C, et al. A 26 week randomised, double blind, placebo controlled exploratory study of sulfasalazine in juvenile onset spondyloar-thropathies. Ann Rheum Dis 2002;61(10):941–2.

[105] Cron RQ, Sharma S, Sherry DD. Current treatment by United States and Canadian pediatric rheumatologists. J Rheumatol 1999;26:2036–8.

[106] Ruperto N, Murray KJ, Gerlon V, et al. A randomized trial of parenteral methotrexate comparing an intermediate dose with a higher dose in children with juvenile idiopathic arthritis who failed to respond to standard doses of methotrexate. Arthritis Rheum 2004;50:2191–201.

[107] Alsufyani K, Ortiz-Alvarez O, Cabral DA, et al. The role of subcutaneous administration of methotrexate in children with juvenile idiopathic arthritis who have failed oral methotrexate. J Rheumatol 2004;31(1):179–82.

[108] Gianinni EH, Cassidy JT. Methotrexate in juvenile rheumatoid arthritis. Do the benefits outweigh the risks? Drug Saf 1993;9(5):325–39.

[109] Hunt PG, Rose CD, McIlvain-Simpson G, et al. The effects of daily intake of folic acid on the efficacy of methotrexate therapy in children with juvenile rheumatoid arthritis. A controlled study. J Rheumatol 1997;24:2230–2.

[110] Passo MH, Hashkes PJ. Use of methotrexate in children. Bull Rheum Dis 1998;47(5):1–5.

[111] Silverman E, Mouy R, Spiegel L, et al. Durability of efficacy, safety and tolerability of leflunomide or methotrexate over 48 weeks of treatment in pediatric patients with juvenile rheumatoid arthritis. Arthritis Rheum 2004;50:S90.

[112] Eberhard BA, Laxer RM, Andersson U, et al. Local synthesis of both macrophage and T cell cytokines by synovial fluid cells from children with juvenile rheumatoid arthritis. Clin Exp Immunol 1994;96:260–6.

[113] Lovell DJ, Giannini EH, Reiff A, et al. Etanercept in children with polyarticular juvenile rheumatoid arthritis. N Engl J Med 2000;342:763–9.

[114] Lovell D, Giannini EH, Reiff A, et al. Long-term efficacy and safety of etanercept in children with polyarticular-course juvenile rheumatoid arthritis. Interim results from an ongoing multicenter, open label, extended-treatment trial. Arthritis Rheum 2003;489(1):218–26.

[115] Haapasaari J, Kautiainen H, Hannula S, et al. Good results from combining etanercept to prevailing DMARD therapy in refractory juvenile idiopathic arthritis. Clin Exp Rheumatol 2002;20(6):867–70.

[116] Mease P. Psoriatic arthritis: the role of THF inhibition and the effect of its inhibition with etanercept. Clin Exper Rheum 2002;20(6 Suppl 28):S116–21.

[117] Lahdenne P, Vähäsalo P, Honkanen V. Infliximab or etanercept in the treatment of children with refractory juvenile idiopathic arthritis: an open label study. Ann Rheum Dis 2003;62(3):245–7.

[118] Lovell DJ, Ruperto N, Cuttica R, et al. Randomized trial of infliximab plus methotrexate for the treatment of polyarticular juvenile rheumatoid arthritis. Presented at the American College of Rheumatology Annual Meeting, San Antonio, TX. October 16–21, 2004.

[119] Lovell DJ, Ruperto N, Goodman S, et al. Preliminary data from the study of adalimumab in children with juvenile idiopathic arthritis. Arthritis Rheum 2004;50(Suppl):S436.

[120] Verbsky JW, White AJ. Effective use of the recombinant interleukin-1 receptor agonist anakinra in therapy resistant systemic onset juvenile rheumatoid arthritis. J Rheumatol 2004; 31:2071–5.

[121] Hendrickson M. Efficacy of anakinra in refractory systemic arthritis. Arthritis Rheum 2004; 50(9):S438.

[122] Irigoyen PI, Olson J, Hom C, et al. Treatment of systemic onset juvenile rheumatoid arthritis with anakinra. Arthritis Rheum 2004;50(9):S437.

[123] Pasquale V, Allantaz F, Arce E, et al. Dramatic clinical response to IL-1 blockade in systemic onset juvenile idiopathic arthritis. Presented at the American College of Rheumatology Annual Meeting, San Antonio, TX. 2004.

[124] Yokota S, Miyama T, Imagawa T, et al. Phase II trial of anti-IL-6 antibody (MRA) for children with systemic onset juvenile idiopathic arthritis. Arthritis Rheum 2003;48(9 Suppl):S429.

[125] Yokota S. Interleukin 6 as a therapeutic target in systemic-onset juvenile idiopathic arthritis. Curr Opin Rheumatol 2003;15(5):581–6.

[126] Choy E. Clinical experience with inhibition of interleukin-6. Rheum Dis Clin North Am 2004; 30:405–15.

[127] De Kleer IM, Brinkman DM, Ferster A, et al. Autologous stem cell transplantation for refractory juvenile idiopathic arthritis: analysis of clinical effects, mortality and transplant related morbidity. Ann Rheum Dis 2004;63:1318–26.

PEDIATRIC CLINICS

OF NORTH AMERICA

Pediatr Clin N Am 52 (2005) 443–467

Systemic Lupus Erythematosus

Susanne M. Benseler, MD, Earl D. Silverman, MD, FRCP*

*Division of Rheumatology, Department of Pediatrics, The Hospital for Sick Children,
555 University Avenue, Toronto, Ontario, M5G IX8, Canada*

Systemic lupus erythematosus in children and adolescents (pSLE) is a multi-system autoimmune disease with a great variability in disease presentation and course. The diagnosis of systemic lupus erythematosus (SLE) is based on the clinical and laboratory features consistent with this illness in the absence of another autoimmune disease that could explain the findings. At time of diagnosis of pSLE, most but not all patients have at least four of the American College of Rheumatology Classification Criteria for SLE (Table 1) [1]. This article summarizes available epidemiologic data, clinical patterns, approaches to investigation and treatment, and recent outcome data.

Incidence

The incidence of SLE varies significantly in different ethnic groups and populations, with annual incidence rates in adults ranging from 1.9 to 5.6 per 100,000 [2–6]. Sex-specific incidence rates differ between men and women, with rates between 0.4 and 0.6 for white males, 3.5 and 4.6 for white females, 0.7 for African American males, and 9.2 for African American females [7,8].

Pediatric data suggest the incidence of SLE with onset before age 19 years is probably between 6 and 18.9 cases per 100,000 in white females and higher in black (20–30 per 100,000) and Puerto Rican females (16–36.7 per 100,000) [9].

* Corresponding author.

E-mail address: Earl.Silverman@sickkids.ca (E.D. Silverman).

Table 1
The 1982 revised criteria for classification of systemic lupus erythematosus*

Criterion	Definition
Malar rash	Fixed erythema, flat or raised, over the malar eminences, tending to spare the nasolabial folds
Discoid rash	Erythematous raised patches with adherent keratotic scaling and follicular plugging; atrophic scarring may occur in older lesions
Photosensitivity	Skin rash as a result of unusual reaction to sunlight, by patient history or physician observation
Oral ulcers	Oral or nasopharyngeal ulceration, usually painless, observed by physician
Arthritis	Nonerosive arthritis involving two or more peripheral joints, characterized by tenderness, swelling, or effusion
Serositis	Pleuritis—convincing history of pleuritic pain or rubbing heard by a physician or evidence of pleural effusion
	or
	Pericarditis—documented by ECG or rub or evidence of pericardial effusion
Renal disorder	Persistent proteinuria greater than 0.5 g/day (or > 3+ if quantitation not performed)
	or
	Cellular casts—may be red cell, hemoglobin, granular, tubular, or mixed
Neurologic disorder	Seizures in the absence of offending drugs or known metabolic derangements (eg, uremia, ketoacidosis, or electrolyte imbalance)
	or
	Psychosis in the absence of offending drugs or known metabolic derangements (eg, uremia, ketoacidosis, or electrolyte imbalance)
Hematologic disorder	Hemolytic anemia with reticulocytosis
	or
	Leukopenia less than 4000/mm^3 total on two or more occasions
	or
	Lymphopenia less than 1500/mm^3 on two or more occasions
	or
	Thrombocytopenia less than 100,000/mm^3 in the absence of offending drugs
Immunologic disorder	Positive lupus erythematosus cell preparation
	or
	Anti-DNA antibody to native DNA in abnormal titer
	or
	Presence of anti-Sm nuclear antigen
	or
	False-positive serologic test for syphilis known to be positive for at least 6 months and confirmed by *Treponema pallidum* immobilization or fluorescent treponemal antibody absorption test
Antinuclear antibody	An abnormal titer of antinuclear antibody by immunofluorescence or an equivalent assay at any point in time and in the absence of drugs known to be associated with drug-induced lupus syndrome

* The proposed classification is based on 11 criteria. For the purpose of identifying patients in clinical studies, a person shall be said to have SLE if any 4 or more of the 11 criteria are present, serially or simultaneously, during any interval of observation.

Incidence rates are higher in Hispanics, blacks, native Americans, and persons from Southeast and South Asia [10–12].

In the authors' Toronto pSLE cohort, the male:female ratio is 1:4.4, consistent with most larger reviews of white and Asian pediatric populations [13,14]. In African-Caribbean and South American populations, the incidence is higher in girls than in boys, with male:female ratios as low as 1:7 [15,16]. The median age at pSLE diagnosis in the authors' cohort was 12.2 years, comparable with other large pSLE series [14]. The time from onset of symptoms to diagnosis varied from 1 month to 3.3 years (median, 4 months) in the authors' cohort. The overall 10-year survival rate for adult patients with SLE is between 85% and 92%; 5-year survival rates are 3% to 5% higher [17,18]. Thirty years ago, the reported survival rates for pSLE patients were 82.6% at 5 years and 76.1% at 10 years [19]. The recent 5-year survival rate for pSLE has been reported to be as high as 100, with 10-year survival rates as high as 86% [20]. Mortality rates are associated with socioeconomic status and individual access to health care, educational background, racial/ethnic background, endemic infection rates, disease activity, and renal or central nervous system (CNS) involvement [15,16, 20–27].

Earlier diagnosis and rapid introduction of aggressive immunosuppressive treatment lead to an improved outcome.

Clinical patterns

Children and adolescents with SLE frequently present with systemic, constitutional symptoms such as fever, diffuse hair loss, fatigue, weight loss, and evidence of diffuse inflammation as demonstrated by lymphadenopathy and hepatosplenomegaly, and these manifestations are seen throughout the course of the disease. Skin, musculoskeletal, and renal systems are the most common organ systems involved in pSLE. Important treatment decisions are based mainly on evidence of major organ involvement, including nephritis, neuropsychiatric disease, and severe hematologic disease. Gastrointestinal disease, including significant liver involvement, myositis, and myocarditis, is rare in children. Table 2 summarizes the frequencies of clinical features of SLE at presentation.

Musculoskeletal disease

Most pSLE patients have musculoskeletal involvement, mainly arthritis, arthralgia, or tenosynovitis. Although myalgia is seen in 20% to 30% of patients, true myositis is seen much less frequently. The arthritis seen in pSLE is commonly a painful, symmetric polyarthritis affecting both large and small joints.

Table 2
Frequencies of clinical features of children and adolescents with SLE at diagnosis and anytime during their disease

Clinical features	At diagnosis		At any time	
	Toronto series (%)	pSLE literature (%)	Toronto series (%)	pSLE literature (%)
Constitutional and generalized symptoms				
Fever	55	60–90	86	80–100
Lymphadenopathy	34	13–45	34	13–45
Hepatosplenomegaly	30	16–42	30	19–43
Organ disease				
Arthritis	78	60–88	80	60–90
Any skin rash	79	60–78	86	60–90
Malar rash	36	22–60	38	30–80
Nephritis	51	20–80	69	48–100
Neuropsychiatric disease	25	5–30	34	26–95
Cardiovascular disease	14	5–30	17	25–60
Pulmonary disease	18	18–40	18	18–81
Gastrointestinal disease	19	14–30	24	24–40

Data from Refs. [16,24,26,28–33].

The affected joints usually have only mild to moderate joint effusions; however, significant joint-line tenderness and painfully reduced ranges of movement are common. The pain is generally more severe than that seen in children with juvenile idiopathic arthritis, and prolonged morning stiffness is common. The arthritis is rarely associated with radiographic changes. Patients with long-standing definite polyarticular or systemic juvenile idiopathic arthritis have been reported to develop pSLE [34–36]. Noninflammatory musculoskeletal pain frequently occurs following treatment and may be the result of a pain amplification syndrome secondary to a sleep disturbance or mood change as a result of the glucocorticoid therapy.

Treatment-induced musculoskeletal complications include avascular necrosis (AVN), osteoporosis (which may be accompanied by fracture or vertebral body collapse), and growth failure. Steroid-induced myopathy is rarely seen.

AVN occurs in approximately 10% of pediatric cases and seems to be more common in children than adults. Typically, the juxta-atricular regions of the large, weight-bearing bones are affected; hips and knees are most commonly affected. In general, AVN is associated with long-term, high-dose steroid therapy, but it may occur with standard therapy for significant renal or neuropsychiatric involvement. It may be seen within weeks of the introduction of steroids. Osteoporosis and vertebral fractures are commonly seen and are frequently asymptomatic. Long bone fractures are rare. A reduction in bone mineral density can result from steroid therapy but also can be secondary to lupus per se, low calcium and vitamin D intake, and reduced physical activity. Preventive strategies for osteoporosis in pSLE include a high calcium intake and adequate doses of vitamin D and exercise. The use of bisphosphonates should be considered after an osteoporosis-induced fracture [37,38].

Treatment

The arthritis frequently occurs at the time of diagnosis of pSLE or with disease flares and usually responds to the therapy of other organ involvement. Isolated arthritis is usually treated with a nonsteroidal anti-inflammatory drug combined with an antimalarial drug (usually hydroxychloroquine at a dose of 5 mg/kg), but frequently steroids are required. In the authors' experience, methotrexate works well as a steroid-sparing agent. The major side effects of hydroxychloroquine are maculopathy and gastrointestinal distress; rare instances of neuromyotoxicity and cardiomyopathy have been described [39]. Ophthalmologic examination is required every 6 months [40].

Mucocutaneous involvement

Skin involvement has been reported in 50% to 80% of patients at the time of diagnosis of pSLE and in up to 85% of patients during the course of the disease. Cutaneous disease may include a malar rash, photosensitive skin rash, vasculitic skin lesions with nodules or ulceration, palmar/plantar erythema, Raynaud's phenomenon, annular erythema, and, less frequently, discoid lupus or lupus profundus (Table 3). Alopecia is common, but scarring alopecia is rare and usually is seen only with discoid lesions.

Table 3
Mucocutaneous involvement children and adolescents with SLE

Features	Toronto series (%)	pSLE literature (%)
Skin involvement	86	50–90
Malar rash[a]	68	40–80
Photosensitive rash	39	35–50
True vasculitic rash	18	10–20
Raynaud's phenomenon	14	10–20
Hair loss	31	20–40
Digital ulcers	6	5–10
Discoid lesions	5	5–10
Mucous membrane involvement		
Oral/nasal ulcers	29	10–30

[a] The malar or "butterfly" rash is a hallmark of SLE. This is a maculopapular rash over the cheeks (malar eminences) extending over the bridge of the nose and sparing the nasolabial folds (Fig. 1).

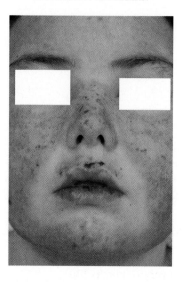

Fig. 1. Malar rash in a patient with pediatric SLE.

The malar or butterfly rash is a hallmark of SLE. This is a maculopapular rash over the cheeks (malar eminences) extending over the bridge of the nose sans spring the nasolabial folds (Fig. 1). In one third of patients, the rash is photosensitive. Other sun-exposed areas may also may a photosensitive rash. Sun exposure may cause a systemic flare as well as exacerbating the skin disease (Fig. 2). Avoidance of sunbathing, and the use of sun-blocking agents with high sun-protecting factor and protective clothing, including long-sleeved shirts and hats, is recommended. A photosensitive rash and, in particular,

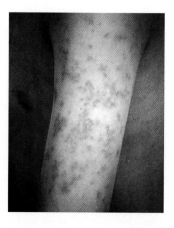

Fig. 2. Photosensitive rash on arms following sun exposure.

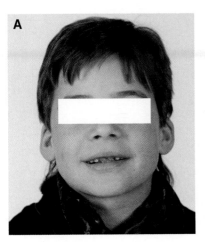
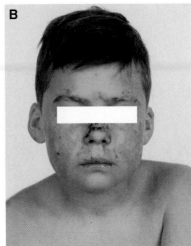

Fig. 3. Effect of sun-exposure in a patient with a photosensitive malar rash. (*A*) Before sun exposure. (*B*) After sun exposure.

annular erythema are frequently associated with anti-Ro and anti-La antibodies (Fig. 3).

Discoid lupus lesions are seen rarely in pSLE but when present tend to heal with a scar (Fig. 4). A true vasculitic skin rash may include ulceration, nodules, or even palpable purpura. These skin lesions are commonly painful, are most frequently located on fingers or toes, and can result in splinter hemorrhages and digital infarcts. These skin lesions may be identical to chilblains, a common cutaneous lesion seen in children, particularly in countries with cold, damp winters. Severe, ulcerating, lesions may signify more significant disease activity in other organs, whereas the appearance of a malar

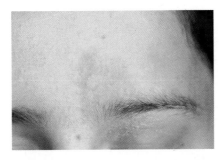

Fig. 4. Discoid lupus erythematosus lesion on the forehead.

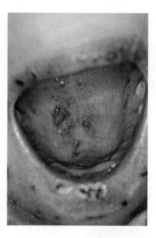

Fig. 5. Painless oral ulceration.

rash often heralds a disease flare. The pinnae of the ears are frequently involved, and the lesions may range from hyperemia to true vasculitis. Raynaud's phenomenon seems to be less common in pediatric than in adult lupus.
Local measures, including avoidance of cold, use of insulated mittens rather
than gloves, and the wearing of multiple layers of clothing, hats, and hand/feet
warmers, are sufficient for most SLE patients. In more severe disease the use
of calcium-channel–blocking agents or other vasodilating medication is required. Involvement of the oral and nasal mucosa ranges from hyperemia,
petechial rashes on the hard palate to true ulceration of the oral or nasal mucosa. The ulcers are painless (Fig. 5).

Patients with complement component deficiencies, in particular C4 deficiencies, often present with prominent cutaneous features that are frequently resistant
to therapy (Fig. 6) [41].

Neuropsychiatric disease

Involvement of the CNS and the peripheral nervous system is referred to as
neuropsychiatric systemic lupus erythematosus (NP-SLE). NP-SLE occurs in
20% to 70% of pSLE patients [31,42–45]. The large differences in the incidence
of NP-SLE among various studies result largely from the differences in the
frequency of lupus-associated headaches. In 1999, the American College of
Rheumatology classified neuropsychiatric involvement into 19 separate disease
entities (Table 4) [46,47]. In the authors' experience, most patients with NP-SLE
fulfill criteria for more than one of these entities. As with other major organ
involvement, most patients with NP-SLE have the initial neuropsychiatric signs
and symptoms within the first year of diagnosis of SLE. Approximately 25% of

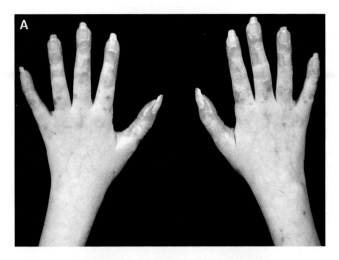

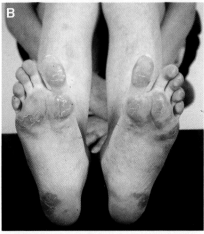

Fig. 6. Therapy-refractory skin rash in a pSLE patient with C4 complement deficiency on (*A*) hands and (*B*) feet.

patients first demonstrate neuropsychiatric disease later during the course of the disease [42].

Headaches

Headache is the most common neuropsychiatric manifestation. A true lupus headache is refractory to standard analgesic treatment [48]. Although the significance of headache in the absence of other neurologic symptoms is controversial, a severe, unremitting headache may reflect active CNS vasculitis,

Table 4
Neuropsychiatric lupus in children and adolescents with pSLE

1999 ACR nomenclature and case definitions for neuropsychiatric SLE	Toronto series (%) N = 56	pSLE literature (%)
Central nervous system		
Aseptic meningitis	NA	NA
Cerebrovascular disease	24	12–30
Demyelinating syndrome	0	4–10
Headache	75	22–95
Isolated headache	27	NA
Movement disorder	11	3–15
Myelopathy	2	1–8
Seizure disorder	18	10–42
Acute confusional state	11	20–40
Anxiety disorder	14	10–28
Cognitive dysfunction	27	20–57
Mood disorder/depression	34	28–57
Psychosis	36	12–50
Peripheral nervous system	NA	3–30
Including Guillain–Barré syndrome, autonomic disorder, mononeuropathy, cranial neuropathy, myasthenia-like syndrome, plexopathy and peripheral neuropathy		

Abbreviation: NA, not available.
Data from Refs. [28,33,45,48–50].

cerebral vein thrombosis (CVT), or raised intracranial pressure caused by CNS infection or pseudotumor cerebri. Headache in pSLE is frequently seen in association with more severe CNS involvement including organic brain syndrome and psychosis. It also may be secondary to CVT. CVT may present in the absence of other CNS manifestations and is almost universally associated

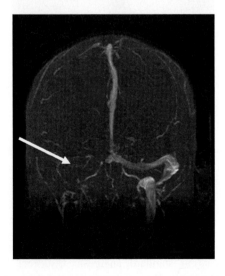

Fig. 7. MR venogram of cerebral vein thrombosis in a patient with pediatric SLE. The arrow shows absence of filling on the right side.

with the presence of the lupus anticoagulant (LAC) [51]. In the authors' series of 56 NP-pSLE patients, 18% developed a CVT. Neuroimaging including either CT or MR venogram (Fig. 7) is required on an urgent basis.

Psychosis

The diagnosis of psychosis is made in 30% to 50% of pediatric patients with neuropsychiatric involvement. Characteristically the hallucinations have features of an organic psychosis including visual or tactile hallucinations. Suicidal ideations are common [42,52]. Frequently headaches, cognitive dysfunction, and confusion are all present. Measures of general disease activity may be normal in approximately one third of patients. Brain parenchymal imaging, including MRI scans, is frequently normal (in up to 67% of patients), making the diagnosis difficult. Although some authors have advocated the use of CNS single photon emission computed tomography (SPECT) imaging, the authors have not found this investigation to be of any benefit in differentiating NP-SLE–associated psychosis from other forms of psychosis, including steroid-induced psychosis. SPECT scans are frequently abnormal in SLE patients in the absence of CNS symptoms and may even be normal in the presence of overt pSLE–associated psychosis [53]. In the authors' experience, steroid-induced psychosis is uncommon and may be differentiated from NP-SLE by the absence of other features of CNS involvement including headache, confusion, and concentration difficulties and the presence of mania, head-banging, and excessive crying (uncommon features of NP-SLE) [54,55].

Cognitive dysfunction

Cognitive impairment, which ranges from concentration difficulties and a decrease in school performance to frank confusion and coma, occurs in 20% to 57% of children with NP-SLE. Inflammatory markers may be normal in one third of patients, and parenchymal imaging may be normal in up to two thirds of patients.

Cerebrovascular disease

Cerebrovascular disease occurs in 12% to 30% of cases. When present, cerebrovascular disease usually involves the microcirculation, and therefore angiographic studies are usually normal except in the presence of a stroke [56]. Headaches and seizures are the most common clinical signs and symptoms of CNS vasculitis. Inflammatory markers are often elevated, and cerebrovascular disease is strongly associated with the presence of antiphospholipid antibodies [57].

Seizures

Seizures occur in approximately 10% to 40% of pediatric cases, frequently at presentation. Patients with seizures frequently have associated headaches, cerebrovascular disease, and cognitive dysfunction. Generalized seizures are more common than focal seizures. Inflammatory markers are often elevated. Parenchymal lesions are seen in 80% of the authors' cohort. Seizures in pSLE may also develop secondary to uremia, hypertension, or CNS infections.

Movement disorders

Movement disorders include chorea, cerebellar ataxia, hemiballismus, tremor, and parkinsonian-like movements and occur in 5% to 10% of cases [58]. Chorea is the most common movement disorder and is more common in pSLE than in adult-onset SLE [59]. Antiphospholipid antibodies are almost universally present in patients with chorea, which may be isolated or occur in conjunction with other manifestations of the antiphospholipid antibody syndrome. With the decline in rheumatic fever in developed countries, the diagnosis of SLE or antiphospholipid antibody syndrome should be considered in all patients presenting with chorea [60].

Peripheral nervous system

Both cranial and peripheral neuropathies occur infrequently in pSLE [61], with cranial nerve involvement being the more common. pSLE patients may present with optic neuropathy [62] and oculomotor palsy [63] and less frequently with facial palsy [64], trigeminal neuropathy, or nystagmus and vertigo [65]. Transverse myelitis may present with acute paraplegia or quadriplegia and may be the presenting sign of SLE [50,66]. Autonomic nerve dysfunction occurs in up to 50% of adults with SLE, and autoantibodies directed against autonomic nervous system tissue may be of etiologic importance [67].

Investigation

The tools for diagnosing NP-SLE in children include cerebrospinal fluid (CSF) cell count, protein, and CNS imaging apart from systemic inflammatory markers and autoantibodies. There is no good diagnostic test for the presence of NP-SLE, however, and the results of investigations frequently are normal. The major reason for performing investigations in patients with presumed SLE-induced CNS involvement is to exclude other non-SLE causes of CNS diseases, especially infection.

Lumbar puncture may show an elevated CSF protein or white blood cell count, in the absence of infection, with an elevated opening pressure. An altered integrity of the blood–brain barrier and immunoglobulin synthesis in the CSF have been implicated in NP-SLE but are not part of routine investigations [68]. Investigational studies have demonstrated elevated soluble interleukin-2 receptor, tumor necrosis factor-alpha, interleukin-1-beta, interleukin-6, matrix metalloproteinase 9, and prolactin levels in the CSF [69–71]. The clinical usefulness of these tests has yet to be proven. Anti-ribosomal P antibodies have been associated with the presence of depression and psychosis but are frequently present in patients without any CNS disease. Similarly, antineuronal antibodies are not specific for cognitive dysfunction. Imaging tools in NP-SLE may include CT, MRI, MR angiogram, MR venogram, conventional angiography, SPECT, and MR spectroscopy. Neuroimaging techniques are best used to demonstrate arterial or venous occlusion and are important investigations in the presence of a stroke, seizures, and to demonstrate CVT. The diagnosis of CVT may be confirmed by the absence of flow on a MR or CT venogram [72]. NP-SLE–related CNS perfusion defects may be assessed by SPECT, but the authors have found this investigation unhelpful in the presence of SLE and no longer use this test [53,73,74]. CNS SPECT scans are more useful in a patient without the diagnosis of SLE to help differentiate an organic psychosis from idiopathic psychosis.

Treatment

The treatment guidance of NP-SLE mandates an interdisciplinary approach involving psychiatrists, psychologists, neurologists, and rheumatologists. Psychosis, acute confusional state, or organic brain syndrome are potentially life-threatening complications. These patients require combination therapy of high-dose steroids and an additional immunosuppressive agent such as azathioprine or cyclophosphamide. In addition, psychotropic drugs frequently are needed. When depression is severe, antidepressants should be added to the immunosuppressive therapy. Treatment of seizures should be directed at finding their cause in addition to anticonvulsive medications. As previously described, headaches resistant to analgesia are frequently caused by significant underlying CNS disease including CVT, vasculitis, or infection. Therefore, the underlying cause must be identified to direct the treatment.

Renal disease

Lupus nephritis has been reported in 29% to 80% of pediatric cases, depending on whether the reporting investigators are rheumatologists or nephrologists [16,24,29,33,75–77]. In the authors' combined rheumatology/

nephrology clinic, renal disease is present in 50% to 55% of patients with pSLE. In approximately 90% of patients with renal lupus, the nephritis is manifested within the first year after diagnosis of SLE. The World Health Organization (WHO) has defined a morphologic classification of kidney biopsies in SLE, and this classification was revised in 2003 by the International Society of Nephrology and the Renal Pathology Society (Table 5) [78]. The histologic classes range from normal by light microscopy (class 1) to advanced sclerotic nephritis (class VI). Although it may be easy to predict the histologic classification in patients who present with severe renal failure and significant hypertension, in less severe cases it is difficult to predict the histologic lesion based on clinical and laboratory parameters including the urine sediment and degree of proteinuria. It is well recognized that patients with class IV nephritis can present with a normal serum creatinine levels and blood pressure and with minimally active urine sediment. Because treatment differs for differing forms of SLE nephritis, the authors suggest that a renal biopsy is warranted at the time of initial presentation in patients with an active urine sediment or abnormal renal function.

The most significant lesions are associated with widespread subendothelial immune deposits and proliferation of the mesangial cells. The spectrum of active lupus nephritis ranges from mild mesangial proliferative lupus nephritis (class II) to global diffuse proliferative glomerulonephritis (class IV-G [A] lupus nephritis). Chronic inactive lupus nephritis ranges from focal glomerular scars on kidney biopsy (class III-C lupus nephritis) to diffuse global sclerosing lupus nephritis (class IV-D). Most patients who develop end-stage renal disease have either class III or class IV lupus nephritis. Although activity and chronicity indices initially were thought to have prognostic significance, most pathologists now use the revised WHO classification instead [79,80].

Class II lupus nephritis is relatively mild lesion requiring significantly less therapy than required for class III or class IV lupus nephritis and is associated with an excellent renal and patient long-term survival. In 20% to 30% of patients, however, transformation from mesangial proliferative lupus nephritis to class III or class IV lupus nephritis may occur after months to years. Long-term patient and renal survival rates are then similar to those of patients initially presenting with this lesion.

Isolated membranous nephritis occurs in 10% to 20% of patients with renal disease. The clinical presentation ranges from mild proteinuria with or without hematuria or casts to nephrotic-range proteinuria. Unlike the presentation of patients with idiopathic membranous nephritis, pSLE patients with class V lupus nephritis frequently have hematuria. The possibility of lupus nephritis should always be considered in patients who present during adolescence with what appears to be idiopathic nephrotic syndrome, nephrotic syndrome with hematuria, or resistant nephrotic syndrome. Class V nephritis may be seen in conjunction with another renal lesion.

Renal vasculitis occurs in less than 10% of patients with renal lupus. When present, it is most commonly a thrombotic microangiopathy and less frequently is true renal vasculitis [81,82].

Table 5
International Society of Nephrology/Renal Pathology Society 2003 classification of lupus nephritis

Lupus nephritis class	Toronto series (%)	Pediatric literature[a] (%)
Class I Minimal mesangial lupus nephritis[b]	NA	NA
Class II Mesangial proliferative lupus nephritis[c]	16	15–25
Class III Focal lupus nephritis[d]	33	12–24
Class III (A) Active lesions, focal proliferative lupus nephritis		
Class III (A/C) Active and chronic lesions, focal proliferative and sclerosing lupus nephritis		
Class III (C) Chronic inactive lesions with glomerular scars: focal sclerosing lupus nephritis		
Class IV Diffuse lupus nephritis[e]	48	44–64
Class IV-S (A) Active lesions, diffuse segmental proliferative lupus nephritis		
Class IV-G (A) Active lesions, diffuse global proliferative lupus nephritis		
Class IV-S (A/C) Active and chronic lesions, diffuse segmental proliferative and sclerosing lupus nephritis		
Class IV-G (A/C) Active and chronic lesions, diffuse global proliferative and sclerosing lupus nephritis		
Class IV-S (C) Chronic inactive lesions with glomerular scars: diffuse segmental sclerosing lupus nephritis		
Class IV-G (C) Chronic inactive lesions with glomerular scars: diffuse global sclerosing lupus nephritis		
Class V Membranous lupus nephritis[f]	18	8–20
VI Advanced sclerosing lupus nephritis[g]	NA	NA

Abbreviation: NA, not available.

[a] Refs. [14,16,24,29,33,75–77].

[b] Normal glomeruli by light microscopy, but mesangial immune deposits by immunofluorescence.

[c] Purely mesangial hypercellularity of any degree or mesangial matrix expansion by light microscopy, with mesangial immune deposits. A few isolated subepithelial or subendothelial deposits may be visible by immunofluorescence or electron microscopy, but not by light microscopy.

[d] Active or inactive focal, segmental or global endo- or extracapillary glomeronephritis involving <50% of all glomeruli, typically with focal subendothelial immune deposits, with or without mesangial alterations.

[e] Active or inactive diffuse, segmental or global endo- or extracapillary glomeronephritis involving ≥50% of all glomeruli, typically with diffuse subendothelial immune deposits, with or without mesangial alterations. This class is divided into diffuse segmental (IV-S) lupus nephritis, when ≥50% of the involved glomeruli have segmental lesions, and diffuse global (IV-G) lupus nephritis, when ≥50% of the involved glomeruli have global lesions. A segmental lesion is defined as a glomerular lesion that involves less than half of the glomerular tuft. This class includes cases with diffuse wire loop deposits but with little or no glomerular proliferation.

[f] Global or segmental subepithelial immune deposits or their morphologic sequelae by light microscopy and by immunofluorescence or electron microscopy, with or without mesangial alterations; class V lupus nephritis may occur in combination with class III or IV in which case both will be diagnosed; class V lupus nephritis may show advanced sclerosis.

[g] Ninety per cent or more of glomeruli globally sclerosed without residual activity.

Data from Weening JJ, D'Agati VD, Schwartz MM, et al. The classification of glomerulonephritis in systemic lupus erythematosus revisited. J Am Soc Nephrol 2004;15:241–50.

Most patients with lupus nephritis have constitutional symptoms including fever, malaise, anorexia, and weight loss. Hypertension before steroid treatment can be found in one third of pediatric lupus nephritis patients. The presence of hypertension and peripheral edema is usually associated with either class III or class IV lupus nephritis [14]. The hypertension frequently is exacerbated following the introduction of steroid treatment. Laboratory investigations may demonstrate a low serum albumin level, decreased C3 or C4 complement levels, high-titer anti-dsDNA antibodies, or other SLE-associated autoantibodies. Urine analysis may reveal proteinuria or hematuria with an active urine sediment with or without evidence of azotemia. Most patients with impaired renal function have either class III or IV lupus nephritis.

Renal flares are common during the disease course of lupus nephritis and frequently can be detected by increasing proteinuria before the recurrence of constitutional symptoms. The overall renal outcome of children with lupus nephritis has improved significantly during the past decades. The recent 5-year renal survival rates for class IV lupus nephritis are 88% to 93% [14,75]. The reported 10-year renal survival rate is 85% [75]. Factors associated with overall adverse renal outcome include class IV lupus nephritis on biopsy [14], initial evidence of nephrotic syndrome [14], and non-white ethnicity [75].

Treatment

Therapy of children with lupus nephritis should be based on the renal histology.

Class II lupus nephritis

Patients with mesangial proliferative lupus nephritis require a relatively short course of treatment with low-dose steroids (0.1–0.5 mg/kg prednisone/day) with a rather fast taper over months. The long-term outcome of these patients is excellent, and the side effects of steroid therapy must be weighed against the excellent prognosis.

Class III and IV lupus nephritis

Historically, patients with class III lupus nephritis have been managed with steroids alone. More recently, it has been recognized that active class III nephritis falls within the spectrum of proliferative nephritis, and many investigators therefore advocate the same therapy as for class IV nephritis. The authors agree with this suggestion. The mainstay of therapy of proliferative nephritis is high-dose steroids (initially 2 mg/kg/day, maximum 60–80 mg/day, in divided doses) with a slow taper and the addition of a second agent at the time of confirmation of the histology. Most centers advocate the use of pulse monthly cyclophosphamide, although daily oral azathioprine has been associated with similar long-term outcome [83,84]. Recent case series suggest that mycophenolate mofetil (MMF) may be as effective as, if not superior to, monthly intravenous pulse cyclophosphamide [85,86]. Large multicentered trials directly comparing MMF and intravenous cyclophosphamide are underway, and the results of these studies will better indicate the role MMF in class III and class IV lupus nephritis [87]. MMF and azathioprine are safer than cyclophosphamide. Based on their published case series and the results of meta-analysis of therapy of class III and class IV lupus nephritis, the authors advocate the use of azathioprine at the time of diagnosis of class III or class IV lupus nephritis [75].

Class V nephritis

Most patients with pure lupus membranous nephritis require only low doses of steroids for a short period. Only a minority of patients requires a prolonged course of steroids or the use of a second immunosuppressive agent. The second agent of choice is cyclosporin, azathioprine, or MMF. Cyclophosphamide is rarely indicated. Many investigators now advocate the use of angiotensin-converting enzyme inhibitors as adjunctive therapy to decrease the proteinuria. In some patients, the renal biopsy shows a mixed lesion with features of class II, III, or IV nephritis in addition to class V nephritis. In these cases, the therapy should be directed by the presence or absence of a proliferative lesion. When class III or IV lesions are present, immunosuppressive agents should be used as outlined in the discussion of therapy for proliferative nephritis.

Hematologic involvement

Anemia, thrombocytopenia, and leukopenia are seen in 50% to 75% of patients. The most common anemia is normochromic normocytic anemia, which, when persistent, usually becomes a microcytic and hypochromic anemia. The Coombs' test is positive in approximately 30% to 40% of patients, but less than 10% of patients have overt hemolysis. Thrombocytopenia is present in 15% to 45% of adults and may be the initial presentation in up to 15% of pediatric cases. Patients with chronic autoimmune idiopathic thrombocytopenic purpura (AITP) should be assessed for the presence of antinuclear antibodies, because they are at high risk developing SLE [88]. In the authors' experience, most, if not all, patients with AITP and Coombs'-positive hemolytic anemia (Evan's syndrome) either have evidence of SLE at presentation of the cytopenia or develop SLE. Many patients with AITP secondary to SLE have resistant thrombocytopenia that usually requires prolonged use of steroids or multiple courses of intravenous immunoglobulin. Splenectomy should be avoided. Case series have suggested that B cell–directed anti-CD20 therapy may be of benefit in patients with resistant AITP or hemolytic anemia [89]. Classic thrombotic thrombocytopenia purpura, presenting with microangiopathic hemolytic anemia and neurologic and renal disease, is an rare diagnosis in children; when it is present, an underlying diagnosis of SLE should be sought.

Leukopenia is seen in 20% to 40% of cases of pSLE. Both lymphopenia and granulocytopenia can be found, although lymphopenia is more common. Lymphopenia is a sensitive marker of general disease activity and does not require specific therapy. When lymphopenia is profound (an absolute count persistently less than $500 \times 10_9$ cells/litre), an underlying infection with the herpes family of viruses should be actively sought. Granulocytopenia is usually secondary to a central depression of granulopoiesis, splenic sequestration or to antigranulocyte antibodies.

Coagulation abnormalities are common in pSLE. LAC is positive in 20% to 30% of pediatric cases. These patients have an increased incidence of deep vein thrombosis or CVT and thromboemboli but rarely have arterial thrombosis [51]. Most patients with an arterial thrombosis have a true vasculitis in addition to the LAC. Treatment with heparin followed by low molecular weight heparin or warfarin is required if a thrombosis occurs. Antiphospholipid antibodies in SLE are common, but in pediatric patients the risk of thrombosis is related to the presence of the LAC and not other currently measured antiphospholipid antibodies [90,91]. A complication of antiphospholipid antibodies is the development of the catastrophic antiphospholipid antibody syndrome characterized by severe microangiopathic thrombotic changes with thrombosis in multiple organs. Other coagulation abnormalities in SLE include prothrombin deficiency and, rarely, an acquired von Willebrand's–factor deficiency [92]. The antiphospholipid syndrome is discussed elsewhere in this issue.

Cardiac involvement

The most common form of cardiac involvement is pericarditis with pericardial effusion. Less commonly, endo- or myocarditis or valvular disease is found, and, rarely, ischemic heart disease may result secondary to coronary artery vasculitis. Valvular heart disease may be associated with the presence of antiphospholipid antibodies or with noninfective or Libman-Sacks endocarditis [93]. Symptomatic pericarditis is the most common cardiac manifestation, occurring in approximately 15% to 25% of patients and in up to 68% of patients with echocardiographic abnormalities [94]. Pericarditis rapidly responds to nonsteroidal anti-inflammatory medication alone or to a low to moderate dose of corticosteroids.

The major cardiac morbidity associated with SLE is premature atherosclerosis. A number of traditional and nontraditional atherosclerotic risk factors, including lipid abnormalities, altered endothelial function, nephritis, and proteinuria, have been implicated in the development of premature atherosclerosis in patients with pSLE [95,96]. Reports of myocardial perfusion deficits, altered vascular reactivity, and carotid intima-media thickness in pSLE patients suggest that even during adolescence pediatric patients are at risk for premature atherosclerosis, myocardial infarction, and cerebral vascular events [95]. It is likely that the major risk factor for premature atherosclerosis is the chronic inflammatory process of pSLE itself. This risk is likely to increase with the use of corticosteroids as the main line of pSLE treatment. One of the added benefits of the use of antimalarial agents in SLE is their lipid-lowering effect. Interdisciplinary approaches involving dieticians and physiotherapists to control classic Framingham risk factors such as obesity, reduced physical exercise, and high blood lipid levels are mandatory for the management of pSLE patients.

Pulmonary involvement

Pulmonary involvement is common in pSLE and occurs in 25% to 75% of cases. The clinical spectrum includes pleuritis, pneumonitis, infectious pneumonia, pulmonary hemorrhage, pulmonary hypertension, and pneumothorax. Uncommon manifestations are diaphragm involvement (including shrinking lung syndrome), vasculitis, and pulmonary embolus.

Severity of pulmonary involvement ranges from asymptomatic abnormalities of pulmonary function tests to severe life-threatening pulmonary hemorrhage. The most common manifestation is pleuritis with or without pericarditis. These patients commonly have respiratory symptoms or chest pain, and the pleuritis may be unilateral. When the pleuritis is mild, treatment can consist of anti-inflammatory doses of nonsteroidal drugs, but prednisone, at a low to moderate dose, may be required.

When patients present with acute respiratory failure and fever, treatment with broad-spectrum antibiotics and high-dose steroids, including pulse therapy, may be required. The use of bronchial washings obtained by bronchoscopy should be considered early, but frequently patients require an open-lung biopsy to determine whether lung involvement is related directly to the SLE or to determine accurately the organism leading to the respiratory failure. Patients with SLE receiving immunosuppressive therapy are at high risk for infection with opportunistic organisms including Herpes viruses, *Pneumocystis carinii*, Legionella, and fungal infections. These infections must be ruled out before the introduction of significant immunosuppressive therapy.

Gastrointestinal and liver disease

Gastrointestinal involvement occurs in 20% to 40% of patients. Abdominal pain can result from peritoneal inflammation (serositis), vasculitis, pancreatitis, malabsorption, pseudo-obstruction, paralytic ileus, or direct bowel wall involvement (enteritis).

Lupus enteropathy may present as acute ischemic enteritis or a protein-losing enteropathy [97]. Bowel wall inflammation presenting as cramping abdominal pain and diarrhea can reflect enteritis or can develop secondary to a mesenteric vasculitis or thrombosis. Patients with gastrointestinal vasculitis are at risk for perforation, and the signs and symptoms may be masked by the use of high-dose steroids.

Pancreatitis is uncommon, with an overall incidence of less than 5%, and may reflect active disease, an infectious complication, or be secondary to drug therapy, in particular steroids or azathioprine [98–100].

Splenomegaly, occurring in 20% to 30% of pediatric cases, usually reflects the generalized inflammatory state. Functional asplenia is common and increases the risk of sepsis. Hepatomegaly occurs in 40% to 50% of patients, and up to 25% have abnormal liver function tests. Markedly elevated liver function tests can be seen in lupoid hepatitis.

Endocrine involvement

The thyroid is the endocrine organ most commonly involved in SLE. Both hypothyroidism and hyperthyroidism are seen, but hypothyroidism is the more common abnormality. Up to 35% of pSLE patients have antithyroid antibodies, with 10% to 15% of patients developing overt hypothyroidism [101]. Steroid-induced diabetes mellitus occurs in 5% to 10% of patients and frequently requires insulin treatment. Delayed puberty and menstrual abnormalities are common. Irregular menses frequently are related to active disease and usually resolve when the disease is controlled. Ovarian failure is a significant complication of cyclophosphamide therapy and is dose dependant [102,103].

Autoantibodies

The hallmark of SLE is the production of autoantibodies directed against histone, non-histone, RNA-binding, cytoplasmic, and nuclear proteins. Antinuclear autoantibodies are seen in up to 100% of patients, and anti-DNA antibodies are seen in 60% to 70% of cases. Antibodies against the RNA-binding proteins, anti-U1 RNP and anti-Sm antibodies, occur in 70% to 90% and in 40% to 50% of patients, respectively. Antibodies against Ro and La occur in 30% to 40% and in 15% to 20% of patients, respectively. The most commonly measured antiphospholipid antibodies are anti-anticardiolipin antibodies, found in approximately 50% of patients, and LAC, present in 20% of cases. Antiphospholipid antibodies are associated with an increased risk of thrombosis, development of chorea, avascular necrosis, epilepsy, migraine headache, and livedo reticularis [104]. Antiribosomal P antibodies are present in approximately 15% of patients; a higher percentage of patients with psychosis have these autoantibodies. Aside from the lupus anticoagulant and the antinuclear autoantibodies, most laboratories use ELISA to detect specific autoantibodies. When anti-Sm antibodies are detected by immunodiffusion, a less sensitive assay than ELISA, these autoanti-

SYSTEMIC LUPUS ERYTHEMATOSUS

bodies have a specificity of 100% for SLE. This specificity is higher than that for anti-DNA antibodies. Rheumatoid factor is seen in 12% to 29% of patients and frequently is seen in association with anti-Ro and anti-La antibodies.

References

[1] Tan EM, Fries JF, Masi AT, et al. The 1982 revised criteria for the classification of systemic lupus erythematosus. Arthritis Rheum 1982;25:1271–7.

[2] Hopkinson ND, Doherty M, Powell RJ. Clinical features and race-specific incidence/prevalence rates of systemic lupus erythematosus in a geographically complete cohort of patients. Ann Rheum Dis 1994;53:675–80.

[3] Ghaussy NO, Sibbitt Jr W, Bankhurst AD, et al. The effect of race on disease activity in systemic lupus erythematosus. J Rheumatol 2004;31:915–9.

[4] Cooper GS, Parks CG, Treadwell EL, et al. Differences by race, sex and age in the clinical and immunologic features of recently diagnosed systemic lupus erythematosus patients in the southeastern United States. Lupus 2002;11:161–7.

[5] Lopez P, Mozo L, Gutierrez C, et al. Epidemiology of systemic lupus erythematosus in a northern Spanish population: gender and age influence on immunological features. Lupus 2003; 12:860–5.

[6] Alamanos Y, Voulgari PV, Siozos C, et al. Epidemiology of systemic lupus erythematosus in northwest Greece 1982–2001. J Rheumatol 2003;30:731–5.

[7] Nossent HC. Systemic lupus erythematosus in the Arctic region of Norway. J Rheumatol 2001;28:539–46.

[8] McCarty DJ, Manzi S, Medsger Jr TA, et al. Incidence of systemic lupus erythematosus. Race and gender differences. Arthritis Rheum 1995;38:1260–70.

[9] Siegel M, Lee SL. The epidemiology of systemic lupus erythematosus. Semin Arthritis Rheum 1973;3:1–54.

[10] Mok CC, Lau CS. Lupus in Hong Kong Chinese. Lupus 2003;12:717–22.

[11] Vilar MJ, Sato EI. Estimating the incidence of systemic lupus erythematosus in a tropical region (Natal, Brazil). Lupus 2002;11:528–32.

[12] Peschken CA, Esdaile JM. Systemic lupus erythematosus in North American Indians: a population based study. J Rheumatol 2000;27:1884–91.

[13] Lo JT, Tsai MJ, Wang LH, et al. Sex differences in pediatric systemic lupus erythematosus: a retrospective analysis of 135 cases. J Microbiol Immunol Infect 1999;32:173–8.

[14] Bogdanovic R, Nikolic V, Pasic S, et al. Lupus nephritis in childhood: a review of 53 patients followed at a single center. Pediatr Nephrol 2004;19:36–44.

[15] Mok CC, Lee KW, Ho CT, et al. A prospective study of survival and prognostic indicators of systemic lupus erythematosus in a southern Chinese population. Rheumatology (Oxford) 2000; 39:399–406.

[16] Balkaran BN, Roberts LA, Ramcharan J. Systemic lupus erythematosus in Trinidadian children. Ann Trop Paediatr 2004;24:241–4.

[17] Cervera R, Khamashta MA, Font J, et al. Morbidity and mortality in systemic lupus erythematosus during a 10-year period: a comparison of early and late manifestations in a cohort of 1,000 patients. Medicine (Baltimore) 2003;82:299–308.

[18] Bellomio V, Spindler A, Lucero E, et al. Systemic lupus erythematosus: mortality and survival in Argentina. A multicenter study. Lupus 2000;9:377–81.

[19] Caeiro F, Michielson FM, Bernstein R, et al. Systemic lupus erythematosus in childhood. Ann Rheum Dis 1981;40:325–31.

[20] Miettunen PM, Ortiz-Alvarez O, Petty RE, et al. Gender and ethnic origin have no effect on longterm outcome of childhood-onset systemic lupus erythematosus. J Rheumatol 2004;31: 1650–4.

[21] Wang LC, Yang YH, Lu MY, et al. Retrospective analysis of mortality and morbidity of pediatric systemic lupus erythematosus in the past two decades. J Microbiol Immunol Infect 2003;36:203–8.

[22] Vyas S, Hidalgo G, Baqi N, et al. Outcome in African-American children of neuropsychiatric lupus and lupus nephritis. Pediatr Nephrol 2002;17:45–9.

[23] Segasothy M, Phillips PA. Systemic lupus erythematosus in Aborigines and Caucasians in central Australia: a comparative study. Lupus 2001;10:439–44.

[24] Alsaeid K, Kamal H, Haider MZ, et al. Systemic lupus erythematosus in Kuwaiti children: organ system involvement and serological findings. Lupus 2004;13:613–7.

[25] Ward MM. Education level and mortality in systemic lupus erythematosus (SLE): evidence of underascertainment of deaths due to SLE in ethnic minorities with low education levels. Arthritis Rheum 2004;51:616–24.

[26] Ali US, Dalvi RB, Merchant RH, et al. Systemic lupus erythematosus in Indian children. Indian Pediatr 1989;26:868–73.

[27] Chen YS, Yang YH, Lin YT, et al. Risk of infection in hospitalised children with systemic lupus erythematosus: a 10-year follow-up. Clin Rheumatol 2004;23:235–8.

[28] Sibbitt Jr WL, Brandt JR, Johnson CR, et al. The incidence and prevalence of neuropsychiatric syndromes in pediatric onset systemic lupus erythematosus. J Rheumatol 2002;29:1536–42.

[29] Barron KS, Silverman ED, Gonzales J, et al. Clinical, serologic, and immunogenetic studies in childhood-onset systemic lupus erythematosus. Arthritis Rheum 1993;36:348–54.

[30] Huong DL, Papo T, Beaufils H, et al. Renal involvement in systemic lupus erythematosus. A study of 180 patients from a single center. Medicine (Baltimore) 1999;78:148–66.

[31] Siamopoulou-Mavridou A, Mavridis AK, et al. Clinical and serological spectrum of systemic lupus erythematosus in Greek children. Clin Rheumatol 1991;10:264–8.

[32] Saurit V, Campana R, Ruiz Lascano A, et al. [Mucocutaneous lesions in patients with systemic lupus erythematosus]. Medicina (B Aires) 2003;63:283–7 [in Spanish].

[33] Chandrasekaran AN, Rajendran CP, Ramakrishnan S, et al. Childhood systemic lupus erythematosus in south India. Indian J Pediatr 1994;61:223–9.

[34] Vuilleumier C, Sauvain MJ, Aebi C, et al. Systemic lupus erythematosus initially presenting as idiopathic juvenile arthritis with positive antinuclear antibodies. Acta Paediatr 2003;92: 512–3.

[35] Saulsbury FT, Kesler RW, Kennaugh JM, et al. Overlap syndrome of juvenile rheumatoid arthritis and systemic lupus erythematosus. J Rheumatol 1982;9:610–2.

[36] Citera G, Espada G, Maldonado Cocco JA. Sequential development of 2 connective tissue diseases in juvenile patients. J Rheumatol 1993;20:2149–52.

[37] Noguera A, Ros JB, Pavia C, et al. Bisphosphonates, a new treatment for glucocorticoid-induced osteoporosis in children. J Pediatr Endocrinol Metab 2003;16:529–36.

[38] Cimaz R. Osteoporosis in childhood rheumatic diseases: prevention and therapy. Best Pract Res Clin Rheumatol 2002;16:397–409.

[39] Mavrikakis I, Sfikakis PP, Mavrikakis E, et al. The incidence of irreversible retinal toxicity in patients treated with hydroxychloroquine: a reappraisal. Ophthalmology 2003;110:1321–6.

[40] Marmor MF. New American Academy of Ophthalmology recommendations on screening for hydroxychloroquine retinopathy. Arthritis Rheum 2003;48:1764.

[41] Berkel AI, Birben E, Oner C, et al. Molecular, genetic and epidemiologic studies on selective complete C1q deficiency in Turkey. Immunobiology 2000;201:347–55.

[42] Steinlin MI, Blaser SI, Gilday DL, et al. Neurologic manifestations of pediatric systemic lupus erythematosus. Pediatr Neurol 1995;13:191–7.

[43] Platt JL, Burke BA, Fish AJ, et al. Systemic lupus erythematosus in the first two decades of life. Am J Kidney Dis 1982;2:212–22.

[44] Yancey CL, Doughty RA, Athreya BH. Central nervous system involvement in childhood systemic lupus erythematosus. Arthritis Rheum 1981;24:1389–95.

[45] Loh WF, Hussain IM, Soffiah A, et al. Neurological manifestations of children with systemic lupus erythematosus. Med J Malaysia 2000;55:459–63.

[46] The American College of Rheumatology. Nomenclature and case definitions for neuro-psychiatric lupus syndromes. Arthritis Rheum 1999;42:599–608.

[47] Ainiala H, Hietaharju A, Loukkola J, et al. Validity of the new American College of Rheumatology criteria for neuropsychiatric lupus syndromes: a population-based evaluation. Arthritis Rheum 2001;45:419–23.

[48] Mitsikostas DD, Sfikakis PP, Goadsby PJ. A meta-analysis for headache in systemic lupus erythematosus: the evidence and the myth. Brain 2004;127:1200–9.

[49] Steens SC, Bosma GP, ten Cate R, et al. A neuroimaging follow up study of a patient with juvenile central nervous system systemic lupus erythematosus. Ann Rheum Dis 2003;62: 583–6.

[50] Olfat MO, Al-Mayouf SM, Muzaffer MA. Pattern of neuropsychiatric manifestations and outcome in juvenile systemic lupus erythematosus. Clin Rheumatol 2004;23:395–9.

[51] Levy DM, Massicotte MP, Harvey E, et al. Thromboembolism in paediatric lupus patients. Lupus 2003;12:741–6.

[52] Karassa FB, Magliano M, Isenberg DA. Suicide attempts in patients with systemic lupus erythematosus. Ann Rheum Dis 2003;62:58–60.

[53] Russo R, Gilday D, Laxer RM, et al. Single photon emission computed tomography scanning in childhood systemic lupus erythematosus. J Rheumatol 1998;25:576–82.

[54] Ingram DG, Hagemann TM. Promethazine treatment of steroid-induced psychosis in a child. Ann Pharmacother 2003;37:1036–9.

[55] Klein-Gitelman MS, Pachman LM. Intravenous corticosteroids: adverse reactions are more variable than expected in children. J Rheumatol 1998;25:1995–2002.

[56] Liem MD, Gzesh DJ, Flanders AE. MRI and angiographic diagnosis of lupus cerebral vasculitis. Neuroradiology 1996;38:134–6.

[57] Sanna G, Bertolaccini ML, Cuadrado MJ, et al. Neuropsychiatric manifestations in systemic lupus erythematosus: prevalence and association with antiphospholipid antibodies. J Rheumatol 2003;30:985–92.

[58] Tan EK, Chan LL, Auchus AP. Reversible parkinsonism in systemic lupus erythematosus. J Neurol Sci 2001;193:53–7.

[59] Bruyn GW, Padberg G. Chorea and systemic lupus erythematosus. A critical review. Eur Neurol 1984;23:435–48.

[60] Besbas N, Damarguc I, Ozen S, et al. Association of antiphospholipid antibodies with systemic lupus erythematosus in a child presenting with chorea: a case report. Eur J Pediatr 1994; 153:891–3.

[61] Campello I, Almarcegui C, Velilla J, et al. [Peripheral neuropathy in systemic lupus erythematosus]. Rev Neurol 2001;33:27–30 [in Spanish].

[62] Al-Mayouf SM, Al-Hemidan AI. Ocular manifestations of systemic lupus erythematosus in children. Saudi Med J 2003;24:964–6.

[63] Genevay S, Hayem G, Hamza S, et al. Oculomotor palsy in six patients with systemic lupus erythematosus. A possible role of antiphospholipid syndrome. Lupus 2002;11:313–6.

[64] Blaustein DA, Blaustein SA. Antinuclear antibody negative systemic lupus erythematosus presenting as bilateral facial paralysis. J Rheumatol 1998;25:798–800.

[65] Liao CH, Yang YH, Chiang BL. Systemic lupus erythematosus with presentation as vertigo and vertical nystagmus: report of one case. Acta Paediatr Taiwan 2003;44:158–60.

[66] al-Mayouf SM, Bahabri S. Spinal cord involvement in pediatric systemic lupus erythematosus: case report and literature review. Clin Exp Rheumatol 1999;17:505–8.

[67] Maule S, Quadri R, Mirante D, et al. Autonomic nervous dysfunction in systemic lupus erythematosus (SLE) and rheumatoid arthritis (RA): possible pathogenic role of autoantibodies to autonomic nervous structures. Clin Exp Immunol 1997;110:423–7.

[68] Abbott NJ, Mendonca LL, Dolman DE. The blood-brain barrier in systemic lupus erythematosus. Lupus 2003;12:908–15.

[69] Gilad R, Lampl Y, Eshel Y, et al. Cerebrospinal fluid soluble interleukin-2 receptor in cerebral lupus. Br J Rheumatol 1997;36:190–3.

[70] Jara LJ, Irigoyen L, Ortiz MJ, et al. Prolactin and interleukin-6 in neuropsychiatric lupus erythematosus. Clin Rheumatol 1998;17:110–4.

[71] Ainiala H, Hietaharju A, Dastidar P, et al. Increased serum matrix metalloproteinase 9 levels in systemic lupus erythematosus patients with neuropsychiatric manifestations and brain magnetic resonance imaging abnormalities. Arthritis Rheum 2004;50:858–65.

[72] Uziel Y, Laxer RM, Blaser S, et al. Cerebral vein thrombosis in childhood systemic lupus erythematosus. J Pediatr 1995;126:722–7.

[73] Reiff A, Miller J, Shaham B, et al. Childhood central nervous system lupus; longitudinal assessment using single photon emission computed tomography. J Rheumatol 1997;24: 2461–5.

[74] Liu FY, Huang WS, Kao CH, et al. Usefulness of Tc-99m ECD brain SPECT to evaluate the effects of methylprednisolone pulse therapy in lupus erythematosus with brain involvement: a preliminary report. Rheumatol Int 2003;23:182–5.

[75] Hagelberg S, Lee Y, Bargman J, et al. Longterm followup of childhood lupus nephritis. J Rheumatol 2002;29:2635–42.

[76] Gupta KL. Lupus nephritis in children. Indian J Pediatr 1999;66:215–23.

[77] Sumboonnanonda A, Vongjirad A, Suntornpoch V, et al. Renal pathology and long-term outcome in childhood SLE. J Med Assoc Thai 1998;81:830–4.

[78] Weening JJ, D'Agati VD, Schwartz MM, et al. The classification of glomerulonephritis in systemic lupus erythematosus revisited. J Am Soc Nephrol 2004;15:241–50.

[79] Austin III HA, Muenz LR, Joyce KM, et al. Prognostic factors in lupus nephritis. Contribution of renal histologic data. Am J Med 1983;75:382–91.

[80] Schwartz MM, Lan SP, Bernstein J, et al. Irreproducibility of the activity and chronicity indices limits their utility in the management of lupus nephritis. Lupus Nephritis Collaborative Study Group. Am J Kidney Dis 1993;21:374–7.

[81] Appel GB, Pirani CL, D'Agati V. Renal vascular complications of systemic lupus erythematosus. J Am Soc Nephrol 1994;4:1499–515.

[82] Wu CT, Fu LS, Wen MC, et al. Lupus vasculopathy combined with acute renal failure in lupus nephritis. Pediatr Nephrol 2003;18:1304–7.

[83] Yee CS, Gordon C, Dostal C, et al. EULAR randomised controlled trial of pulse cyclophosphamide and methylprednisolone versus continuous cyclophosphamide and prednisolone followed by azathioprine and prednisolone in lupus nephritis. Ann Rheum Dis 2004; 63:525–9.

[84] Houssiau FA, Vasconcelos C, D'Cruz D, et al. Immunosuppressive therapy in lupus nephritis: the Euro-Lupus Nephritis Trial, a randomized trial of low-dose versus high-dose intravenous cyclophosphamide. Arthritis Rheum 2002;46:2121–31.

[85] Hu W, Liu Z, Chen H, et al. Mycophenolate mofetil vs cyclophosphamide therapy for patients with diffuse proliferative lupus nephritis. Chin Med J (Engl) 2002;115:705–9.

[86] Buratti S, Szer IS, Spencer CH, et al. Mycophenolate mofetil treatment of severe renal disease in pediatric onset systemic lupus erythematosus. J Rheumatol 2001;28:2103–8.

[87] Ginzler E, Aranow C, Buyon J, et al. A multicenter study of mycophenolate mofetil (MMF) vs. intravenous cyclophosphamide (IVC) as induction therapy for severe lupus nephritis (LN): preliminary results [abstract 1690]. Proceedings of the annual meeting of the American College of Rheumatology. Arthritis Rheum 2003;48:S647.

[88] Zimmerman SA, Ware RE. Clinical significance of the antinuclear antibody test in selected children with idiopathic thrombocytopenic purpura. J Pediatr Hematol Oncol 1997;19:297–303.

[89] ten Cate R, Smiers FJ, Bredius RG, et al. Anti-CD20 monoclonal antibody (rituximab) for refractory autoimmune thrombocytopenia in a girl with systemic lupus erythematosus. Rheumatology (Oxford) 2004;43:244.

[90] Berube C, Mitchell L, Silverman E, et al. The relationship of antiphospholipid antibodies to thromboembolic events in pediatric patients with systemic lupus erythematosus: a cross-sectional study. Pediatr Res 1998;44:351–6.

[91] McClain MT, Arbuckle MR, Heinlen LD, et al. The prevalence, onset, and clinical significance

of antiphospholipid antibodies prior to diagnosis of systemic lupus erythematosus. Arthritis Rheum 2004;50:1226–32.

[92] Eberhard A, Sparling C, Sudbury S, et al. Hypoprothrombinemia in childhood systemic lupus erythematosus. Semin Arthritis Rheum 1994;24:12–8.

[93] Chan YK, Li EK, Tam LS, et al. Intravenous cyclophosphamide improves cardiac dysfunction in lupus myocarditis. Scand J Rheumatol 2003;32:306–8.

[94] Guevara JP, Clark BJ, Athreya BH. Point prevalence of cardiac abnormalities in children with systemic lupus erythematosus. J Rheumatol 2001;28:854–9.

[95] Falaschi F, Ravelli A, Martignoni A, et al. Nephrotic-range proteinuria, the major risk factor for early atherosclerosis in juvenile-onset systemic lupus erythematosus. Arthritis Rheum 2000; 43:1405–9.

[96] Soep JB, Mietus-Snyder M, Malloy MJ, et al. Assessment of atherosclerotic risk factors and endothelial function in children and young adults with pediatric-onset systemic lupus erythematosus. Arthritis Rheum 2004;51:451–7.

[97] Molina JF, Brown RF, Gedalia A, et al. Protein losing enteropathy as the initial manifestation of childhood systemic lupus erythematosus. J Rheumatol 1996;23:1269–71.

[98] Duncan HV, Achara G. A rare initial manifestation of systemic lupus erythematosus–acute pancreatitis: case report and review of the literature. J Am Board Fam Pract 2003;16:334–8.

[99] Swol-Ben J, Bruns CJ, Muller-Ladner U, et al. Leukoencephalopathy and chronic pancreatitis as concomitant manifestations of systemic lupus erythematosus related to anticardiolipin antibodies. Rheumatol Int 2004;24:177–81.

[100] Ikura Y, Matsuo T, Ogami M, et al. Cytomegalovirus associated pancreatitis in a patient with systemic lupus erythematosus. J Rheumatol 2000;27:2715–7.

[101] Eberhard BA, Laxer RM, Eddy AA, et al. Presence of thyroid abnormalities in children with systemic lupus erythematosus. J Pediatr 1991;119:277–9.

[102] Katsifis GE, Tzioufas AG. Ovarian failure in systemic lupus erythematosus patients treated with pulsed intravenous cyclophosphamide. Lupus 2004;13:673–8.

[103] Flanc RS, Roberts MA, Strippoli GF, et al. Treatment of diffuse proliferative lupus nephritis: a meta-analysis of randomized controlled trials. Am J Kidney Dis 2004;43(2):197–208.

[104] Ravelli A, Caporali R, Di Fuccia G, et al. Anticardiolipin antibodies in pediatric systemic lupus erythematosus. Arch Pediatr Adolesc Med 1994;148:398–402.

ELSEVIER
SAUNDERS

PEDIATRIC CLINICS
OF NORTH AMERICA

Pediatr Clin N Am 52 (2005) 469–491

Antiphospholipid Syndrome

Angelo Ravelli, MD[a],*, Alberto Martini, MD[a,b]

[a]Pediatria II, Istituto di Ricovero e Cura a Carattere Scientifico G. Gaslini,
Largo G. Gaslini, 5, 16147, Genoa, Italy
[b]Department of Pediatrics, University of Genova, Largo G. Gaslini, 5, 16147, Genoa, Italy

The description of the antiphospholipid syndrome (APS) has been one of the most striking developments in the field of clinical immunology in the last 2 decades. APS is a systemic autoimmune disorder characterized by a combination of arterial or venous thrombosis and recurrent fetal loss, accompanied by elevated titers of antiphospholipid antibodies (aPL), namely the lupus anticoagulant (LA) and anticardiolipin antibodies (aCL) [1,2]. The syndrome may occur in isolation (primary APS) or in association with an underlying systemic disease, particularly systemic lupus erythematosus (SLE) (secondary APS).

Because aPL-related thrombosis can occur anywhere in the body, the recognition of APS has had a major impact on several medical specialties, including pediatrics. The earliest descriptions of the association between a circulating anticoagulant and vascular thrombosis in the pediatric population are those of Olive et al in 1979 [3] and St Clair et al in 1981 [4]. In recent years, the features of APS have been increasingly recognized in children [5,6]. Most information on APS in the pediatric population, however, comes from individual case reports or small patient series; large-scale multicenter studies are lacking.

The following case highlights some of the important clinical and laboratory features of the APS.

Case report

A previously normal 6-year-old boy developed pain in the left lower limb, limping, and increasing calf swelling. One week after onset of symptoms, he was

---

* Corresponding author. Pediatria II, Istituto G. Gaslini, Largo G. Gaslini, 5, 16147, Genoa, Italy.
E-mail address: angeloravelli@ospedale-gaslini.ge.it (A. Ravelli).

brought to the local hospital, where Doppler ultrasonography disclosed an extensive thrombosis in his left iliac and femoral veins. Family history was negative for autoimmune diseases or coagulation disorders. He was transferred to the authors' institute 1 day later for further examination.

On admission, the boy had low-grade fever but was in good general health. Physical examination revealed swelling, heat, and redness of the left calf, which had a circumference 3 cm greater than the contralateral one; there were mild cervical, axillary, and inguinal lymphadenopathy and slight spleen enlargement. Laboratory investigations were as follows: white blood cell count, $9.6 \times 10^9/L$; hemoglobin, 103 g/L; platelet count, $138 \times 10^9/L$; erythrocyte sedimentation rate, 32 mm/hour; C-reactive protein, 2.2 mg/dL; prothrombin time 65%; partial thromboplastin time, 64 seconds (normal, < 32 seconds); and fibrinogen, 2.3 g/L. Liver and kidney function tests, viral serologies, serum complement fractions, rheumatoid factor, and urinalysis were normal or negative. Antinuclear antibodies (ANA) were positive at 1:160, whereas anti-DNA and anti-extractable nuclear antigen antibodies were negative. The direct Coombs test was weakly positive. IgG and IgM aCLs were detected, using ELISA, at a titer of 66 G phospholipid (GPL) (normal, < 20) and 42 M phospholipid (MPL) (normal, < 20), respectively, and LA was positive by kaolin clotting time. Protein C, protein S, antithrombin III, and homocysteine levels were within normal limits, and factor V Leiden mutation was absent. Based on the association of deep vein thrombosis with the presence of aPL, a diagnosis of APS was made.

The boy was treated with low molecular weight heparin for 2 weeks and then placed on long-term warfarin prophylaxis to maintain the international normalized ratio (INR) between 2.0 and 3.0 Repeated Doppler ultrasonography after 1 and 2 weeks showed progressive recanalization of involved vessels. Six months later, angiographic MRI revealed complete recovery of the vascular occlusion.

One year after the occurrence of thrombosis, several papular and plaque lesions were noted over the dorsal surface of the hands and the extensor aspect of both elbows and knees. The erythrocyte sedimentation rate was raised to 48 mm/hour, and ANA were still detectable at 1:320, but anti-DNA antibodies and urinalysis were negative, and serum complement fractions were within normal limits. Cutaneous biopsy led to a histologic diagnosis of lupus panniculitis. Treatment with prednisone (0.5 mg/kg/day) and hydroxychloroquine was started, which led to considerable improvement of skin disease.

After 18 months the patient was readmitted because of the development of a full-blown clinical and laboratory picture of SLE, with proteinuria (1.2–2.6 g/24 hours), microhematuria, decreased C3 (48 mg/dL; normal, 84–192 mg/dL) and C4 (4 mg/dL; normal, 10–42 mg/dL), and high-titer anti-DNA antibodies (1:2560).

This boy was diagnosed as having APS based on the association of vascular thrombosis with the presence of elevated titers of circulating aCL, a positive LA test, and the exclusion of other congenital or acquired thrombophilic conditions. In the early stages of his disease, no evidence of a systemic autoimmune syndrome was found, except for the presence of low-titer ANA, weakly-positive Coombs test, and mild lymphadenopathy. The disease therefore was labeled as primary APS. After successful treatment of the acute thrombotic event, the boy was placed on long-term antithrombotic prophylaxis with intermediate-intensity warfarin, and no further vascular thrombosis was seen in the 2.5-year follow-up. One year after onset of symptoms, he presented with skin lesions consistent with lupus panniculitis, and 1.5 years later he developed full-blown SLE.

Laboratory detection of antiphospholipid antibodies

The presence of aPL is the central serologic finding of APS [7]. aPL tests detect a heterogeneous group of antibodies, which possess different pathogenic properties. Those more strongly associated with clinical manifestations react predominantly against serum phospholipid-binding proteins (initially called "cofactors") rather than against phospholipids per se. The most common of these proteins are anti-β2-glycoprotein I (aβ2-GPI) and prothrombin, although other phospholipid-binding proteins, such as protein C, protein S, and annexin V, have been involved [8]. In addition to these antibodies, there are aPL that bind directly to negatively charged phospholipid themselves. They occur in patients with infections, such as syphilis, infectious mononucleosis, and HIV infection, and following exposure to certain medications and usually are not pathogenic. Routine assays, however, do not readily distinguish between these major antibody subsets.

The most commonly detected subgroups of aPL are LA, aCL, and aβ2-GPI. Placement into these subgroups is based on the method of determination. LA is identified by coagulation assays, in which it prolongs clotting times. In contrast, aCL and aβ2-GPI are demonstrated by immunoassays that measure immunologic reactivity against a phospholipid or a phospholipid-binding protein (cardiolipin and β2-GPI, respectively). In general, LA is more specific for APS, whereas aCL is more sensitive. The specificity of aCL for APS increases with titer and is higher for the IgG than for the IgM and IgA isotype. There is no definitive association between specific clinical manifestations and particular subgroups of aPL, however. Therefore, multiple tests for aPL should be used, because patients may be negative according to one test but positive according to another.

aCL test results are reported according to isotype (IgG, IgM, or IgA) and level. Levels of IgG, IgM, and IgA aCL are reported in GPL, MPL, or A phospholipid (APL) units, respectively, as defined by the First International Workshop on aCL [9]. Because of the relatively wide error range of absolute levels, the use of semiquantitative measures to report results (normal or low positive, 20–80 units; moderate positive, 20–80 units; high positive, above 80 units) is preferable [1].

The LA test is a functional assay that measures the ability of this subgroup of aPL to prolong clotting tests such as the partial thromboplastin time, the

Russell viper venom time, or the kaolin clotting time. Inhibition of clotting in vitro is caused by blocking the conversion of prothrombin to thrombin in the presence of a phospholipid template. This process delays the formation of fibrin and, therefore, prolongs the time to clot formation, hence the name of LA. In vivo, however, the presence of LA is paradoxically associated with thrombotic events rather than with bleeding. Current criteria for the detection of LA require prolongation of coagulation in at least one phospholipid-dependent coagulation assay. According to established guidelines, two or more assays that are sensitive to this antibody must be negative to rule out the presence of LA [10].

The observation that many aCL are directed at an epitope on β2-GPI led to the development of aβ2-GPI immunoassays [11]. Although the use of these assays is not currently included in the criteria for APS, aβ2-GPI are strongly associated with thrombosis and other features of APS. The clinical utility of aPL assays for autoantibodies other than aCL and of phospholipid-binding proteins other than β2-GPI remains unclear. A significant minority of patients with APS have a biologic false-positive standard test for syphilis, which measures the ability of aPL to precipitate an antigen (eg, the VDRL antigen) containing a mixture of cardiolipin, phosphatidylcholine, and cholesterol.

Classification criteria and diagnostic issues

In 1998, a set of criteria for classification of patients with APS (the Sapporo criteria) was proposed (Box 1) [7].

Although these criteria are intended to provide a basis for including patients with the syndrome in research protocols, they are used in practice as a guide to diagnosing the syndrome in individual patients. There are, however, patients with probable APS who do not meet the Sapporo criteria because of the presence of clinical and laboratory features that are not accepted universally as part of the syndrome. These manifestations include livedo reticularis, chorea, cardiac valve disease, transient cerebral ischemia, transverse myelitis, migraine, hemolytic anemia, and thrombocytopenia [12].

Because pregnancy morbidity is not a pediatric problem, and coincident thrombotic risk factors that are common in adults (as discussed below) have little or no impact in the pediatric population, it is likely that the sensitivity and specificity of the Sapporo criteria for aPL-related thrombosis is higher in children than in adults.

In clinical practice, a diagnostic workup for aPL should be considered in all children and adolescents with venous or arterial thrombosis for which there is no alternative explanation, particularly in the presence of recurrent manifestations. Likewise, unexplained thrombocytopenia, hemolytic anemia, chorea, livedo reticularis, and prolongation of any phospholipid coagulation test should lead to determination of aPL status.

Box 1. Preliminary criteria for the classification of APS

Clinical criteria

1. Vascular thrombosis: One or more clinical episodes of arterial, venous, or small vessel thrombosis, in any tissue or organ. Thrombosis must be confirmed by imaging or Doppler studies or histopathology, with the exception of superficial venous thrombosis. For histopathologic confirmation, thrombosis should be present without significant evidence of inflammation in the vessel wall.
2. Pregnancy morbidity
   A. One or more unexplained deaths of a morphologically normal fetus at or beyond the tenth week of gestation, with normal fetal morphology documented by ultrasound or by direct examination of the fetus, or
   B. One or more premature births of a morphologically normal neonate at or before the thirty-fourth week of gestation because of severe preeclampsia or eclampsia, or severe placental insufficiency, or
   C. Three or more unexplained consecutive spontaneous abortions before the tenth week of gestation, with maternal anatomic or hormonal abnormalities and paternal and maternal chromosomal causes excluded

Laboratory criteria

1. aCL of IgG and/or IgM isotype in blood, present in medium or high titer, on two or more occasions at least 6 weeks apart, measured by a standardized ELISA for β2-GPI–dependent aCL.
2. Lupus anticoagulant present in plasma, on two or more occasions at least 6 weeks apart, detected according to the guidelines of the International Society on Thrombosis and Hemostasis (Scientific Subcommittee on Lupus Anticoagulant/Phospholipid-Dependent Antibodies), in the following steps:
   A. Prolonged phospholipid-dependent coagulation demonstrated on a screening test (eg, activated partial thromboplastin time [aPTT], kaolin clotting time, dilute Russell's viper venom time, dilute prothrombin time, Texarin time)
   B. Failure to correct the prolonged coagulation time on the screening test by mixing with normal platelet-poor plasma

> C. Shortening or correction of the prolonged coagulation time
>   on the screening test by the addition of excess phospholipid
> D. Exclusion of other coagulopathies (eg, factor VIII inhibitor
>   or heparin) as appropriate
>
> Definite APS is considered to be present if at least one of the
> clinical criteria and one of the laboratory criteria are met.

Pathogenetic mechanisms

Despite the strong association between aPL and thrombotic complications, the in vivo mechanisms responsible for thrombosis in patients with APS have not been fully elucidated. Proposed pathophysiologic mechanisms may be categorized in at least four types (reviewed in [13] and [14]). First, aPL may interfere with or modulate the function of phospholipid-binding proteins involved in the regulation of the coagulation cascade, leading to a procoagulant state. Examples include interference with β2-GPI, inhibition of activated protein C and antithrombin III pathways and fibrinolysis, and increased tissue factor activity. Other proteins that are important in regulating coagulation, such as prothrombin, proteins C and S, and annexin V, may also be targeted by aPL. A second theory focuses on the activation of endothelial cells. Binding of aPL, which recognize β2-GPI on resting endothelial cells, induces activation of the same cells, which is manifested by increased expression of cell-surface adhesion molecules and increased secretion of cytokines and prostaglandins. It is well known that activated endothelial cells promote coagulation. A third theory proposes an oxidant-mediated injury of the vascular endothelium. Oxidized low-density lipoproteins (LDL), which are leading contributors to atherosclerosis, are taken up by macrophages, causing macrophage activation and consequent damage to endothelial cells. Autoantibodies to oxidized LDL are known to occur in association with aCL, and some aCL have been shown to cross-react with oxidized LDL. A fourth route by which aPL may promote thrombosis is by platelet activation, leading to enhanced platelet adhesion or increased thromboxane synthesis. Thrombosis in APS has also been likened to that of heparin-induced thrombocytopenia, which may also induce vascular thrombosis [15].

Recent evidence in animal models indicates that viral and bacterial peptides, perhaps through a molecular mimicry mechanism, may induce aPL production, which in turn may promote thrombosis [16].

Whatever the pathogenetic mechanisms, it is likely that other factors play a role in determining whether patients develop the clinical manifestations of APS. Most patients with persistently elevated antibody levels never experience thrombosis. A second hit may, therefore, be necessary for thrombosis to occur. For instance, several other prothrombotic factors, such as smoking, contraception, hypertension, obesity, and atherosclerosis, may increase the risk of vascular occlusion in aPL-positive patients. Notably, a recent study found that about half of patients with acute thrombosis that led to a diagnosis of APS had coincident risk factors for thrombosis [17]. Furthermore, an association between the number of prothrombotic risk factors and history of thrombotic events has been observed in individuals with positive IgG aCL [18].

Although the pathogenetic mechanisms involved in pediatric APS have not been thoroughly investigated, it is assumed that they are similar to those operating in adults. The frequency of vascular thrombosis is much lower in children than in adults, however, and other risk factors for thrombosis, such as cigarette smoking and atherosclerosis, are not applicable in the pediatric population. Therefore, children with aPL-associated thrombosis constitute a relatively "clean" sample to assess the clinical relevance of aPL and to provide pathogenic aPL to be studied for their specificity.

Clinical features

With the obvious exception of pregnancy morbidity, most of the clinical features that can occur in adults with APS have also been described in children. The thrombotic process can involve virtually any organ, and a wide spectrum of

Table 1
Sites of vascular thrombosis associated with aPL in children

Vessel involved	Clinical manifestations
Veins	
Limbs	Deep vein thrombosis
	Superficial vein thrombosis
Large veins	Superior or inferior vena cava thrombosis
Lungs	Pulmonary thromboembolism
	Pulmonary hypertension
Skin	Livedo reticularis
Brain	Cerebral venous sinus thrombosis
Liver	
Large vessels	Budd-Chiari syndrome
Small vessels	Hepatomegaly, enzyme elevation
Eyes	Retinal vein thrombosis
Adrenal glands	Addison's disease
Arteries	
Brain	Stroke, transient ischemic attacks
Kidney	
Large vessels	Renal artery thrombosis
Small vessels	Renal thrombotic microangiopathy
Limbs	Ischemia, gangrene
Heart	Myocardial infarction
Liver	Hepatic infarction
Gut	Mesenteric artery thrombosis

manifestations may be seen within any organ system. Thrombotic episodes associated with aPL may occur in vascular beds that are infrequently affected in other prothrombotic states. Some years ago, by reviewing the case histories of 50 pediatric patients with aPL-positive thrombosis reported in the literature [5], the authors found that this condition was more common in females, and that the age at first symptom ranged from 8 months to 16 years. Many patients had secondary APS associated with systemic autoimmune disease, particularly SLE, but some patients had primary APS. The clinical features, however, seemed to be the same in primary and secondary APS. Although most of the reported patients had involvement of the venous circulation, arterial thrombosis seemed relatively more common in younger children. A few patients had a family history of aPL-positive clinical events. The thrombotic manifestations reported in pediatric patients with APS are presented in Table 1.

Venous thrombosis

As in adults with APS, the deep and superficial veins of the lower limbs are the most frequently reported sites of venous thrombosis in children (Fig. 1). Some of these patients may develop pulmonary embolism. Thromboembolic pulmonary hypertension, caused by either recurrent pulmonary emboli or in situ thrombosis, is exceedingly rare in the pediatric population. Other reported sites of venous thrombosis in pediatric patients include the renal, mesenteric, hepatic, and retinal veins, as well as the superior and inferior vena cava (Fig. 2).

Arterial thrombosis

Cerebral arteries are the most frequent site of arterial thrombosis in children, with most patients presenting with stroke or transient ischemic attacks, as discussed later. Other arterial sites of thrombosis include the retinal, coronary, hepatic, mesenteric, and peripheral arteries.

Nervous system manifestations

Stroke and transient ischemic attacks are the most frequent neurologic complications of APS. Strokes occur more often in the region supplied by the middle cerebral artery (Fig. 3). Cerebral infarction may be silent, however, and when multiple events occur, patients may develop seizures or dementia secondary to widespread cerebral damage. Notably, a high prevalence of aPL has been reported in children with idiopathic cerebral ischemia, suggesting that these antibodies may play a major pathogenetic role in children who lack the other prothrombotic factors [19]. Thrombosis of the cerebral sinus has been observed in

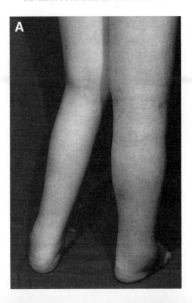

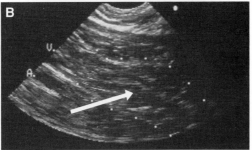

Fig. 1. Right limb deep vein thrombosis in a 16-year-old boy with systemic JIA who had circulating aPL and was exposed to another thrombophilic factor (a prolonged plaster immobilization for a tibial fracture. (*A*) Diffuse edema of the right limb. (*B*) Doppler ultrasonography showing complete occlusion of a popliteal vein by a thrombus (*arrow*).

both primary and SLE-associated APS [20]. Ocular ischemic events, including anterior ischemic optic neuropathy, central retinal artery occlusion, amaurosis fugax, and occlusion of retinal veins, and sensorineural hearing loss, often presenting as sudden deafness, have been described in patients with APS. Several other neurologic abnormalities have been linked to aPL but are not clearly related to thrombosis. They include chorea, transverse myelopathy, Guillain-Barré syndrome, psychosis, and migraine headaches. It has been suggested that these complications may result from direct interaction between aPL and the nervous tissue, or from immune complex deposition in cerebral or spinal cord vessels. Seizures have also been reported in association with aPL, but cerebral infarction should be excluded as a cause.

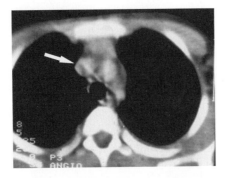

Fig. 2. Chest CT scan showing superior vena cava thrombosis (*arrow*) in a 13-year-old boy with primary APS.

Cardiac valve abnormalities

Cardiac valve abnormalities resembling Libman-Sacks endocarditis can be observed by Doppler echocardiography in a number of adults with APS. Valvular thickening has been reported most commonly, but valvular vegetations, regurgitation, and stenosis may occur. Although any of the four heart valves may be affected, the mitral valve is most frequently involved, followed by the aortic valve; tricuspid and pulmonary valve involvement is uncommon. Valvular abnormalities in APS are different from hose seen in rheumatic heart disease: valvular thickening is diffuse in the former condition, whereas in rheumatic carditis it is more localized, is detected at leaflet tips, and is often accompanied by thickening, fusion, and calcification of the chordae tendinae. The frequency of this complication in pediatric APS is unknown.

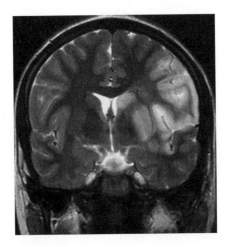

Fig. 3. Brain MRI revealing a stroke in the territory of the middle cerebral artery in a 12-year-old girl with SLE and antiphospholipid syndrome.

Skin manifestations

Several cutaneous manifestations have been associated with APS, including leg ulcers, livedo reticularis, cutaneous necrosis, gangrene of the digits or extremities, thrombophlebitis, necrotizing purpura, and nailfold infarcts. Leg ulcers, which occur more often in the pretibial area and ankle, can be multiple and focal, are painful and sharply marginated, have a necrotic center or base, and leave a white atrophic scar on healing. Livedo reticularis is the most frequently reported skin manifestation of APS. Although its pathogenesis is unknown, it results from the stagnation of blood in dilated superficial capillaries and venules and primarily affects the skin of the tights, shins, and forearms. The clinical triad of livedo reticularis, cerebrovascular disease, and hypertension (Sneddon's syndrome), which is frequently accompanied by the detection of aPL, is exceedingly rare in children.

Thrombocytopenia and hemolytic anemia

A decrease in platelet count, usually in the range of 100 to 150×10^9/L is observed in about one third of patients with APS. Thrombocytopenia is rarely severe enough to cause hemorrhage (ie, $< 50 \times 10^9$/l), however. The pathogenesis of thrombocytopenia in APS is unclear. Proposed mechanisms include binding of aPL to platelet membrane phospholipids, β2-GPI/phospholipid complexes, or coexisting antibodies to platelet membrane glycoprotein. About 10% to 20% of patients with APS have a positive Coombs' test, but hemolytic anemia is relatively uncommon. The association of hemolytic anemia and thrombocytopenia (Evans' syndrome) has been reported occasionally in patients with APS. Differentiation of primary APS from classic idiopathic thrombocytopenic purpura is important to indicate closer follow-up for future manifestations related to the aPL or for progression to frank SLE (as discussed later).

Catastrophic antiphospholipid syndrome

In most patients with APS, thrombotic events develop singly, and recurrence usually occurs months or years after the initial episode. Occasionally, however, aPL-positive patients may present with an acute and devastating syndrome characterized by multiple and simultaneous vascular occlusions throughout the body. This syndrome is termed "catastrophic APS" and is defined as clinical involvement of at least three different organ systems over a period of days or weeks with histopathologic evidence of multiple occlusions of large and small vessels [21]. Thrombosis of large vessels is less common in patients with this syndrome, who tend to develop an acute microangiopathy affecting small vessels of multiple organs. The kidney is the organ most commonly affected, followed by the lung, the central nervous system, the heart, and the skin. Disseminated intravascular coagulation is observed in approximately 25% of cases. Patients may present with a medical collapse with severe thrombocytopenia, adult respiratory distress syndrome, and multiorgan failure, often accompanied by severe hypertension. The mortality rate is 50%, and death is usually caused by multiorgan failure. Precipitating factors of catastrophic APS include infections, surgical procedures, neoplasms, lupus flares, withdrawal of warfarin therapy, and the use of oral contraceptives [22]. Catastrophic APS, which has been occasionally reported in children [23,24], should be distinguished from severe lupus vasculitis, sepsis, thrombotic thrombocytopenic purpura, macrophage activation syndrome [25], and disseminated intravascular coagulation.

Differential diagnosis

Thrombosis in children can be caused by many other conditions (Box 2).

Few clinical clues differentiate APS from other types of thrombophilia. A careful history, physical examination, and appropriate laboratory studies are, therefore, essential to make the proper diagnosis. Leukopenia, thrombocytopenia, livedo reticularis, arthralgia or a rheumatic illness, or a family history of rheumatic illness (particularly SLE) increases the likelihood that APS is the cause of the newly diagnosed thrombosis. In some patients with APS, however, the sole abnormality may be the existence of aPL. Because a normal aPTT does not exclude the presence of LA, a patient presenting with a first thrombotic event should be screened for aCL and with other assays that are sensitive to LA.

Box 2. Disease states beside APS that should be considered in children and adolescents with unexplained venous or arterial thrombosis

Factor V Leiden (activated protein C resistance)
Protein C deficiency
Protein S deficiency
Antithrombin III deficiency
Homocysteinemia
Nephrotic syndrome
Estrogen-containing oral contraceptives
Myeloproliferative disorders
Behçet's syndrome
Systemic vasculitis
Heparin-induced thrombosis

Acquired coagulation factor inhibitors and antiphospholipid antibodies

The acquired hypoprothombinemia–lupus anticoagulant syndrome

Although the presence of LA confers an increased risk for thrombosis, this antibody has been occasionally associated with a bleeding tendency. This condition, which has been termed "acquired hypoprothombinemia–LA syndrome" and is usually preceded by a viral infection, is characterized by serious bleeding, profound decrease of prothrombin level, and presence of circulating high-affinity antibodies that bind prothrombin without neutralizing its coagulant activity; hypoprothombinemia probably results from the rapid clearance of prothrombin antigen-antibody complexes [26–28]. Prompt recognition of this syndrome is critical because corticosteroid therapy is effective.

The varicella-autoantibody syndrome

Another condition in which aPL are associated with the presence of acquired coagulation factor inhibitors is a syndrome occasionally observed in children with acute varicella zoster virus infection [29]. It is characterized by purpura fulminans, thromboembolism, or disseminated intravascular coagulation secondary to an acquired, transient, isolated deficiency of protein S caused by the presence of circulating autoantibodies to the same protein. These antibodies have no direct inhibitory effect on the activity of protein S; the decrease of protein S antigen levels presumably results from rapid clearance of circulating immune complexes. In most children with this complication, the presence of LA and, less commonly, aCL has been identified, although the specificity of these aPL has not been demonstrated. Recently, significantly increased prevalence of LA and transiently reduced plasma level of free protein S have been demonstrated in children with varicella in the absence of thrombotic complications, suggesting that this common infectious disease is characterized by a marked hyper-coagulability state [30].

Neonatal antiphospholipid syndrome

It is well known that the presence of aPL during pregnancy is accompanied by a high incidence of obstetric and fetal complications, including first-trimester miscarriage, second-trimester pregnancy loss, preeclampsia, intrauterine growth retardation, and prematurity. Careful obstetric monitoring of pregnant women with circulating aPL and appropriate treatment can improve pregnancy outcome considerably, although fetal complications such as intrauterine growth retardation and prematurity may occur despite treatment.

Evidence exists that in pregnant women with APS, aCL can cross the placenta and can be detected in cord blood [31]. Follow-up of infants born to mothers with APS has shown that aCL levels are detectable in newborns' sera and decrease progressively, disappearing within 6 months. However, neonatal thrombosis related to the transplacental transfer of aPL seems to be very uncommon. In general, vascular thrombosis in neonates is rare and, with the exception of spontaneous renal venous thrombosis, is usually associated with indwelling catheters. Several studies of the outcome of infants born to mother with APS have revealed that, except for prematurity and its complications, these neonates did not develop occlusive events (reviewed in [31]). This finding is surprising because it is known that the thrombotic risk is much greater in the first month of life than at any other age in childhood. Furthermore, thrombotic occlusions have been detected in experimental mouse models of aPL-induced fetal loss. Premature infants are also known to have diminished antithrombin III levels, which may further increase the risk of thrombotic events. It has been hypothesized that the unexpected low frequency of thrombosis in infants born to mother with APS may result from the different capacity of the aPL IgG subclasses to cross the placenta (ie, to the low placental transfer of the more pathogenic IgG2); alternatively, the intact neonatal vessel wall may not favor thrombus formation [31].

A few instances of thrombosis in infants born to aPL-positive mothers have been reported, however. In some cases aPL were not detected or looked for in the neonate, whereas in others the presence of aPL both in the mother and the baby has been documented (reviewed in [5] and [31]). These reports suggest that aPL acquired transplacentally may promote the development of neonatal thrombosis; however, these antibodies may simply constitute a second hit, leading to thrombosis in a neonate who is exposed to another thrombophilic factor, such as an indwelling catheter. In addition, these antibodies may explain the pathogenesis of renal venous thrombosis, which is a poorly understood disease, often with antenatal onset. Given the rarity of neonatal thrombosis, multicenter studies are needed to establish the true pathogenetic effect of transplacentally acquired aPL.

On clinical grounds, although the precise risk of thrombosis in infants born to mother with APS is unknown (and probably very low), it is advisable to monitor these infants closely for any possible aPL-related clinical manifestations, at least until transplacentally acquired aPL become undetectable [32]. Furthermore, the clinical evaluation of all neonates with vascular thrombosis should include testing for aPL, irrespective of the presence of other risk factors or a positive family history of thrombosis or autoimmune disease.

The clinical significance of antiphospholipid antibodies in juvenile systemic lupus erythematosus

The reported prevalence of aCL and LA in juvenile SLE ranges from 19% to 87% and from 10% to 62%, respectively (reviewed in [33–43]) (Table 2). This wide variability may reflect either the different sensitivities and specificities of the assays used for the detection of aPL or a diversity in the clinical features of the patient populations. It may also depend, at least in part, on differences in the disease activity, because some investigators have observed a relationship between

Table 2
Prevalence of aPL and frequency of thrombotic events in juvenile SLE

Authors (year)	No. of patients	aCL (%)	LA (%)	aβ2-GPI (%)	Thrombosis (%)
Shergy et al (1988) [33]	32	50	ND	ND	0
Montes de Oca et al (1991) [34]	120	ND	19	ND	9
Molta et al (1993) [35]	37	19	11	ND	8
Ravelli et al (1994) [36]	30	87	20	ND	3
Gattorno et al (1995) [37]	19	79	42	ND	16
Seaman et al (1995) [38]	29	66	62	ND	24
Berube et al (1998) [39]	59	19	24	ND	17
Gedalia et al (1998) [40]	36	37	ND	ND	8
von Scheven et al (2002) [41]	57	53	23	48	5
Campos et al (2003) [42]	57	70	29	ND	9
Levy et al (2003) [43]	149	39	16	ND	9

Abbreviations: aCL, anticardiolipin antibodies; aβ2-GPI, anti-β2-glycoprotein I antibodies; LA, lupus anticoagulant; ND, not determined.

the presence and titer of these antibodies and selected indicators of lupus activity: the lowest prevalence was observed in a cohort of samples obtained during periods of clinical remission. In some series, high levels of aCL have been associated with the occurrence of neuropsychiatric manifestations, but this association was not found in other series. The observed frequency of vascular thrombosis in juvenile SLE ranges from 0 to 24% (Table 2). As reported in adults, LA seems to be correlated more strictly with thrombotic events than aCL [43,44]. In the only study that investigated aβ2-GPI in juvenile SLE, a prevalence of 48% was found [41]. These antibodies were not seen as frequently as aCL or LA and, with the exception of stroke, demonstrated weaker correlation with APS features than other aPL assays.

Recently, the presence of aPL in lupus patients has been associated with the development of ischemic microangiopathic nephropathy [45]. Clinically, this condition is manifested by hypertension (often malignant), proteinuria, and renal failure. Histopathologic study of kidney biopsy samples shows vaso-occlusive lesions of intrarenal vessels associated with acute thrombosis and intra-arteriolar lesions as well as with zones of cortical ischemic atrophy. Awareness of aPL-related nephropathy is important because its treatment may require anticoagulation instead of immunosuppressive medications. Because lupus nephritis and aPL-associated ischemic nephropathy cannot be distinguished clinically, renal biopsy is essential.

Antiphospholipid antibodies in other systemic disorders

The presence of aCL in juvenile idiopathic arthritis (JIA) has been investigated in several cross-sectional studies, which found a prevalence ranging from 7% to 53% (reviewed in [5] and [31]). Most studies identified no association between the presence of aCL and disease activity, and no clinical manifestation of APS was observed. Only two reports exist on the development of aPL-associated thrombosis in JIA patients [46,47]; one of these patients, however, was exposed to another thrombophilic factor (a prolonged plaster immobilization for a tibial fracture) (Fig. 1) [46]. It seems, therefore, that despite an apparently significant prevalence of aCL, thrombotic complications are rare in JIA, suggesting that these antibodies may have different pathogenetic potential and, possibly, antigen specificity as compared with SLE. On the other hand, the frequency of LA and aβ2-GPI in JIA is much lower than that of aCL [31]. Notably, aPL have been preferentially found in serum of children with JIA who were previously infected with parvovirus B19 and had established, persistent infection [48].

The presence of circulating aPL has been observed in a variety of other pediatric autoimmune and nonautoimmune syndromes, including juvenile dermatomyositis, rheumatic fever, insulin-dependent diabetes mellitus, HIV infection, and atopic dermatitis. In most of these conditions, APS is uncommon, and the significance of aPL deserves further confirmation.

Outcome of primary antiphospholipid syndrome

The relationship between primary APS and SLE is unclear. Although most authors agree that the primary syndrome is a distinct clinical entity with its own genetic, immunologic, clinical, and serologic characteristics, other investigators believe that primary APS, lupuslike disease, and SLE may represent three different facets of a unique clinical spectrum of disease [49]. In recent years, some cases of primary APS that evolved into SLE have been reported, and a survey of 90 adult patients with primary APS showed that 12 of them (13.3%) developed SLE or lupuslike disease during a median follow-up of 8.3 years [50]. The authors investigated the long-term outcome of 14 pediatric patients with primary APS who were followed for a median of 9 years in three Italian pediatric rheumatology centers [51]. At the time of the presenting clinical manifestation, no patient fulfilled more than one of the updated criteria for SLE [52], except for the presence of aPL and low-titer ANA. During follow-up, two patients developed 4 or more of the 11 1982 revised criteria for SLE [53] and were thus diagnosed as having a frank SLE, and one patient displayed the features of a lupuslike syndrome. The percentage of progression to SLE or lupuslike syndrome observed in the authors' pediatric cohort of primary APS (21.4%) was almost double than that found by Gomez et al [50] in the previously mentioned study on adult patients with primary APS. Of note, in the authors' two patients who developed SLE, the features of this disease occurred soon after the presentation of APS (after 9 and 14 months, respectively), and in the patient with lupuslike syndrome the more widespread clinical manifestations developed as early as 6 months after APS onset. These findings suggest that a significant proportion of children who present with the features of primary APS may progress in a relatively short time to SLE or to a lupuslike syndrome.

Management

Asymptomatic antiphospholipid antibody–positive individuals

Both aCL and LA can be found in children without any underlying disease. Such naturally occurring aPL are usually present in low titer and may result from previous infections or vaccinations. A wide range of frequency of aCL, from 2% to 82%, has been reported in healthy children [31]. This variability mainly results from methodological problems, including choice of inappropriate study groups, differently defined cut-off values, and lack of uniformity of the assays employed. Because aPL have been observed in association with various infections, and because postinfectious aPL tend to be transient, aPL positivity should always be verified with a further determination after the infection has cleared. The incidental discovery of LA usually is reported in children who undergo preoperative evaluations for tonsillectomy who are found to have prolonged aPTT. In most cases, no definite disease is found, and the aPTT corrects spontaneously within a few months.

Despite the established association between aPL and thrombosis, most asymptomatic persons who are found incidentally to have positive aPL tests do not develop thrombosis. The aCL test has been found to be positive in low titers in about 2% of a healthy obstetric population, but this finding does not seem to be associated with an adverse outcome [54]. A recent study has shown that no patient with asymptomatic aPL (that is, an aPL detected as a result of investigations for an unexpected prolongation of the aPTT) experienced thrombosis or pregnancy morbidity [17]. These findings suggest that screening-detected aPL in asymptomatic persons are of limited clinical relevance.

There is considerable controversy, however, as to whether prophylactic treatment is indicated for individuals with persistently positive aPL who have no history of thrombosis, because the thrombotic risk of these persons is unknown. At present, these patients generally receive either no treatment or prophylactic low-dose aspirin, although there is no evidence yet to support the usefulness of the latter. On the other hand, a panel of experts has recently recommended the use of low-dose aspirin for prevention of thrombosis in patients with aPL but without prior history of thrombosis [55]. Prospective studies that are under way should provide definitive, evidence-based answers. Hydroxychloroquine, which has modest anticoagulant properties and is widely used in SLE, may be useful in preventing thrombosis in asymptomatic aPL-positive patients with this disease [56].

Because children are less exposed than adults to coincident risk factors, the thrombotic risk in asymptomatic aPL-positive children is probably much lower than in adults. Nevertheless, secondary risk factors that increase the tendency to thrombosis should be pursued. For instance, prophylaxis of venous thrombosis with subcutaneous heparin should be considered to cover higher-risk situations, such as prolonged immobilization or surgery. Furthermore, particular attention should be paid to children who carry a heritable procoagulant state. Adolescents with circulating aPL must be advised to avoid other risk factors, such as smoking and use of oral contraceptives.

Another unresolved issue concerns patients with aPL who do not have recurrent thrombosis but do have livedo reticularis, thrombocytopenia, hemolytic anemia, chorea, cardiac valve vegetations, or cognitive dysfunction and, thus, do not fulfill the criteria for APS. It is unknown whether anticoagulation treatment is indicated in these patients.

Antiphospholipid antibody–positive patients with thrombosis

The management of acute thrombosis in patients with APS is no different from that of thrombosis arising from other causes.

Treatment with high-dose corticosteroids, cyclophosphamide, and plasmaphe-resis to reduce transiently the levels of circulating aPL, together with adequate anticoagulation, is indicated only in life-threatening situations such as the cata-strophic antiphospholipid syndrome, as discussed later. Otherwise, immuno-suppressive treatment, unless required for other accompanying features, is not advised, because aPL rapidly return to previous levels upon cessation of therapy, and these drugs do not prevent further thrombotic events.

Retrospective studies in adults have clearly shown that aPL-associated throm-boses tend to recur. There is, therefore, consensus about the need to treat patients who experience an aPL-related thrombosis to prevent recurrences. The duration and intensity of antithrombotic therapy are not yet clearly established, however. Some authors suggest that it should be continued until aPL are present, whereas others believe that life-long prophylaxis is needed. A 1995 report of a retro-spective study concluded that anticoagulant therapy producing an INR of 3.0 or higher affords better protection against recurrence than does less intense anti-coagulant therapy [57]. Twenty-nine of the 81 patients with INR of 3 or higher had a significant hemorrhagic complication, however, and the complication was severe in 7 of them. A high rate of recurrent thrombosis (1.30 per patient/year), greater than that of untreated patients, was observed within 6 months after cessation of warfarin treatment, suggesting that, once established, warfarin therapy should be long-term. The results of this study led to the recommendation of using high-intensity warfarin prophylaxis (target INR ≥ 3.0) to prevent thrombotic recurrence in patients with APS.

These recommendations were recently challenged by two prospective, ran-domized, controlled trials in patients with APS who were assigned to moderate (target INR, 2.0–3.0) or high-intensity (target INR, 3.0–4.0) warfarin therapy [58,59]. Both studies found that the overall risk of recurrent thrombosis was very low and was unexpectedly lower in patients who received moderate-intensity warfarin than in those who were given high-intensity warfarin. Based on these results, it was suggested that warfarin administered with a target INR of 2.0 to 3.0 should be considered standard therapy in all patients with APS who have not had recurrent thrombosis while receiving warfarin prophylaxis [60]. Another recent large, randomized trial showed that the presence of aPL (either LA or aCL) among patients with ischemic stroke does not predict increased risk for subsequent thrombotic events, and that warfarin therapy is not superior to aspirin therapy for secondary prevention of stroke in aPL-positive patients [61]. Other investigators, who expressed several concerns about the study methodology, questioned the results of this study [62–64]. These arguments demonstrate that consensus on the approach to prevent thrombosis associated with APS is far from being reached. In addition, the existing studies have failed to address several crucial questions, such as whether arterial and venous thromboses require the same intensity of anticoagulation, whether and when warfarin prophylaxis should be stopped, whether patients who develop thrombosis in the presence of other risk factors should be treated like those without any risk factor other than aPL, and how to manage patients with recurrent thrombosis despite high-intensity coagulation. Monitoring the level of anticoagulation in patients with APS is complicated by the lack of standardized reagents for the determination of the INR and the potential interference of aPL in this measurement.

Concerning APS in pediatric patients, only a few data are available on the recurrence rate of thrombosis or on the optimal anticoagulation regimen [43,51]. Thrombosis seems to be less common in juvenile than in adult-onset SLE, and the general risk of recurrence is probably lower in children than in adults. Specific problems with the use of warfarin in children are that the dose of this drug is age and weight dependent and that its administration requires close monitoring because of changing requirements. Furthermore, long-term anticoagulation at high therapeutic level may expose the younger patients to a high risk of bleeding during play and sport.

Based on these considerations, it is the authors' present policy to perform moderate-intensity anticoagulation therapy (target INR, 2.0–3.0) in children who had an aPL-related thrombotic event. A similar therapeutic approach has been proposed by other investigators [65]. In the authors' experience, this protocol has not been associated with recurrence of thrombosis or with bleeding.

Given the rarity of aPL-related thrombosis in childhood, the optimal therapeutic approach can be defined only through a large, controlled, prospective multicenter trial.

Catastrophic antiphospholipid syndrome

Recommendations for treatment of catastrophic APS are based entirely on case reports or on expert consensus [66]. Because thromboses tend to be self-perpetuating, an aggressive therapeutic approach, including prompt treatment of any precipitating factor, is warranted. The use of a combination of anticoagulants and steroids plus either plasmapheresis or intravenous immunoglobulins and, in case of lupus flare, cyclophosphamide has been suggested. The fibrinolytic agents streptokinase and urokinase also have been used with varying success. Other reported management options include prostacyclin, defibrotide, danazol, cyclosporine, azathioprine, hemodialysis, and splenectomy.

Thrombocytopenia

The thrombocytopenia of APS is usually mild and does not require treatment. For severe thrombocytopenia, the usual treatment is corticosteroid therapy. Anecdotal reports have shown improvement of corticosteroid-resistant thrombocytopenia with dapsone, danazol, chloroquine, warfarin, and low-dose aspirin. Aspirin administration is, however, potentially dangerous, especially in patients with very low platelet counts. Splenectomy is not advisable because theoretically the postsplenectomy thrombocytosis may increase the thrombotic risk; moreover, in some instances splenectomy has been ineffective in increasing the platelet count [67]. Intravenous immunoglobulins may raise the platelet count temporarily and may be useful before surgery.

Summary

APS is recognized increasingly as a leading cause of vascular thrombosis in the pediatric population. With the obvious exception of pregnancy morbidity, most of the clinical features that may occur in adults with APS have been described also in children. Because the coincident prothrombotic factors that are common in adults have little or no impact in children, pediatric patients with APS constitute a suitable sample to investigate the relationship of aPL with the associated clinical manifestations, such as thrombocytopenia, hemolytic anemia, chorea, and livedo reticularis, and the specificities of aPL that are more linked to thrombosis. On the other hand, because of the high frequency of infectious processes in early life, children may have a greater prevalence of nonpathogenic and transient aPL. For these reasons, the diagnostic and therapeutic approach to APS in childhood may be different from that for adults. Because of the rarity of aPL-related thrombosis in children, the natural history and optimal management can be defined only through large, multicenter, controlled studies.

References

[1] Harris NE, Khamashta MA. Antiphospholipid syndrome. In: Hochberg MC, Silman AJ, Smolen JS, Weinblatt ME, Weisman MH, editors. Rheumatology. 3rd edition. Philadelphia: Elsevier; 2003. p. 1445–53.

[2] Levine JS, Branch DW, Rauch J. The antiphospholipid syndrome. N Engl J Med 2002; 346(10):752–63.

[3] Olive D, André E, Brocard O, Labrude P, Alexandre P. Lupus érythémateux disséminé revélé par des thrombophlébites des membres inferieurs. Arch Fr Pediatr 1979;36(9):959–60.

[4] St Clair W, Jones B, Rogers JS, Crouch M, Hrabovsky E. Deep venous thrombosis and a circulating anticoagulant in systemic lupus erythematosus. Am J Dis Child 1981;135(3):230–2.

[5] Ravelli A, Martini A. Antiphospholipid antibody syndrome in pediatric patients. Rheum Dis Clin N Am 1997;23(3):657–76.

[6] von Scheven E, Athreya BH, Rose CD, Goldsmith DP, Morton L. Clinical characteristics of antiphospholipid antibody syndrome in children. J Pediatr 1996;129(3):339–45.

[7] Wilson WA, Gharavi AE, Koike T, Lockshin MD, Branch DW, Piette J-C, et al. International consensus statement on preliminary classification criteria for definite antiphospholipid syndrome. Report of an international workshop. Arthritis Rheum 1999;42(7):1309–11.

[8] Hanly JG. Antiphospholipid syndrome: an overview. CMAJ 2003;168(13):1675–82.

[9] Harris EN, Gharavi AE, Patel S, Hughes GRV. Evaluation of the anti-cardiolipin antibody test. Report of an International Workshop held 4 April 1986. Clin Exp Immunol 1987;68:215–22.

[10] Brandt JT, Triplett DA, Alving B, Scharrer I. Criteria for the diagnosis of lupus anticoagulants: an update. On behalf of the Subcommittee on Lupus Anticoagulant/Antiphospholipid Antibody of the Scientific and Standardisation Committee of the ISTH. Thromb Haemost 1995;74(4): 1185–90.

[11] Matsuura E, Igarashi Y, Yasuda T, Triplett DA, Koike T. Anticardiolipin antibodies recognize beta 2-glycoprotein I structure altered by interacting with an oxygen modified solid phase surface. J Exp Med 1994;179(2):457–62.

[12] Cervera R, Piette JC, Font J, Khamashta MA, Shoenfeld Y, Camps MT, et al. Antiphospholipid syndrome: clinical and immunologic manifestations and patterns of disease expression in a cohort of 1,000 patients. Arthritis Rheum 2002;46(4):1019–27.

[13] Espinosa G, Cervera R, Font J, Shoenfeld Y. Antiphospholipid syndrome: pathogenic mechanisms. Autoimmun Rev 2003;2(2):86–93.

[14] Mackworth-Young CG. Antiphospholipid syndrome: multiple mechanisms. Clin Exp Immunol 2004;136(3):393–401.

[15] Arnout J. The pathogenesis of the antiphospholipid syndrome: a hypothesis based on parallelisms with heparin-induced thrombocytopenia. Thromb Haemost 1996;75(4):536–41.

[16] Gharavi AE, Wilson W, Pierangeli S. The molecular basis of antiphospholipid syndrome. Lupus 2003;12(8):579–83.

[17] Giron-Gonzalez JA, Garcia Del Rio E, Rodriguez C, Rodriguez-Martorell J, Serrano A. Antiphospholipid syndrome and asymptomatic carriers of antiphospholipid antibody: prospective analysis of 404 individuals. J Rheumatol 2004;31(8):1560–7.

[18] Hudson M, Herr A-L, Rauch J, Neville C, Chang E, Ibrahim R, et al. The presence of multiple prothrombotic risk factors is associated with a higher risk of thrombosis in individuals with anticardiolipin antibodies. J Rheumatol 2003;30(11):2385–91.

[19] Angelini L, Ravelli A, Caporali R, Rumi V, Nardocci N, Martini A. High prevalence of antiphospholipid antibodies in children with idiopathic cerebral ischemia. Pediatrics 1994; 94(4 Pt 1):500–3.

[20] Uziel Y, Laxer RM, Blaser S, Andrew M, Schneider R, Silverman ED. Cerebral vein thrombosis in childhood systemic lupus erythematosus. J Pediatr 1995;126(5 Pt 1):722–7.

[21] Asherson RA, Cervera R, Piette JC, Font J, Lie JT, Burcoglu A, et al. Catastrophic antiphospholipid syndrome. Clinical and laboratory features of 50 patients. Medicine (Baltimore) 1998;77(3):195–207.

[22] Erkan D, Cervera R, Asherson RA. Catastrophic antiphospholipid syndrome. Where do we stand? Arthritis Rheum 2003;48(12):3320–7.

[23] Falcini F, Taccetti G, Ermini M, Trapani S, Matucci Cerinic M. Catastrophic antiphospholipid antibody syndrome in pediatric systemic lupus erythematosus. J Rheumatol 1997;24(2): 389–92.

[24] Orsino A, Schneider R, DeVeber G, Grant R, Massisotte P, Canning Carcao M. Childhood acute myelomonocytic leukaemia (AML-M4) presenting as catastrophic antiphospholipid antibody syndrome. J Pediatr Hematol Oncol 2004;26(5):327–30.

[25] Ravelli A. Macrophage activation syndrome. Curr Opin Rheumatol 2002;14(5):548–52.

[26] Bernini JC, Buchanan GR, Ashcraft J. Hypoprothombinemia and severe hemorrhage associated with a lupus anticoagulant. J Pediatr 1993;123(6):937–9.

[27] Eberhard A, Sparling C, Sudbury S, Ford P, Laxer R, Silverman E. Hypoprothombinemia in childhood systemic lupus erythematosus. Semin Arthritis Rheum 1994;24(1):12–8.

[28] Hudson N, Duffy CM, Rauch J, Paquin JD, Esdaile JM. Catastrophic haemorrhage in a case of paediatric primary antiphospholipid syndrome and factor II deficiency. Lupus 1997;6(1):68–71.

[29] Josephson C, Nuss R, Jacobson L, Hacker MR, Murphy J, Weinberg A, et al. The varicella-autoantibody syndrome. Pediatr Res 2001;50(3):345–52.

[30] Kurugol Z, Vardar F, Ozkinay F, Kavakli K, Ozkinay C. Lupus anticoagulant and protein S deficiency in otherwise healthy children with acute varicella infection. Acta Paediatr 2000; 89(10):1186–9.

[31] Avcin T, Cimaz R, Meroni PL. Recent advances in antiphospholipid antibodies and antiphospholipid syndromes in pediatric populations. Lupus 2002;11(1):4–10.

[32] Motta M, Tincani A, Lojacono A, Faden D, Gorla R, Airo P, et al. Neonatal outcome in patients with rheumatic disease. Lupus 2004;13(9):718–23.

[33] Shergy WJ, Kredich DW, Pisetsky DS. The relationship of anticardiolipin antibodies to disease manifestations in pediatric systemic lupus erythematosus. J Rheumatol 1988;15(9):1389–94.

[34] Montes de Oca MA, Babron MC, Bletry O, Broyer M, Courtecuisse V, Fontaine JL, et al. Thrombosis in systemic lupus erythematosus: a French collaborative study. Arch Dis Child 1991; 66(6):713–7.

[35] Molta C, Meyer O, Dosquet C, Montes de Oca M, Babron MC, Danon F, et al. Childhood-onset systemic lupus erythematosus: antiphospholipid antibodies in 37 patients and their first-degree relatives. Pediatrics 1993;92(6):849–53.

[36] Ravelli A, Caporali R, Di Fuccia G, Zonta L, Montecucco C, Martini A. Anticardiolipin antibodies in pediatric systemic lupus erythematosus. Arch Pediatr Adolesc Med 1994;148(4): 398–402.

[37] Gattorno M, Buoncompagni A, Molinari AC, Barbano GC, Morreale G, Stalla F, et al. Antiphospholipid antibodies in paediatric systemic lupus erythematosus, juvenile chronic arthritis and overlap syndromes: SLE patients with both lupus anticoagulant and high-titre anticardiolipin antibodies are at risk for clinical manifestations related to the antiphospholipid syndrome. Br J Rheumatol 1995;34(9):873–81.

[38] Seaman DE, Londino Jr AV, Kwoh CK, Medsger Jr TA, Manzi S. Antiphospholipid antibodies in pediatric systemic lupus erythematosus. Pediatrics 1995;96(6):1040–5.

[39] Berube C, Mitchell L, Silverman E, David M, Saint Cyr C, Laxer R, et al. The relationship of antiphospholipid antibodies to thromboembolic events in pediatric patients with systemic lupus erythematosus: a cross-sectional study. Pediatr Res 1998 Sep;44(3):351–6.

[40] Gedalia A, Molina JF, Garcia CO, Doggett S, Espinoza LR, Gharavi AE. Anticardiolipin antibodies in chidlhood rheumatic disorders. Lupus 1998;7(8):551–3.

[41] von Scheven E, Glidden DV, Elder ME. Anti-beta2-glycoprotein I antibodies in pediatric systemic lupus erythematosus and antiphospholipid syndrome. Arthritis Rheum 2002;47(4): 414–20.

[42] Campos LM, Kiss MH, D'Amico EA, Silva CA. Antiphospholipid antibodies and antiphospholipid syndrome in 57 children and adolescents with systemic lupus erythematosus. Lupus 2003;12(11):820–6.

[43] Levy DM, Massicotte MP, Harvey E, Hebert D, Silverman ED. Thromboembolism in paediatric lupus patients. Lupus 2003;12(10):741–6.

[44] Schmugge M, Revel-Vilk S, Hiraki L, Rand ML, Blanchette VS, Silverman ED. Thrombocytopenia and thromboembolism in pediatric systemic lupus erythematosus. J Pediatr 2003; 143(5):666–9.

[45] Daugas E, Nochy D, Huong du LT, Duhaut P, Beaufils H, Caudwell V, et al. Antiphospholipid syndrome nephropathy in systemic lupus erythematosus. J Am Soc Nephrol 2002;13(1): 42–52.

[46] Caporali R, Ravelli A, Ramenghi B, Montecucco C, Martini A. Antiphospholipid antibody associated thrombosis in juvenile chronic arthritis. Arch Dis Child 1992;67(11):1384–5.

[47] Andrews A, Hickling P. Thrombosis associated with antiphospholipid antibody in juvenile chronic arthritis. Lupus 1997;6(6):556–7.

[48] Von Landenberg P, Lehmann HW, Knoll A, Dorsch S, Modrow S. Antiphospholipid antibodies in pediatric and adult patients with rheumatic disease are associated with parvovirus B19 infection. Arthritis Rheum 2003;48(7):1939–47.

[49] Ravelli A, Martini A, Burgio GR. Antiphospholipid antibodies in paediatrics. Eur J Pediatr 1994;153(7):472–9.

[50] Gomez JA, Martin H, Amigo MC, Aguirre MA, Cuadrado MJ, Khamashta MA, et al. Long-term follow-up in 90 patients with primary antiphospholipid syndrome (PAPS). Do they develop lupus? [abstract]. Arthritis Rheum 2001;44(Suppl):S146.

[51] Gattorno M, Falcini F, Ravelli A, Zulian F, Buoncompagni A, Martini G, et al. Outcome of primary antiphospholipid syndrome in childhood. Lupus 2003;12(6):449–53.

[52] Hochberg MC. Updating the American College of Rheumatology criteria for the classification of systemic lupus erythematosus [letter]. Arthritis Rheum 1997;40(9):1725.

[53] Tan EM, Cohen AS, Fries JF, Masi AT, McShane DJ, Rothfield NF, et al. The 1982 revised criteria for the classification of systemic lupus erythematosus. Arthritis Rheum 1982;25(11): 1271–7.

[54] Harris EN, Spinnato JA. Should anticardiolipin tests be performed in otherwise healthy pregnant women? Am J Obstet Gynecol 1991;165(5 Pt 1):1272–7.

[55] Alarcon-Segovia D, Boffa MC, Branch W, Cervera R, Gharavi A, Khamashta M, et al. Prophylaxis of the antiphospholipid syndrome: a consensus report. Lupus 2003;12(7):499–503.

[56] Petri M. Hydroxychloroquine use in the Baltimore Lupus Cohort: effects on lipids, glucose and thrombosis. Lupus 1996;5(Suppl 1):S16–22.

[57] Khamashta MA, Cuadrado MJ, Mujic F, Taub NA, Hunt BJ, Hughes GR. The management of thrombosis in the antiphospholipid-antibody syndrome. N Engl J Med 1995;332(15):993–7.

[58] Crowther MA, Ginsberg JS, Julian J, Denburg J, Hirsh J, Douketis J, et al. A comparison of two intensities of warfarin for the prevention of recurrent thrombosis in patients with the antiphospholipid antibody syndrome. N Engl J Med 2003;349(12):1133–8.

[59] Finazzi G, Marchioli R, Barbui T. A randomized clinical trial of oral anticoagulant therapy in patients with antiphospholipid antibody syndrome: the WAPS study [abstract]. J Thromb Haemost 2003;1(Suppl 1):OC365.

[60] Crowther MA. Antiphospholipid antibody syndrome: further evidence to guide clinical practice? J Rheumatol 2004;31(8):1474–5.

[61] Levine SR, Brey RL, Tilley BC, Thompson JL, Sacco RL, Sciacca RR, et al. APASS Investigators. Antiphospholipid antibodies and subsequent thrombo-occlusive events in patients with ischemic stroke. JAMA 2004;291(5):576–84.

[62] Wahl D, Regnault V, de Moerloose P, Lecompte T. Antiphospholipid antibodies and risk for recurrent vascular events [letter]. JAMA 2004;291(22):2701–2.

[63] Cabral AR. Antiphospholipid antibodies and risk for recurrent vascular events [letter]. JAMA 2004;291(22):2701.

[64] Ruiz-Irastorza G, Khamashta MA, Hughes GR. Antiphospholipid antibodies and risk for recurrent vascular events [letter]. JAMA 2004;291(22):2701.

[65] Silverman E. What's new in the treatment of pediatric SLE? J Rheumatol 1996;23(9):1657–60.

[66] Asherson RA, Cervera R, de Groot PG, Erkan D, Boffa MC, Piette JC, et al. Catastrophic antiphospholipid syndrome: international consensus statement on classification criteria and treatment guidelines. Lupus 2003;12(7):530–4.

[67] Hunt BJ, Khamashta MA. Management of the Hughes syndrome. Clin Exp Rheumatol 1996; 14(2):115–7.

ELSEVIER
SAUNDERS

PEDIATRIC CLINICS
OF NORTH AMERICA

Pediatr Clin N Am 52 (2005) 493–520

Inflammatory Myopathies in Children

Sandrine Compeyrot-Lacassagne, MD[a],
Brian M. Feldman, MD, MSc, FRCPC[a,b],*

[a]Division of Rheumatology, The Hospital for Sick Children, 555 University Avenue,
Toronto, ON, M5G 1X8 Canada
[b]University of Toronto, 555 University Avenue, Toronto, ON, M5G 1X8 Canada

Juvenile idiopathic inflammatory myopathies (JIIM) are rare conditions that
are probably autoimmune in nature. Childhood myositis is relatively more
homogeneous than adult myositis; juvenile dermatomyositis (JDM) is by far
the most common inflammatory myopathy, followed by far fewer cases of juvenile polymyositis, amyopathic dermatomyositis, overlap myositis, and inclusion
body myositis. Childhood myositis differs also in the higher incidence of vasculopathy, often with intimal proliferation of small blood vessels, thrombosis, and
sometimes infarction [1,2]. Although JDM is the most common presentation
(with primarily skin and muscle manifestations), the underlying systemic
vasculopathy can involve many systems. Treatment is directed toward reducing
inflammation through immunosuppression. The disorders have a good outcome
with favorable prospects for normal school and work performance, but many
of the affected children will have a chronic disease and will require long-
term therapy.

This article describes a recent patient who presented with typical JDM
and uses her case to discuss aspects of the childhood inflammatory myopathies.

The case

Kathryn is a 13-year-old white girl (Fig. 1) who met the diagnostic criteria
of Bohan and Peter [1] at presentation. She initially was referred to the authors'

* Corresponding author. 555 University Avenue, Toronto, ON, M5G 1X8, Canada.
E-mail address: Brian.Feldman@sickkids.ca (B.M. Feldman).

0031-3955/05/$ – see front matter © 2005 Elsevier Inc. All rights reserved.
doi:10.1016/j.pcl.2005.01.004
pediatric.theclinics.com

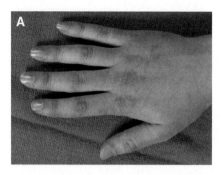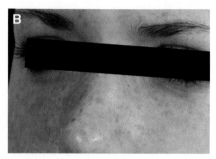

Fig. 1. (*A*) Patient's hand at the time of diagnosis showing a papulosquamous eruption on the extensor surface of the metacarpophalangeal and proximal interphalangeal joints (Gottron's papules). (*B*). Patient at diagnosis showing a malar (crossing the nasal bridge) and forehead rash as well as a heliotrope discoloration of the upper eyelids with mild edema.

by a dermatologist for typical Gottron's papules on her knuckles that developed within the 2 months before presentation. During 1 month she had developed progressive proximal muscle weakness associated with intermittent knee pain. On initial assessment, she had low-grade fever with malar rash and a heliotrope rash over the upper eyelids. She had evidence of Gottron's papules over her knuckles and elbows. Capillaroscopy (microscopic examination) of the nail beds showed capillary changes with decreased capillary density, dilatation, tortuosity, and dropout. She had symmetrical proximal muscle weakness, stress pain in the right knee, and an effusion in the left knee associated with pain and limited range of motion. Her laboratory results were in keeping with JDM. She had a significant increase of all the muscle enzymes and high-titer anti-nuclear antibodies (1/1280) with a speckled pattern; other measured autoantibodies were all negative. An MRI of the proximal muscles (upper and lower limb girdles) confirmed diffuse acute myositis with some atrophy of the paraspinal and gluteal muscles (Fig. 2). An electromyogram (EMG) was consistent with a myopathic

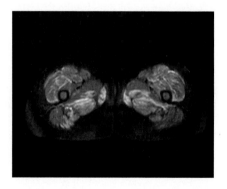

Fig. 2. Fat-suppressed T2 MRI of patient at diagnosis. The bright areas reflect edema and inflammation in the quadriceps and hamstring muscles bilaterally.

process. Because her presentation and laboratory findings were typical, she did not undergo muscle biopsy. The rest of the clinical and laboratory examination was normal, ruling out any other organ involvement. She initially was treated with high-dose oral corticosteroids (approximately 2 mg/kg divided into three doses) and experienced some improvement, but significant proximal muscle weakness persisted. Because of her incomplete response, she received three pulses of high-dose intravenous methylprednisolone (30 mg/kg/dose) 6 weeks after presentation with an excellent clinical response. She had also started treatment with methotrexate (MTX) at presentation. Now, a few months later, her corticosteroids are being tapered; she will probably discontinue prednisone at about 10 months after presentation but will continue taking MTX. She is doing well clinically. Her strength is normal, the rash has cleared, and her muscle enzyme tests are all normal, but she continues to have a mildly elevated erythrocyte sedimentation rate.

Epidemiology

Kathryn's presentation suggests several questions of an epidemiologic nature. How common is a case like this? Does ethnicity play a role in the frequency of JIIM? Is 13 years a typical age of presentation? Is it unusual to see JDM presenting in a girl?

It would seem from the literature that JIIM are quite rare. Several recent studies have demonstrated an incidence of about two to three cases per million children per year. For example, a survey study in Great Britain suggested that the incidence of JDM is about 1.9 per million children below 16 years of age [3]. More recently, data from a National Institutes of Health–sponsored registry have suggested that the incidence rate of JDM in the United States, between 1995 and 1998, ranged in different states from 2.5 to 4.1 per million children, with an average annual incidence rate of 3.2 per million children below the age of 17 years [4]. Childhood myositis is much more rare than the inflammatory myopathies in adults; in one series of 124 patients with myositis, only 21% of the patients were under 15 years of age at diagnosis [5]. At the Hospital for Sick Children Myositis Clinic in Toronto, a city with a population in the metropolitan area of about 4.5 million persons, the authors have followed 137 children with JIIM (121 with JDM, 5 with amyopathic JDM, 5 with juvenile polymyositis, and 6 with overlap connective tissue diseases) in the last 14 years. Worldwide, it seems that JIIM are quite rare.

Unlike some other autoimmune diseases, (eg, systemic lupus erythematosus) there does not seem to be an over-representation of black or Asian patients. In the American registry study, there was a predominance of white non-Hispanic children (65.1%), followed by Hispanic (14.2%) and African-American non-Hispanic (11.4%) children [4]. At the Hospital for Sick Children, about 81% of the patients are white, 6% are East Indian, 6% are Asian, 5% are African-

Canadian, and 2% are Native Canadian. Given the small numbers of patients, these figures probably reflect the ethnic distribution of the population served.

JIIM often develops during the school-age years. For example, in the British nation-wide study, the median age at onset was 6.8 years [3]. Likewise, at the Hospital for Sick Children, the median age at diagnosis is 7 years. The youngest patient was 1.2 years of age at diagnosis (patients younger than this would probably be given the diagnosis of infantile myositis, which is not included in the authors' series). Two thirds of the authors' patients were diagnosed between the ages of 4 and 11.5 years.

Girls are usually affected more often than boys. The sex ratio has varied greatly in the reported studies, however, ranging from 1:1 in Singapore for children under the age of 5 years [6] to 5:1 (girls:boys) in the British series [3]. At the Hospital for Sick Children, the sex ratio has consistently been about 2:1 (girls:boys) over the years.

This patient, then, although a bit older than most newly diagnosed children, is not otherwise unusual, considering the rarity of the disorder overall.

Etiology and pathogenesis

Why did Kathryn develop JDM? She did not have a family history, nor did she have a personal history of a clear exposure to an infectious or environmental agent.

The etiology and pathogenesis of JIIM are unknown. Many potential pathogenic mechanisms have been suggested, including a genetic predisposition, the role of triggering factors such as infectious agents, and the role of complement and soluble adhesion molecules [7,8]. Like other presumably autoimmune diseases, the JIIM probably result from interactions with environmental agents in a genetically predisposed host.

Genetic predisposition

Three lines of evidence suggest that children who develop JIIM have a genetic predisposition. First, there is a relatively strong association with certain major histocompatibility complex (MHC) alleles and the development of myositis. Second, maternal microchimerism has been discovered at a higher frequency in children with myositis. Third, children who inherit high-producing tumor necrosis factor (TNF) genes have a more severe and longer-lasting form of juvenile myositis than those who do not have these genes.

The MHC antigens determine, among other things, the antigens to which an individual's immune system can react. It is possible that only certain people inherit MHC molecules that can present the autoantigens important in the development of JIIM. For example, the MHC antigen HLA-DQA1*0501 has been proved to be important in JIIM susceptibility in several ethnic groups. Reed and Stirling [9] studied 70 patients with JDM and found that 87% of African-American patients, 92% of Hispanic patients, and 86% of white patients had this allele (versus 33%, 28%, and 46% of controls, respectively). Other MHC class I and II alleles have been shown to be involved in disease susceptibility [10]. The HLA-DMA*0103 and HLA-DMB*0102 alleles are significantly more frequent in patients with JDM [11].

Maternal microchimerism (ie, the persistence of maternal blood cells transferred by the placenta during fetal development) has been identified in CD4 or CD8 peripheral blood cells and in the inflammatory lesions of the skin and the muscle of children with JIIM. Microchimerism, which seems to be involved in the pathogenesis of systemic sclerosis, might be responsible for inducing a graft-versus-host response manifesting as autoimmune disease [12–15]. Mothers' HLA genotypes may facilitate the transfer and the persistence of chimeric cells in the circulation of their children with JDM [15]. Contradictory data have been reported about the association of HLA-DQA1*0501 and microchimerism, however [14–16]. Artlett et al [16] did not find any association between the DQA1*0501 allele (in the donor or in the recipient) and the existence of microchimerism in children with JIIM, whereas Reed et al [15] recently demonstrated that the presence of microchimerism in the JDM patients is associated with the DQA1*0501 allele in the mother. Either way, chimeric cells may play an important role in JIIM pathogenesis. For example, maternal-derived chimeric T cells have been shown to develop a memory response to the children's lymphocytes.

TNF-α is an immunomodulator and proinflammatory cytokine that has been implicated in the pathogenesis of autoimmune diseases. TNF-α gene polymorphisms have been reported to be associated with several rheumatic diseases [17]. The first polymorphism described raised the hypothesis that this polymorphism may contribute to autoimmunity [18]. It has been shown more recently that this polymorphism, identified by a G-to-A substitution at the NCOI restriction site, is a strong transcriptional activator that has direct effects on TNF-α gene regulation and is associated with a high-producing TNF-α phenotype [19]. The association between increased production of TNF-α, long disease duration, and pathologic calcification has been investigated in JIIM. A long disease course (> 36 months) and the development of calcification were found to be associated with the TNF-α allele substitution (along with an increased TNF-α production, which may lead to the perpetuation of the inflammatory response) [20]. TNF-α expression in the muscle fibers of affected patients has been recently investigated. An untreated JDM patient who had the TNF-α-308A allele had an increased number of TNF-α stained muscle fibers. It has been suggested that increased local TNF-α production may prolong muscle fiber damage [21]. It has also been demonstrated that the TNF-α-308A allele is associated with increased circulating concentrations of thrombospondin-1, an anti-angiogenic factor that may play a role in the increased vascular occlusion seen in children with JDM who have the TNF-α-308A allele [22].

Taken together, these findings suggest that some children inherit a number of genes that, perhaps in combination, predispose them to the development of JIIM.

Role of infectious agents and environmental factors

A number of infectious agents and other environmental triggers have been suspected in the pathogenesis of JIIM. Rider et al [23] have summarized some of these agents (Table 1). At present, there is not strong epidemiologic or clinical evidence to support any environmental agent in the pathogenesis of JIIM.

Massa et al [24] have suggested a mechanism of molecular mimicry that might act as a trigger of an abnormal immune response leading to JDM: an abnormal response to a microbial antigen that is homologous to a self-antigen may induce the disease. It has been shown that self-epitopes in the human skeletal myosin heavy chain are homologous to specific amino acid sequences in the M5 protein of *Streptococcus pyogenes*. Recognition of these self-epitopes in skeletal muscle triggers activation of disease-specific cytotoxic T cells; these cells are responsible for a cytotoxic response to the M5–Myo peptide pair and may be associated with active disease. Other common pathogens, such as *Borrelia Burgdorferi*, *Mycoplasma hominis*, *Haemophilus influenzae*, *Helicobacter pylori*, *Escherichia coli*, and *Bacillus subtilis*, share sequence homologies with the Myo peptide of human skeletal myosin [24].

Finally, gene-expression profiles have been studied in patients with untreated JDM who were positive for the DQA1*0501 allele. Interferon-inducible genes were dysregulated in the muscle biopsies of these patients compared with controls. This pattern of gene expression is consistent with an interferon (IFN)-$\alpha\beta$ transcription cascade supporting the hypothesis of a host defense mechanism against infection. Both IFN-$\alpha\beta$ and IFN-γ cascades may lead to muscle ischemia and increased production of TNFα and nitric oxide and may potentially inhibit regeneration of necrotic muscle fibers [25].

Table 1
Triggering factors associated with juvenile idiopathic inflammatory myopathies

Bacteria	A hemolytic streptococcus, *Borellia* spp
Virus	Hepatitis B, RNA picornaviruses, Coxsackie virus B, Echovirus, Influenza, Parainfluenza, Parvovirus B19, HTLV-1
Parasites	*Toxoplasma gondii*, trichinosis, filiarisis
Vaccines	Hepatitis B, MMR, typhoid, cholera
Medications	D-penicillamine, carnitine, GH
Bone marrow transplantation	Graft-versus-host myositis
Ultraviolet light	Unusual sun exposure

Abbreviations: GH, growth hormone; HTLV-1, human t cell lymphotropic virus type 1; MMR, measles, mumps, rubella.
From Rider LG, Miller FW. Classification and treatment of the juvenile idiopathic inflammatory myopathies. Rheum Dis Clin North Am 1997;23(3):619–55; with permission.

Although unproven, it certainly seems plausible that infectious or other environmental agents can trigger JIIM. Studies suggest that if genetically susceptible patients are exposed to one or several of these agents, they may develop the disease.

Some of the immune mechanisms that seem to be responsible for the inflammatory change seen in JIIM are now known. Complement-mediated damage of vessels seems to occur uniformly in JDM patients. Adhesion molecules are overexpressed and may lead to recruitment of inflammatory cells around vessels and in muscle. MHC class I molecules are expressed early in JIIM muscle and may lead to further development of an inflammatory reaction locally.

Role of complement

Complement-induced injury seems to be a major mechanism in JDM. Activated complement, which has been shown to occur in JIIM, might induce further cytokine release and vessel injury. The activation of the complement cascade leads to cellular damage mediated by the membrane attack complex (MAC) and is probably responsible for capillary damage in JDM [26]. The factors triggering vascular damage, antibody deposition, and complement activation are not known. CD59 is present in the sarcolemma of human skeletal muscle fibers. CD59 regulates MAC by preventing its full assembly and its deposition in vessels. In JDM, the expression of CD59 is decreased in the muscle fibers and vessels, potentially leading to increased local activation, vessel damage, and muscle ischemia; deposition of MAC is increased in the vessels but not in non-necrotic muscle fibers [27].

Role of soluble adhesion molecules

Adhesion molecules such as intracellular adhesion molecule (ICAM)-1 and vascular cell adhesion molecule (VCAM-1) belong to the immunoglobulin gene superfamily. These molecules may encourage local recruitment of inflammatory cells. ICAM-1 expression on endothelial cells seems to be increased consistently in capillaries and perimysial large vessels; it is increased occasionally in the endomysial large vessels. VCAM-1 expression is increased inconsistently, mostly in the perimysial large vessels, and is usually surrounded by an inflammatory infiltrate [28]. This phenomenon might be linked to complement activation, because the binding of C5a to endothelial cells may increase the expression of adhesion molecules.

Role of major histocompatibility complex class I expression

Constitutive MHC class I expression in normal muscle is low. A recent study has shown that MHC class I heavy-chain and α2 microglobulin are both overexpressed in the muscle fibers of children with JDM. (This finding is also seen in adults with myositis.) MHC class I expression seems to be an early phenomenon, occurring in the muscle before significant inflammatory changes are seen [29]. Although the pathogenic role of MHC class I in JIIM patients is not yet clear, some believe that expression of these molecules is an important early step in the initiation of a local inflammatory response.

Classification and diagnostic criteria

When Kathryn was referred to the Hospital for Sick Children, a diagnosis had not yet been made. It is appropriate to discuss how best to make a diagnosis of the JIIM and how best to classify these disorders.

Most centers still use the diagnostic criteria and classification system proposed in 1975 [1,30]. There have been and continue to be attempts to update these criteria to take into account a broader understanding of the clinical and immunologic heterogeneity of the JIIMs and to incorporate newer diagnostic technologies.

Bohan and Peter [1,30] proposed five major diagnostic criteria for polymyositis and dermatomyositis in 1975. These five criteria, summarized in Table 2, are still widely used as standard criteria.

Table 2
Diagnostic criteria for the inflammatory myopathies in adults and children

Criteria	Description
Muscle involvement	Symmetrical and progressive proximal muscle weakness ($\pm$ dysphagia and respiratory involvement)
Muscle biopsy	Necrosis of type I and II fibers
	Phagocytosis
	Regeneration with basophilia
	Large vesicular sarcolemmal nuclei
	Prominent nucleoli
	Atrophy in a perifascicular distribution
	Variation in fiber size
	Inflammatory exudates, often perivascular
Elevation of muscle enzymes	Particularly creatine phosphokinase
	Often aldolase
	AST, lactate dehydrogenase
Electromyogram	Short, small, polyphasic motor units, fibrillations, positive sharp waves
	Insertional irritability
	Bizarre, high-frequency repetitive discharges
Dermatologic features	Lilac discoloration of the eyelids (heliotrope) with periorbital edema
	Scaly and erythematous dermatitis over the dorsum of the hands (Gottron's sign)
	Involvement of the knees, elbows and medial malleoli, face, neck and upper torso

Adapted from Bohan A, Peter JB. Polymyositis and dermatomyositis [part 1 of 2]. N Engl J Med 1975;292(7):34–7; with permission.

According to the 1975 criteria, a diagnosis is considered definite if a patient presents with three or four criteria (plus the rash) for dermatomyositis and four criteria for polymyositis. The diagnosis is considered probable if the patient presents two criteria plus the rash for dermatomyositis and three for polymyositis. The diagnosis is considered possible if fewer criteria are present.

In this schema, IIM are classified into five groups: group I, primary idiopathic polymyositis; group II, primary idiopathic dermatomyositis; group III, dermatomyositis (or polymyositis) associated with neoplasia; group IV, childhood dermatomyositis (or polymyositis) associated with vasculitis (vasculopathy); and group V, polymyositis or dermatomyositis associated with collagen-vascular disease (overlap polymyositis) [1].

More recently, Rider et al [23] have proposed a clinico-pathologic classification (Table 3) along with a serologic classification of JIIM. The serologic classification is used in adult patients, in whom myositis-specific antibodies (MSA) are more common and in whom these MSA may define more homogeneous subsets of patients. Some evidence suggests that, when present, MSA

Table 3
Clinicopathologic classification suggested for juvenile idiopathic inflammatory myopathies

Disorder	Description
Juvenile dermatomyositis	Most common juvenile idiopathic inflammatory myopathy
	Pathogenesis humorally mediated with CD4+ T cells and B cells in a perivascular distribution
	Characterized by small vessel thrombosis
Juvenile polymyositis	Pathogenesis cellularly mediated with CD8+ T-cell endomysial inflammation
Overlap myositis	Usually mild myositis with polycyclic course
Orbital or ocular myositis	Reported rarely in children
	Frequent association with other autoimmune disease
Cancer-associated myositis	Reported rarely in children
Focal and nodular myositis	Focal pain and swelling
	Reported rarely in children
Proliferative myositis	Pseudosarcomatous proliferation of giant cells and fibroblasts with associated inflammation and necrosis
	Rare in childhood
Inclusion-body myositis	Proximal and distal muscle weakness
	Low creatinine phosphokinase
	Rimmed vacuoles on trichrome muscle biopsy
	Reported rarely in children
Dermatomyositis sine myositis	Myositis may be sub-clinical
Eosinophilic myositis	Reported rarely in children
Granulomatous myositis	Idiopathic or in association with sarcoidosis
	Rare in childhood

Adapted from Rider LG, Miller FW. Classification and treatment of the juvenile idiopathic inflammatory myopathies. Rheum Dis Clin North Am 1997;23(3):619–55; with permission.

may define clinical subsets in children as well. Similarly, MSA that are associated with other connective tissue diseases may define more homogeneous groups of patients [23]. The serologic classification for children is somewhat controversial, however, because no specific autoantibodies are found in most patients with JIIM [31].

MRI has been recently proposed to detect skin, fascia, and subcutaneous abnormalities along with subclinical muscle involvement, providing potential help in classifying the difficult cases. MRI may become one of the diagnostic criteria, possibly replacing more invasive and painful investigations (such as EMG and muscle biopsy) in otherwise straightforward cases. Its cost and restricted availability makes its use in routine practice difficult in some parts of the world [32,33].

Diagnostic work-up

Kathryn had a number of tests at the time of diagnosis that allowed the authors to reach a diagnosis within the context of the Bohan and Peter criteria. What other tests should be done at diagnosis?

The initial assessment includes the recognition of a therapeutic emergency, such as respiratory distress or swallowing difficulties related to severe muscle weakness. Once these issues have been ruled out, the goal of the work-up is to confirm the first clinical impression and to classify the JIIM to start the treatment as soon as possible. (Because the management of most JIIM is the same, classification in some cases is a somewhat academic exercise.) The usual diagnostic work-up in the Myositis Clinic of the Hospital for Sick Children includes

1. Clinical examination (with recognition of the diagnostic criteria of Bohan and Peter along with other organ involvement)
2. Exclusion of mimics and other conditions in the differential diagnosis (Table 4)
3. Laboratory investigations including
   a. Serum levels of muscle enzymes
   b. Markers of inflammation (eg, erythrocyte sedimentation rate, C-reactive protein)
   c. Autoantibodies (ie, anti-nuclear antibodies as well as antibodies specific for other diseases, such as anti-ds-DNA, anti-Sm, anti-RNP)
   d. Infectious studies and serology as indicated
   e. MRI of the proximal muscles (fat-suppressed T2 or short tau inversion recovery sequences)
   f. EMG
   g. Muscle biopsy (considered when the results of the preliminary work-up are not conclusive)
4. Chest radiograph

5. Pulmonary function tests with measurement of maximal pressures and diffusing capacity
6. ECG
7. Nailfold capillaroscopy (If specialized microscopy is not available, the nailfold capillaries can be visualized by placing water-soluble gel on the skin just proximal to the nail and using a magnified light source such as an otoscope or ophthalmoscope at a setting of +20 or +40.) (Fig. 3)
8. Consultation by the neuromuscular service and rheumatology

Table 4
Differential diagnoses for juvenile idiopathic inflammatory myopathy

Category	Possible entities
Muscular dystrophies (X-linked, autosomal dominant or recessive)	Duchenne's disease Becker's
Congenital myopathies	Congenital muscular dystrophy
Myotonic disorders	Congenital myotonic dystrophy
Metabolic disorders	Glycogen storage disease Certain enzyme deficiencies Familial periodic paralysis Endocrinopathies (Cushing's, hypothyroidism) Chronic dialysis
Infectious/postinfectious myopathies	Viral (Influenza B, Coxsackie B, Echovirus, and Poliomyelitis) Toxoplasmosis Trichinosis, cysticercosis Septic (staphylococcus and other pyogenic myositis) Tetanus
Other connective tissue diseases	Scleroderma Mixed connective tissue disease Systemic lupus erythematosis Systemic arthritis
Genetic disorders	Osteogenesis imperfecta Ehlers–Danlos syndrome Mucopolysaccharidoses
Trauma/toxic	Physical Toxic: drugs (glucocorticoids, hydroxychloroquine, diuretics, alcohol, D-penicillamine, cimetidine, vincristine)
Spinal, muscular, and anterior horn-cell dysfunction	Infantile and juvenile muscle atrophy Arthrogryposis multiplex congenital Amyotrophic lateral sclerosis
Peripheral nerve dysfunction	Charcot–Marie–Tooth disease Neurofibromatosis Guillain–Barré syndrome
Disorders of neuromuscular transmission	Congenital myasthenia gravis Botulism

Adapted from Cassidy JT, Petty RE. Juvenile dermatomyositis. In: Textbook of pediatric rheumatology. 4th edition. 2001. p. 465–504, with permission; Pachman LM. Juvenile dermatomyositis. Pathophysiology and disease expression. Pediatr Clin North Am 1995;42(5):1071–98.

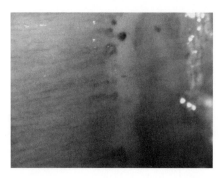

Fig. 3. Photomicrograph (magnification ×20) of the distal nailfold vessels of a patient with JDM, showing an avascular strip just proximal to the nail with more proximal dilated capillary vessels and some dot hemorrhage.

An upper gastrointestinal series and swallowing study may be of interest if there is any clinical suspicion of gastrointestinal involvement.

Clinical features

Kathryn presented with mild systemic symptoms and more marked musculoskeletal and dermatologic complaints. What other clinical signs and symptoms might have been seen?

Constitutional signs and symptoms

In some series, fever at onset has been described as a frequent occurrence. Only about 20% of the authors' patients have presented this way, but fatigue (probably related to muscle weakness), malaise, anorexia, and weight loss have been frequent early complaints. In young children, irritability and developmental regression have been described [8].

Musculo-skeletal manifestations

JDM is characterized by weakness; the weakness, which probably affects all muscle groups, is most obvious in the limb-girdle musculature, the anterior neck flexors, and the trunk muscles. The muscle groups that seem to be the most affected are the shoulders, the hips, the neck flexors, and the abdominal musculature. The affected muscles may be occasionally tender, edematous, or indurated. Gower's and Trendelenberg's signs are typical early findings on examination. Distal muscle weakness is more obvious in the children who overall are more severely affected. Almost one fourth of the authors' patients present with involvement of the pharyngeal, hypopharyngeal, and palatal muscles. This involvement manifests clinically by difficulty in swallowing, dysphonia, nasal speech, and regurgitation of liquids through the nose. The risk of aspiration in this state seems to be high, and great care must be taken with feeding. Parenteral feeding is sometimes needed until pharyngeal weakness has resolved.

Arthralgia and mild, transient, nondeforming, nonerosive arthritis has been described [34–36]. The arthritis usually occurs early in the course of the disease (within the first 6 months) and frequently involves knees, wrists, elbows, and fingers. The initial arthritis can be pauciarticular (67%) or polyarticular (33%). The arthritis generally shows a good response to JIIM therapy, but recurrences are seen during corticosteroid tapers [37]. The evolution into chronic polyarthritis occurs less often [38]. Tenosynovitis or flexor nodules may be present. Flexion contractures are common but in many cases seem to reflect muscle tightening rather than joint capsule disease. In the presence of significant arthritis, an overlap syndrome (with features of lupus, juvenile rheumatoid arthritis, or scleroderma) should be considered.

Cutaneous manifestations

The rash seen in JDM is the hallmark of the disease and is present in all cases [8,34,39]. The most typical features (heliotrope eyelid rash and Gottron's papules) are pathognomonic and are seen in about 80% of patients. The rash may occur before or after the occurrence of clinical weakness [40].

Gottron's papules are sometimes also called collodion patches [41]. They are flat-topped, violaceous or red papules, which can be scaly. A similar non-palpable (macular) rash is called Gottron's sign. This papulosquamous rash is located over the extensor aspect of the knuckles (metacarpophalangeal, proximal, and distal interphalangeal joints), elbows, knees, and the medial malleoli. Over time, the lesions may develop an atrophic white center with telangiectasia. The rash usually spares the interphalangeal spaces [40]. Early in the disease, Gottron's papules over the knuckles may be confused with flat warts [39].

The heliotrope rash over the upper eyelids (with or without edema of the eyelids or the face) is highly characteristic of JDM [41]. It may be a component of a more diffuse malar or facial rash that does not seem to spare the nasolabial folds (which may help differentiate the JDM rash from lupus).

Nailfold capillary and cuticular changes are characteristic of JDM and are part of the systemic vasculopathy. Capillary changes can also lead to gingival telangiectasia [42]. Endothelial cell proliferation and capillary basement membrane thickening leads to vascular occlusion and decreased tissue perfusion [39]. Direct visualization of the capillary beds may reveal areas of new vessel growth in response to these processes. The nailfold capillary changes seen in JIIM include capillary dropout (ischemia leading to capillary loss) leading to end row capillary loss, dilated capillary loops (hemodynamic changes leading to change in vascular morphology), and branching arboreal capillary loops (neovascularization leading to bushy loops). These changes are positively correlated with disease activity [43] and duration of untreated disease [44]. In one study, the loss of end row nailfold capillary loops was related to skin disease activity, suggesting that skin involvement is mainly a reflection of the vasculopathy [44]. The vasculopathic lesions are more common in JDM than in adult dermatomyositis, as are cutaneous calcinosis and lipodystrophy [41]. Almost 100% of the children with JDM have decreased capillary density at the nailfold. Cuticular hypertrophy may also be present in JDM [39].

A photosensitive macular erythematous or violaceous rash may involve the upper chest (V-sign), neck, shoulders (shawl-sign), extremities, hands, scalp, and face. It may evolve into poikiloderma (hyper- or hypo-pigmentation with atrophy and fine telangiectasia) [39].

Other skin rashes may be seen. Mechanic's hands (scaly hand dermatitis) may be present even though it seems to be more common in adult myositis [41]. Pruritus and psoriasiform scalp dermatitis may be seen at presentation. Periungual infarcts and cutaneous and mucosal ulcers may be present at or a few months after the initial presentation [40]. Ulcers at the corners of the eyes, in the axillae, over the elbows, or at pressure points may be signs of systemic vasculitis. Children who have a generalized rash and cutaneous ulceration at onset may have the worst prognosis [45], because the ulceration presumably reflects a more extensive vasculopathy. Edema and induration of the skin and of the sub-cutaneous tissue may be seen, particularly in the periorbital area, the face, and the distal extremities. (When edema is present at the distal extremities, there may be the appearance of "Popeye" arms.)

Calcinosis

Dystrophic calcinosis (Fig. 4) is a characteristic complication of JDM reported in 30% to 70% of the patients in various series [35]. Cutaneous calcifications are often located on the elbows, knees, and other acral parts but can be located anywhere. These lesions can lead to local pain, joint contracture, and overlying skin ulcers.

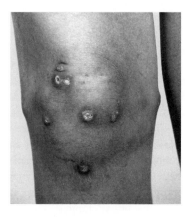

Fig. 4. Superficial calcinosis with some skin ulceration around the right knee of a patient with JDM.

The mechanism of calcinosis is thought to be dystrophic. Damaged muscles release mitochondrial calcium into matrix vesicles that promote mineralization. Histologic study has shown that calcinosis is related to hydroxyapatite accumulation [46].

Dystrophic calcification can also be located at sites of trauma and may result in more severe disease or disease of longer duration. Calcinotic lesions are rarely present at diagnosis but are seen later during the course of the disease [34,39]. Calcinosis can occur as superficial lumps, deep tumorous deposits around joints, or plates along fascial planes, or the lesions may have a widespread exoskeleton distribution. Delayed treatment and severe disease are risk factors for developing calcinosis [34,47]. Aggressive treatment of JDM is hoped to result in a decreased frequency of calcinosis [48–50].

Lipodystrophy

Lipodystrophy and associated metabolic abnormalities are well-known complications of JDM. It is less clear that this problem arises in the other JIIM. Rarely seen at presentation, these changes develop later in the course of the disease in 14% to 25% of patients [39,51]. Lipodystrophy is characterized by a progressive, slow, and symmetrical loss of subcutaneous fatty tissue that mainly involves the upper body. There may be a female preponderance. Lipodystrophy belongs to a wider condition including generalized or localized partial loss of subcutaneous fat, hirsutism, and acanthosis nigricans associated with hepatomegaly, insulin-resistant diabetes mellitus, and hyperlipidemia, especially hypertriglyceridemia [52]. It has been reported recently that 20% of 20 patients in Vancouver had lipodystrophy and either diabetes mellitus or impaired glucose tolerance, whereas 40% had abnormal glucose or lipid studies without lipodystrophy [51]. The physiopathology of this condition is currently unknown, although it is likely that hyperinsulinemia results in many of the clinical features. Hyperinsulinemia in JDM is probably multifactorial, but muscle inflammation with resulting metabolic derangements and prolonged exposure to corticosteroids are probably involved. (Counter-regulatory hormones may play a role in this setting.)

Gastrointestinal involvement

Esophageal dysmotility and malabsorption with decreased absorption of nutrients, and perhaps of oral medications, have been described. Case reports of pancreatitis, cholestasis, and hepatomegaly have been reported in JDM. Clinically severe vasculopathy of the gastrointestinal tract leading to functional problems, pain, altered stool patterns, and gastrointestinal bleeding or even perforation can be one of the most serious manifestations of JIIM, especially JDM.

Vasculitis

The presence of visceral vasculopathy, although rare, is associated with poor prognosis. It is unclear whether true vasculitis (ie, necrotizing arteritis, or leukocytoclastic small vessel vasculitis) occurs in JIIM. In any case, the vasculopathy that is seen can lead to diffuse ischemia of the gastrointestinal mucosa (responsible for ulceration, perforation, or hemorrhage) or to acute mesenteric infarction. Rarely, the vasculopathy can also affect the gallbladder, the urinary bladder, uterus, vagina or testes, and central and peripheral sensorimotor systems. Retinitis with cotton-wool exudates is a rare ophthalmologic manifestation of vasculopathy.

Pulmonary involvement

Lung manifestations are seen much less often in JIIM than in adult myositis. The authors have had very few cases of parenchymal disease at the Hospital for Sick Children (2 of 137 patients). Respiratory weakness and resultant symptoms are more common: one third of their patients had some degree of pulmonary signs or symptoms during the course of the disease [39]. In one recently reported series, the pattern of pulmonary involvement was an asymptomatic restrictive pattern with impairment of diffusion seen in 5 of 12 patients at presentation [53]. Reduction in ventilatory capacity has been found in up to 78% of asymptomatic JDM patients, probably in keeping with respiratory muscle weakness [54]. Decreased diffusion capacity as an early sign of interstitial lung disease has been reported in children who develop anti-Jo-1 antibodies (a type of MSA) [55]. Serious pulmonary disease can occur but fortunately is seldom seen.

Pulmonary disease may occur by two other mechanisms. Pharyngeal weakness may allow pathologic aspiration of food or secretions that can lead to atelectasis or pneumonia. In addition, children with JIIM are treated with immunosuppressive medications; in the setting of pulmonary disease, one must always consider the possibility of opportunistic lung infection. Although rare (the authors have not had a case of opportunistic pneumonia in the Myositis Clinic at the Hospital for Sick Children), fatal opportunistic infections have been reported in children with other autoimmune diseases [56].

Neurologic involvement

Peripheral and central neurologic manifestations have been described in JIIM but are rare. When seen, central nervous system (CNS) disease has been in the setting of severe and refractory disease [57–59]. It is unclear whether CNS involvement is caused by vasculopathy or by specific vasculitis, because the series published so far have failed to demonstrate the presence of true vasculitis on brain autopsy. The symptoms that have been reported have mainly been generalized tonic-clonic seizures with or without subsequent abnormal neurologic signs such as ptosis, hypertonia, flaccid hemiplegia, motor aphasia, and bulbar paresis or coma [57,58]. Other nonspecific symptoms, such as emotional lability and depression, have been reported; in the setting of a chronic disease, it may be difficult to relate these findings specifically to JIIM. Imaging findings in reported patients have ranged from normal to lacunar changes or multiple ischemic infarctions with severe emboli in the cortex on MRI. Several mechanisms have been evoked to explain this CNS involvement, including vasculopathy, CNS vasculitis, hypoxic-ischemic encephalopathy (hypoperfusion), hypertensive encephalopathy, or drug-induced toxicity [58].

Cardiac involvement

Specific cardiac involvement has not been well described in JIIM and is probably rare. In adult series, which have included some JIIM, nonspecific murmurs and ECG abnormalities as well as pericarditis have been reported and seem to be the most common cardiac findings [60]. There have been reports of ECG myocardial infarction, congestive heart failure, and more widespread cardiac vasculopathy in adults and children with JIIM [61–63].

Ophthalmologic involvement

Eye disease is unusual. Isolated case reports of retinopathy and bilateral membranous conjunctivitis have been published. Transient retinal exudates and cotton-wool spots may occur, leading potentially to optic atrophy and visual loss. Side effects of corticosteroids use, such as cataracts and glaucoma, may be seen [39]. The authors no longer recommend ophthalmologist follow-up for their patients; retinal disease is exceptional, and side effects of treatment that affect the eye can easily be detected by non-ophthalmologists (Akikusa, submitted for publication, 2004).

Malignancy and juvenile idiopathic inflammatory myopathies

Unlike adult DM, JDM is rarely associated with malignancy; there have been only a few case reports. The authors do not search for occult malignancy in their patients.

Juvenile polymyositis

Juvenile polymyositis (JPM) is a rare condition. Although the term is used to describe idiopathic myositis without any skin rash, it is possible that some children should really be labeled as having adermatitic dermatomyositis. That is, although there is no skin rash, these patients have a muscle pathology that is identical to JDM (eg, vasculopathy, perifascicular atrophy) rather than to adult polymyositis. JDM and JPM patients are managed similarly and for the most part seem to respond similarly.

Amyopathic juvenile dermatomositis

The term amyopathic JDM refers to a disorder in which the characteristic skin rash of JDM is seen without apparent muscle inflammation. It is still not clear whether amyopathic JDM is a separate entity or is the extreme end of the spectrum of JDM with minimal muscle involvement. Diagnostic criteria for amyopathic DM have been proposed in adults by Euwer and Sontheimer [64] and include absence of proximal muscle weakness and normal muscle enzymes for 2 years after presentation, while skin lesions and skin biopsy are typical. Thirty-nine cases of suspected amyopathic JDM were reported in a survey across North America, but 13 patients had abnormal tests suggesting very mild myositis and therefore were not considered truly amyopathic. The incidence of calcinosis was very low in this population of patients [65]. El-Azhary et al [66] conducted a survey investigating the progression of amyopathic dermatomyositis to myositis and associated malignancy in adults. Only 2 of the 25 patients who could be reached at follow-up developed muscle weakness within 5 years after diagnosis, but 5 patients developed malignancies. None of the seven pediatric patients in this study had progression to myopathy.

Outcome measures

To follow patients in the clinic and to compare patients in clinical studies, it is helpful to use accurate and reliable outcome measurement tools. The Juvenile Dermatomyositis Disease Activity Collaborative Study Group, along with the International Myositis Assessment and Clinical Studies (IMACS) group, has worked to develop and validate new tools to assess disease activity and damage in JIIM. The tools most currently used are the Childhood Health Assessment Questionnaire (CHAQ), Manual Muscle Testing (MMT), the Childhood Myositis Assessment Scale (CMAS), the physician and patient global assessment of disease and skin activity, the physician and patient global assessment of disease and skin damage, and the parent global assessment of disease severity.

MMT is a score that putatively assesses only muscle strength. Seven proximal and five distal muscle groups are assessed bilaterally using a defined scoring system. MMT has been shown to be a significant predictor of disease activity. The CMAS, a measure that incorporates function as well as strength, may be more informative than MMT [67].

The CHAQ was initially developed to measure physical function in children with arthritis. It is a 30-item parent- or self-reporting questionnaire that reflects the child's (or parent's) perceptions of physical abilities or disabilities [68]. This score has undergone validation in JDM; the CHAQ has shown good construct validity and responsiveness [69,70].

The CMAS is a 14-activity observational, performance-based assessment of physical function, strength, and endurance. It has been recently validated in JIIM and has been shown to be a valid assessment of muscle outcome [67,71]. The CMAS9, which includes nine CMAS maneuvers, has been evaluated in normal, healthy children between 4 and 9 years of age to generate normative data. These sex- and age-related normative data provide important information in the interpretation of the CMAS in children with JIIM [72].

Two different groups have recently proposed core sets of measures for disease activity and damage assessment in JDM. The goal of this work is to provide the clinician with standardized outcome measurements for use in clinical practice and in studies. Although MRI is widely used to assess disease activity and damage, it is not always easily available, so the core sets do not require imaging. The proposed core sets are summarized in Table 5 [73–75].

A growth and development domain has been added to the damage core set to assess growth retardation and delayed puberty. These areas are thought to be complications of chronic disease in many children. Candidate tools, including physician global damage assessments and CHAQ, have been proposed along with T1-weighted MRI to evaluate muscle damage and a cutaneous assessment

Table 5
Juvenile dermatomyositis disease activity core set

| Domain | Item used to measure the domain | |
	PRINTO/PRCSG	IMACS
Global assessment by physicians	VAS or Likert scale	VAS or Likert scale
Muscle strength assessment	CMAS and MMT	MMT
Laboratory assessment: muscle enzymes	Creatinine phosphokinase, LDH, aldolase, AST/ALT	At least two of the following: creatinine phosphokinase, aldolase, LDH, AST/ALT
Functional ability assessment	CHAQ	CHAQ and CMAS
Global assessment by parents/patients	VAS or Likert scale	VAS or Likert scale
Global juvenal dermatomyositis disease activity tool	Disease activity score (DAS) and myositis disease activity assessment (MDAA)	

Abbreviations: CHAQ, Childhood Health Assessment Questionnaire; CMAS, Childhood Myositis Assessment Scale; LDH, lactate dehydrogenase; MMT, Manual Muscle Testing; PRCSG, Pediatric Rheumatology Collaborative Study Group (PRCSG); PRINTO, Pediatric International Trials Organization; VAS, visual analogue scale.

From Ruperto N, Ravelli A, Murray KJ, et al. Preliminary core sets of measures for disease activity and damage assessment in juvenile systemic lupus erythematosus and juvenile dermatomyositis. Rheumatol 2003;42:1452–9; with permission (PRINTO/PRCSG); Miller FW, Rider LG, Chung YL, et al. Proposed preliminary core set measures for disease outcome assessment in adult and juvenile idiopathic inflammatory myopathies. Rheumatology (Oxford) 2001;40(11):1262–73 (IMACS).

Table 6
Juvenile dermatomyositis disease damage core set

Domain of damage	Item used to measure domain
Global assessment by physician	VAS or Likert scale
Functional ability assessment	CHAQ
Growth and development	Height and weight
	Menses
	Tanner puberty stage
Global JDM damage tool	Myositis Damage Index (MDI)
Muscle strength assessment	CMAS

Abbreviaitons: CHAQ, Childhood Health Assessment Questionnaire; CMAS, Childhood Myositis Assessment Scale; JDM, juvenile dermatomyositis; VAS, visual analog scale.

tool able to evaluate skin damage [75]. The core set proposed by Ruperto et al [73] is summarized in Table 6.

Therapy

Kathryn was treated with MTX and oral and, later, intravenous corticosteroids. What are the best therapies for children with JIIM? Is the oral or intravenous route of corticosteroids better? What other agents are available for these disorders?

Corticosteroids have been the traditional mainstay of therapy for the JIIM; onset is rapid, and clinical efficacy is seen within days to weeks. Toxicity with chronic use of corticosteroids is high, however. MTX seems to work well in JIIM, especially at maintaining remission, but the onset is slow: MTX may take as long as 12 weeks before a clinical effect is seen. The approach at the Hospital for Sick Children has been to start treatment with corticosteroids and MTX together in patients with JIIM and to use the MTX to allow a much more rapid withdrawal of corticosteroids than had been traditionally done in the past.

Worldwide, corticosteroids remain the main medication used in the treatment of inflammatory myopathy. The authors initially use high-dose oral corticosteroids and subsequently adjust the treatment to the clinical response of the patient. They generally start a new patient with 2 mg/kg/day of prednisone divided into three equal doses (maximum daily dose rarely to exceed 80 mg). At 6 weeks, when clinical improvement is seen in strength, rash is improving, and muscle enzyme tests have normalized, they consolidate the prednisone into a twice-daily, and shortly afterwards a single-daily dose. The prednisone is then tapered by about 10% every 2 weeks.

In the case of incomplete or absent response (steroid resistance), intravenous methylprednisolone pulses (IVMP) (30 mg/kg per treatment, maximum 1000 mg) are given to gain a rapid control of the systemic inflammation. In the presence of dysphagia and dysphonia, pulmonary disease, or suspected gastrointestinal vasculopathy, IVMP is often the initial treatment.

Several groups have proposed the use of IVMP in combination with daily oral corticosteroids for all patients [48,76,77]. The rationale is to achieve early remission to allow the daily oral corticosteroid dose to be decreased sooner and to prevent the side effects of long-term corticosteroid use and the complications related to prolonged disease activity, such as calcinosis. A group at Northwestern University conducted a cost-identification and cost-effectiveness analysis to compare oral and intermittent high-dose corticosteroids [78]. The investigators compared two groups of five patients: patients treated with oral corticosteroids (2 mg/kg/day) and patients who received intermittent IVMP along with low-dose daily oral corticosteroids (0.5 mg/kg/day). Patients treated with IVMP achieved a remission at a median of 2 years earlier, suggesting to the investigators that this approach is cost-effective. IVMP exposes the patient to possible adverse reactions, however [79].

Despite the excellent response to corticosteroids in this condition, the risk that long-term corticosteroid use may lead to growth retardation, cataracts, and secondary osteoporosis has resulted in the more widespread use of steroid-sparing agents.

MTX was first proposed as a second-line agent for refractory JDM along with corticosteroids [80]. It is now more widely prescribed early as a steroid-sparing agent. Treatment combining high-dose corticosteroids and MTX started within 4 weeks after the beginning of treatment in the absence of improvement in muscle enzymes may decrease the incidence of long-term complications such as calcinosis [49]. In a 12-patient pilot study, treatment with oral MTX in combination with intermittent IVMP was started within 6 weeks after diagnosis in six children. This group of patients improved clinically, and the oral corticosteroid dose could be decreased in five patients. None of these patients developed calcinosis. The results of this small study suggest that early use of MTX in combination with IVMP may be useful in JDM [81]. The authors have reported their use of MTX as a first-line treatment for JDM along with corticosteroids in 31 children and compared the clinical course and outcome with that of a control group treated primarily with corticosteroids. The two groups had similar clinical improvement, but the study group had much less exposure to corticosteroids because of an aggressive taper and a lower cumulative dose. The patients in the study group experienced fewer side effects with a greater height velocity and smaller weight gain [82]. Early use of MTX seems to be a safe and efficacious strategy.

Not all patients respond to the combination of MTX and corticosteroids. In some cases, the disease is so severe that additional agents are needed at the outset. In other cases, there is an early response but an inability to taper therapy. A number of additional agents have been proposed for use in JDM. The authors' practice has been to use intravenous immunoglobulin (IVIG) in both of these clinical settings. Very severe initial disease with severe vasculopathy (lungs, skin, or gastrointestinal or nervous system) probably warrants more aggressive immunosuppression with cyclophosphamide.

Many groups have used IVIG with an apparently good response. The IVIG in these reports was given for different indications, including relapse, incomplete response, or for steroid-sparing purposes. The dose, the number of courses, and the time interval varied greatly among the different studies published [83–85]. Only one controlled trial (with adult patients) has conclusively demonstrated efficacy: 15 adult patients were treated with monthly infusions of IVIG for 3 months and improved objectively in strength, neuromuscular symptoms, skin rash, and histopathologic findings [86]. It is difficult to draw definite conclusions about the efficacy of IVIG, because the series published so far are small ($\leq$ 18 patients), and almost all the patients continued to receive corticosteroids along with another second-line agent, such as azathioprine, MTX, or cyclophosphamide, concomitantly. The authors' protocol has been to start treatment with IVIG at a dose of 2 g/kg per infusion (up to a maximum of 70 g) given every 2 weeks for five infusions. If this treatment is associated with clinical improvement, IVIG treatment continues monthly for up to a year. After 12 months of infusion, the authors taper the medication by lengthening the interval between infusions to 6 weeks, 8 weeks, and then to 12 weeks. Patients who can tolerate infusions spaced 12 weeks apart seem to be able to discontinue the therapy completely without flare of symptoms.

Cyclophosphamide has been used in severe and refractory JDM. In the authors' experience, the existence of prominent vasculopathic features such as skin ulcers may be an indication for monthly cyclophosphamide infusions. Twelve patients treated this way have been reported recently. They had refractory disease, and two of them died shortly after the first infusion of cyclophosphamide. The 10 remaining patients had a significant improvement in muscle function at 6 months of therapy without any serious short-term toxicity [87].

Other medications that have been used in treating JIIM include cyclosporin A [88–90] and hydroxychloroquine [91]. There is little published evidence to support either of these treatments. In the authors' experience, cyclosporine seems to be effective, but its use is often complicated by hypertension and hirsutism. Their patients have not seemed to respond noticeably to hydroxychloroquine. Topical FK506 (tacrolimus 0.1% ointment) has been tried in adult patients with refractory skin disease with a reported substantial benefit [92–94]. Therefore, topical tacrolimus seems to be an attractive adjunct given the good safety data in children [95].

Clinical outcome

Kathryn is currently doing well, but what is her future prognosis? What will her school and work experience be? How long will she have her disease?

A few studies have reported the medium- and long-term functional outcomes of patients with JDM [40,45,50,96,97]. Bowyer et al [50] have reported that delayed treatment leads to poorer outcome in terms of disease course and calcinosis. Huber et al [97] looked at the outcomes of patients with JDM in an inception cohort using validated tools. These children were diagnosed between 1984 and 1994 at four Canadian pediatric referral centers with a median follow-up period of 7.2 years. The median age at follow-up was 13 years. Sixty-five of 80 patients could be contacted. Most of the patients had no delay in the initiation of their treatment. Thirty-seven percent of the patients had a monocyclic course (disease that went into permanent remission after about 2 years of activity); the remaining 63% had a chronic continuous or polycyclic course. Physical function was assessed using the CHAQ score. More than two thirds of the patients had a CHAQ score of 0, suggesting no or minimal disability, and only 8% had a score higher than 1.0, representing moderate to severe disability. The predictive factors of higher (worse) CHAQ scores were female gender, chronic continuous course, and presence of calcinosis at some point during the disease course. Growth was analyzed by predicting height based on the mid-parental height. Twenty patients (31%) were more than 1 SD below their predicted height, and 10 (16%) were more than 2 SD below their predicted height. In terms of educational and vocational achievement, some of the patients had failed a single grade because of disease-related absences from school, but they all seemed to have caught up academically. None of the patients had the impression that their disease had interfered with their ability to work. Calcinosis was observed in 22 patients (34%). In those patients, calcinosis developed a median 3.41 years after disease onset. No predictive factors were found for the development of calcinosis in this cohort [97]. At the time of follow-up, 40% of the patients continued to have a rash, and 23% reported weakness. Most of the patients had no pain, but children with a chronic continuous course had higher pain scores. About one third of the patients continued to take medications. In terms of comorbidity and mortality, three patients developed diabetes, and two developed an additional connective tissue disease (one with scleroderma and one with an overlap syndrome) after achieving remission of their JDM. No malignancy was reported. One patient died of acute myocardial failure secondary to multiple myocardial infarctions [61]. This recent study shows that the prognosis and outcome of JDM seem to be good. Patients with a chronic continuous course, however, have a significant long-term functional impairment and more frequently develop side effects of the therapy.

As demonstrated by Kathryn's case, JIIM are rare conditions that require somewhat aggressive anti-inflammatory and immunosuppressive therapy. JDM is by far the most common presentation, with most of the manifestations limited to skin and muscle. Rarely, however, any system can be involved by the underlying vasculopathy. The disorders have a good functional outcome, but many of the affected children will have chronic disease and will require long-term therapy. The outlook for Kathryn and other children with JIIM is bright. The recently expanded understanding of the genetic and immunopathologic underpinnings of the JIIM may result soon in improved, targeted therapies and an even better prognosis.

References

[1] Bohan A, Peter JB. Polymyositis and dermatomyositis [part 1 of 2]. N Engl J Med 1975; 292(7):34–7.

[2] Banker BQ, Victor M. Dermatomyositis (systemic angiopathy) of childhood. Medicine (Baltimore) 1966;45(4):261–89.

[3] Symmons DPM, Sills JA, Davis SM. The incidence of juvenile dermatomyositis: results from a nation-wide study. Br J Rheumatol 1995;34:732–6.

[4] Mendez EP, Lipton R, Ramsey-Goldman R, et al. US incidence of juvenile dermatomyositis, 1995–1998: results from the National Institute of Arthritis and Musculoskeletal and Skin Diseases Registry. Arthritis Rheum 2003;49(3):300–5.

[5] Medsger TAJ, Dawson WN, Masi AT. The epidemiology of polymyositis. Am J Med 1970;48: 715–23.

[6] Ang P, Sugeng MW, Chua SH. Classical and amyopathic dermatomyositis seen at the national centre of Singapore: a 3-year retrospective review of their clinical characteristics and association with malignancy. Ann Acad Med Singapore 2000;29(2):219–23.

[7] Pachman LM. Juvenile dermatomyositis: immunogenetics, pathophysiology and disease expression. Rheum Dis Clin North Am 2002;28:579–602.

[8] Cassidy JT, Petty RE, editors. Juvenile dermatomyositis. In: Textbook of pediatric rheumatology. 4th edition. p. 465–504.

[9] Reed AM, Stirling JD. Association of the HLA-DQA1*0501 allele in multiple racial groups with juvenile dermatomyositis. Hum Immunol 1995;44:131–5.

[10] Shamim EA, Rider LG, Miller FW. Update on the genetics of the idiopathic inflammatory myopathies. Curr Opin Rheumatol 2000;12:482–91.

[11] West JE, Reed AM. Analysis of HLA-DM polymorphism in juvenile dermatomyositis (JDM) patients. Hum Immunol 1999;60:255–8.

[12] Artlett CM, Ramos R, Jiminez SA, et al. Chimeric cells of maternal origin in juvenile idiopathic inflammatory myopathies. Childhood Myositis Heterogeneity Collaborative Group. Lancet 2000;356(9248):2155–6.

[13] Artlett CM, Miller FW, Rider LG. Persistent maternally derived peripheral microchimerism is associated with the juvenile idiopathic inflammatory myopathies. Rheumatology (Oxford) 2001;40(11):1279–84.

[14] Reed AM, Picornell YJ, Harwood A, et al. Chimerism in children with juvenile dermatomyositis. Lancet 2000;356:2156–7.

[15] Reed AM, McNallan K, Wettstein P, et al. Does HLA-dependent chimerism underlie the pathogenesis of juvenile dermatomyositis. J Immunol 2004;172:5041–6.

[16] Artlett CM, O'Hanlon TP, Lopez AM, et al. HLA-DQA1 is not an apparent risk factor for microchimerism in patients with various autoimmune diseases and in healthy individuals. Arthritis Rheum 2003;48(9):2567–72.

[17] Verweij CL, Huizinga TWJ. Tumor necrosis factor alpha gene polymorphisms and rheumatic diseases. Br J Rheumatol 1998;37:923–9.

[18] Wilson AG, de Vries N, Pociot F, et al. An allelic polymorphism within the human tumor necrosis factor alpha promoter region is strongly associated with HLA A1, B8, and DR3 alleles. J Exp Med 1993;177:557–60.

[19] Wilson AG, Symons JA, McDowell TL, et al. Effects of a polymorphism in the human tumor necrosis factor alpha promoter on transcriptional activation. Proc Natl Acad Sci U S A 1997;94: 3195–9.

[20] Pachman LM, Liotta-Davis MR, Hong DK, et al. TNFalpha-308A allele in juvenile

dermatomyositis: association with increased production of tumor necrosis factor alpha, disease duration, and pathologic calcifications. Arthritis Rheum 2000;43(10):2368–77.

[21] Fedczyna TO, Lutz J, Pachman LM. Expression of TNFalpha by muscle fibers in biopsies from children with untreated juvenile dermatomyositis: association with the TNFalpha-308A allele. Clin Immunol 2001;100(2):236–9.

[22] Lutz J, Huwiler KG, Fedczyna T, et al. Increased plasma thrombospondin-1 (TSP-1) levels are associated with the TNF alpha-308A allele in children with juvenile dermatomyositis. Clin Immunol 2002;103:260–3.

[23] Rider LG, Miller FW. Classification and treatment of the juvenile idiopathic inflammatory myopathies. Rheum Dis Clin North Am 1997;23(3):619–55.

[24] Massa M, Costouros N, Mazzoli F, et al. Self epitopes shared between human myosin and Streptococcus pyogenes M5 protein are targets of immune responses in active juvenile dermatomyositis. Arthritis Rheum 2002;46(11):3015–25.

[25] Tezak Z, Hoffman EP, Lutz JL, et al. Gene expression profiling in DQA1*0501 + children with untreated dermatomyositis: a novel model of pathogenesis. J Immunol 2002;168(8): 4154–63.

[26] Wargula JC. Update on juvenile dermatomyositis: new advances in understanding its etiopathogenesis. Curr Opin Rheumatol 2003;15(5):595–601.

[27] Goncalves FGP, Chimelli L, Sallum ME, et al. Immunohistological analysis of CD59 and membrane attack complex of complement in muscle in juvenile dermatomyositis. J Rheumatol 2002;29:1301–7.

[28] Sallum AM, Marie SK, Wakamatsu A, et al. Immunohistochemical analysis of adhesion molecule expression on muscle biopsy specimens from patients with juvenile dermatomyositis. J Rheumatol 2004;31(4):801–7.

[29] Li CKC, Varsani H, Holton JL, et al. MHC class I overexpression on muscles in early juvenile dermatomyositis. J Rheumatol 2004;31(3):605–9.

[30] Bohan A, Peter JB. Polymyositis and dermatomyositis [part 2 of 2]. N Engl J Med 1975; 292(8):403–7.

[31] Feldman BM, Reichlin M, Laxer RM, et al. Clinical significance of specific autoantibodies in juvenile dermatomyositis. J Rheumatol 1996;23(10):1794–7.

[32] Kimball AB, Summers RM, Turner M, et al. Magnetic resonance imaging detection of occult skin and subcutaneous abnormalities in juvenile dermatomyositis. Arthritis Rheum 2000;43(8): 1866–73.

[33] Maillard SM, Jones R, Owens C, et al. Quantitative assessment of MRI T2 relaxation time of thigh muscles in juvenile dermatomyositis. Rheumatology 2004;43(5):603–8.

[34] Pachman LM, Hayford JR, Chung A, et al. Juvenile dermatomyositis at diagnosis: clinical characteristics of 79 children. J Rheumatol 1998;25(6):1198–204.

[35] Pachman LM. Juvenile dermatomyositis. Pathophysiology and disease expression. Pediatr Clin North Am 1995;42(5):1071–98.

[36] Miller LC, Michael AF, Kim Y. Childhood dermatomyositis: clinical course and long-term follow-up. Clin Pediatr 1987;26:561–6.

[37] Tse S, Lubelsky S, Gordon M, et al. The arthritis of inflammatory childhood myositis syndromes. J Rheumatol 2001;28(1):192–7.

[38] Hollister JR. The evolution of juvenile dermatomyositis into chronic arthritis. Arthritis Rheum 1998;41(Suppl):S203.

[39] Ramanan AV, Feldman BM. Clinical features and outcomes of juvenile dermatomyositis and other childhood onset myositis syndromes. Rheum Dis Clin North Am 2002;28(4):833–57.

[40] Peloro TM, Miller OF, Hahn TF, et al. Juvenile dermatomyositis: a retrospective review of a 30-year experience. J Am Acad Dermatol 2001;45(1):28–34.

[41] Santmyire-Rosenberger B, Dugan EM. Skin involvement in dermatomyositis. Curr Opin Rheumatol 2003;15(6):714–22.

[42] Ghali FE, Stein LD, Fine J, et al. Gingival telangiectases. An underappreciated physical sign of juvenile dermatomyositis. Arch Dermatol 1999;135:1370–4.

[43] Feldman BM, Rider LG, Dugan L, et al. Nailfold capillaries as indicators of disease activity in juvenile idiopathic inflammatory myopathies (JIIM). Arthritis Rheum 1999;42(9):S181.

[44] Smith RL, Sundberg J, Shamiyah E, et al. Skin involvement in juvenile dermatomyositis is associated with loss of end row nailfold capillary loops. J Rheumatol 2004;31(8):1644–9.

[45] Ramanan AV, Feldman BM. Clinical outcomes in juvenile dermatomyositis. Curr Opin Rheumatol 2002;14(6):658–62.

[46] Eddy MC, Leelawattana R, McAlister WH, et al. Calcinosis universalis complicating juvenile dermatomyositis: resolution during Probenecid therapy. J Clin Endocrinol Metab 1997;82(11): 3536–42.

[47] Ansell BM. Juvenile dermatomyositis. Rheum Dis Clin North Am 1991;17:931–42.

[48] Pachman LM, Callen AM, Hayford J, et al. Juvenile dermatomyositis: decreased calcinosis with intermittent high-dose intravenous methylprednisolone (IV pulse). Arthritis Rheum 1994; 37(Suppl 9):S429.

[49] Fisler RE, Liang MG, Fuhlbrigge RC, et al. Aggressive management of juvenile dermatomyositis results in improved outcome and decreased incidence of calcinosis. J Am Acad Dermatol 2002;47:505–11.

[50] Bowyer SL, Blane CE, Sullivan DB, et al. Childhood dermatomyositis: factors predicting functional outcome and development of dystrophic calcification. J Pediatr 1983;103:882–8.

[51] Huemer C, Kitson H, Malleson PN, et al. Lipodystrophy in patients with juvenile dermatomyositis-evaluation of clinical and metabolic abnormalities. J Rheumatol 2001;28(3): 610–5.

[52] Senior B, Gellis SS. The syndromes of total lipodystrophy and partial lipodystrophy. Pediatrics 1964;33:593–612.

[53] Trapani S, Camiciottoli G, Vierucci A, et al. Pulmonary involvement in juvenile dermatomyositis: a two-year longitudinal study. Rheumatol 2001;40:216–20.

[54] Pachman LM, Cooke N. Juvenile dermatomyositis: a clinical and immunologic study. J Pediatr 1980;96(2):226–34.

[55] Rider LG, Miller FW, Targoff IN. Myositis specific autoantibodies (MSA) in children: a broadened spectrum of juvenile myositis. Arthritis Rheum 1993;36:S258.

[56] Fortenberry JD, Shew ML. Fatal Pneumocystis carinii in an adolescent with systemic lupus erythematosus. J Adolesc Health Care 1989;10(6):570–2.

[57] Elst EF, Kamphuis SSM, Prakken BJ, et al. Severe central nervous system involvement in juvenile dermatomyositis. J Rheumatol 2003;30(9):2059–63.

[58] Ramanan AV, Sawhney S, Murray KJ. Central nervous system complications in two cases of juvenile onset dermatomyositis. Rheumatology (Oxford) 2001;40(11):1293–8.

[59] Regan M, Haque U, Pomper M, et al. Central nervous system vasculitis as a complication of refractory dermatomyositis. J Rheumatol 2001;28:207–11.

[60] Askari AD, Huettner TL. Cardiac abnormalities in polymyositis/dermatomyositis. Semin Arthritis Rheum 1982;12(2):208–19.

[61] Jimenez C, Rowe PC, Keene D. Cardiac and central nervous system vasculitis in a child with dermatomyositis. J Child Neurol 1994;9(3):297–300.

[62] Bitnum S, Daeschner CWJ, Travis LB. Dermatomyositis. J Pediatr 1964;64:101–31.

[63] Haupt HM, Hutchins GM. The heart and cardiac conduction system in polymyositis-dermatomyositis: a clinicopathologic study of 16 autopsied patients. Am J Cardiol 1982;50(5): 998–1006.

[64] Euwer RL, Sontheimer RD. Amyopathic dermatomyositis: a review. J Invest Dermatol 1993; 100(1):124S–7S.

[65] Plamondon S, Dent PB. Juvenile amyopathic dermatomyositis: results of a case finding descriptive survey. J Rheumatol 2000;27(8):2031–4.

[66] El-Azhary RA, Pakzad SY. Amyopathic dermatomyositis: retrospective review of 37 cases. J Am Acad Dermatol 2002;46(4):560–5.

[67] Huber AM, Feldman BM, Rennebohm RM, et al. Validation and clinical significance of the Childhood Myositis Assessment Scale for assessment of muscle function in the juvenile idiopathic inflammatory myopathies. Arthritis Rheum 2004;50(5):1595–603.

[68] Singh G, Athreya BH, Fries JF, Goldsmith DP. Measurement of health status in children with juvenile rheumatoid arthritis. Arthritis Rheum 1994;37:1761–9.

[69] Feldman BM, Ayling-Campos A, Luy L, et al. Measuring disability in juvenile dermatomyositis: validity of the childhood health assessment questionnaire. J Rheumatol 1995;22(2): 326–31.

[70] Huber AM, Hicks JE, Lachenbruch PA, et al. Validation of the Childhood Health Assessment Questionnaire in the juvenile idiopathic myopathies. Juvenile Dermatomyositis Disease Activity Collaborative Study Group. J Rheumatol 2001;28(5):1106–11.

[71] Lovell DJ, Lindsley CB, Rennebohm RM, et al. Development of validated disease activity and damage indices for the juvenile idiopathic inflammatory myopathies. II. The Childhood Myositis Assessment Scale (CMAS): a quantitative tool for the evaluation of muscle function. The Juvenile Dermatomyositis Disease Activity Collaborative Study Group. Arthritis Rheum 1999;42(10):2213–9.

[72] Rennebohm RM, Jones K, Huber AM, et al. Normal scores for nine maneuvers of the Childhood Myositis Assessment Scale. Arthritis Rheum 2004;51(3):365–70.

[73] Ruperto N, Ravelli A, Murray KJ, et al. Preliminary core sets of measures for disease activity and damage assessment in juvenile systemic lupus erythematosus and juvenile dermatomyositis. Rheumatol 2003;42:1452–9.

[74] Isenberg DA, Allen E, Farewell V, et al. International consensus outcome measures for patients with idiopathic inflammatory myopathies. Development and initial indices in patients with adult onset disease. Rheumatol 2004;43:49–54.

[75] Miller FW, Rider LG, Chung YL, et al. Proposed preliminary core set measures for disease outcome assessment in adult and juvenile idiopathic inflammatory myopathies. Rheumatology (Oxford) 2001;40(11):1262–73.

[76] Laxer RM, Stein LD, Petty RE. Intravenous pulse methylprednisolone treatment of juvenile dermatomyositis. Arthritis Rheum 1987;30(3):328–34.

[77] Paller AS. The use of pulse corticosteroid therapy for juvenile dermatomyositis. Pediatr Dermatol 1996;13(4):347–8.

[78] Klein-Gitelman MS, Waters T, Pachman LM. The economic impact of intermittent high-dose intravenous versus oral corticosteroid treatment of juvenile dermatomyositis. Arthritis Care Res 2000;13(6):360–8.

[79] Klein-Gitelman MS, Pachman LM. Intravenous corticosteroids (IV CS): adverse reactions are more variable than expected in children. J Rheumatol 1998;25:1995–2002.

[80] Miller LC, Sisson BA, Tucker LB, et al. Methotrexate treatment of recalcitrant childhood dermatomyositis. Arthritis Rheum 1992;35(10):1143–9.

[81] Al-Mayouf S, Al-Mazyed A, Bahabri S. Efficacy of early treatment of severe juvenile dermatomyositis with intravenous methylprednisolone and methotrexate. Clin Rheumatol 2000;19: 138–41.

[82] Ramanan A, Campbell-Webster N, Tran D, et al. Initial treatment of juvenile dermatomyositis (JDM) using methotrexate (MTX) and aggressively tapered prednisone (PRED). Pediatric Rheumatology Online Journal;1(4):120. Available at http://www.pedrheumonlinejournal.org/ July/derm/123.htm. Accessed February 8, 2005.

[83] Al-Mayouf SM, Laxer RM, Schneider R, et al. Intravenous immunoglobulin therapy for juvenile dermatomyositis: efficacy and safety. J Rheumatol 2000;27(10):2498–503.

[84] Sansome A, Dubowitz V. Intravenous immunoglobulin in juvenile dermatomyositis—four year review of nine cases. Arch Dis Child 1995;72:25–8.

[85] Lang B, Murphy G. Treatment of dermatomyositis with intravenous globulin. Am J Med 1991; 91:169–72.

[86] Dalakas MC, Illa I, Dambrosia JM, et al. A controlled trial of high-dose intravenous immune globulin infusions as treatment for dermatomyositis. N Engl J Med 1993;329(27):1993–2000.

[87] Riley P, Maillard SM, Wedderburn LR, et al. Intravenous cyclophosphamide pulse therapy in juvenile dermatomyositis. A review of efficacy and safety. Rheumatol 2004;43(4):491–6.

[88] Heckmatt J, Hasson N, Saunders C, et al. Cyclosporin in juvenile dermatomyositis. Lancet 1989:1063–6.

[89] Zeller V, Cohen P, Prieur A, et al. Cyclosporin A therapy in refractory juvenile derma-tomyositis. Experience and longterm followup of 6 cases. J Rheumatol 1996;23(8):1424–7.

[90] Kobayashi I, Yamada M, Takahashi Y, et al. Interstitial lung disease associated with juvenile dermatomyositis: clinical features and efficacy of cyclosporin A. Rheumatology (Oxford) 2003;42(2):371–4.

[91] Olson NY, Lindsley CB. Adjunctive use of hydroxychloroquine in childhood dermatomyositis. J Rheumatol 1989;16(12):1545–7.

[92] Yoshimasu T, Ohtani T, Sakamoto T, et al. Topical FK506 (tacrolimus) therapy for facial erythematous lesions of cutaneous lupus erythematosus and dermatomyositis. Eur J Dermatol 2002;12:50–2.

[93] Hollar CB, Jorizzo JL. Topical tacrolimus 0.1% ointment for refractory skin disease in dermatomyositis: a pilot study. J Dermatolog Treat 2004;15(1):35–9.

[94] Ueda M, Makinodan R, Matsumura M, et al. Successful treatment of amyopathic derma-tomyositis with topical tacrolimus. Br J Dermatol 2003;148:593–611.

[95] Paller A, Eichenfield LF, Leung DYM. A 12-week study of tacrolimus ointment for the treatment of atopic dermatitis in pediatric patients. J Am Acad Dermatol 2001;44(1 Suppl): S47–57.

[96] Shehata R, Al-Mayouf S, Al-Dalaan A, et al. Juvenile dermatomyositis: clinical profile and disease course in 25 patients. Clin Exp Rheumatol 1999;17(1):115–8.

[97] Huber AM, Lang B, LeBlanc CMA, et al. Medium- and long-term functional outcomes in a multicenter cohort of children with juvenile dermatomyositis. Arthritis Rheum 2000;43(3): 541–9.

ELSEVIER
SAUNDERS

PEDIATRIC CLINICS
OF NORTH AMERICA

Pediatr Clin N Am 52 (2005) 521–545

Scleroderma in Children

Francesco Zulian, MD

Pediatric Rheumatology Unit, Department of Pediatrics, University of Padova,
Via Giustiniani 3 35128, Padua, Italy

Juvenile scleroderma syndromes are multisystem autoimmune rheumatic diseases whose unifying characteristic is the presence of hard skin and onset before 16 years of age. They can be separated into two main categories: localized scleroderma (morphea) in which there is skin sclerosis but no vascular or internal organ involvement, and systemic sclerosis, in which there is diffuse skin sclerosis involving many sites of the body together with internal organ involvement.

Juvenile systemic sclerosis

Juvenile systemic sclerosis is a chronic multisystem connective tissue disease characterized by sclerodermatous skin changes and widespread abnormalities of the viscera. In this condition the symmetrical fibrous thickening and hardening of the skin accompany fibrous changes in internal organs, such as esophagus, intestinal tract, heart, lungs, and kidneys.

Classification

According to of the 1980 American College of Rheumatology classification criteria for adults, the diagnosis of systemic sclerosis requires the presence of either the major criterion (diffuse scleroderma involving areas proximal to the metacarpophalangeal or metatarsophalangeal joints) or of two minor criteria (sclerodactyly, digital pitting scars, bibasilar pulmonary fibrosis) [1]. This classification was designed to be specific rather than sensitive to minimize false-

---

E-mail address: zulian@pediatria.unipd.it

positive ascertainment. Subsequently, the widespread use of nailfold capillary microscopy, more precise autoimmune serologic tests, and early detection of Raynaud's phenomenon in patients who, years later, developed systemic sclerosis, have shown the need for a more comprehensive classification.

Because of these issues and the lack of an acceptable classification for pediatric patients, a multicenter multinational project, sponsored by the Pediatric Rheumatology European Society (PRES), was organized to define nomenclature and criteria that allow the classification of homogeneous groups of patients with juvenile systemic sclerosis on the basis of clinical features and laboratory parameters. As a final step of this 3-year project, a consensus conference, including pediatric and adult rheumatologists and dermatologists, was convened in Padua, Italy, June 3 through 6, 2004. By using both Delphi and Nominal Group Technique methodologies, the preliminary classification criteria that define a patient as having juvenile systemic sclerosis were identified and are in the process of being validated (Box 1) [2].

Epidemiology

In general, systemic sclerosis has an estimated annual incidence from 0.45 to 1.9 per 100,000 and a prevalence of approximately 15 to 24 per 100,000 [3]. Onset in childhood is uncommon: children under 10 years account for fewer than 2% of all cases, and it has been estimated that fewer than 10% of all patients develop systemic sclerosis before the age of 20 years [4–7]. No racial predilection or peak age of onset has been determined for children [8]. More accurate epidemiologic data are lacking.

Etiology and pathogenesis

The cause of systemic sclerosis is unknown despite significant advances in the understanding of the pathogenetic mechanisms [9]. The disease can be represented as tripartite process in which dysfunction of the immune system, endothelium, and fibroblasts are mutually involved in a complex process characterized prominently by fibrosis.

Cellular immunity plays a major role in the initiation of scleroderma. This role is clearly indicated by the presence of mononuclear cell infiltrates in early lesions, altered function of T-helper and natural killer cells, and release of various cytokines, chemokines, and growth factors. The early infiltrates of mononuclear cells release several cytokines and chemokines that in turn have effects on both endothelial cells and fibroblasts. Several growth factors, such as transforming growth factor β (TGF-β) and connective tissue growth factor, have also been noted in scleroderma skin. They stimulate the synthesis of extracellular matrix components and promote fibrosis [10–13]. Several cytokines (interleukins [IL]-1, -2, -4, -6, -8, and -12) are increased in scleroderma serum or in scleroderma

---

Box 1. Preliminary criteria for the classification of juvenile systemic sclerosis

Major criteria

 Sclerosis/induration
 Sclerodactyly
 Raynaud's phenomenon

Minor criteria

 Vascular
  Nailfold capillaries changes
  Digital ulcers
 Gastrointestinal
  Dysphagia
  Gastroesophageal reflux
 Renal
  Renal crisis
  New-onset hypertension
 Cardiac
  Arrhythmias
  Heart failure
 Respiratory
  Pulmonary fibrosis (High-resolution CT/radiograph)
  Pulmonary diffusion (DLCO)
  Pulmonary hypertension
 Muskuloskeletal
  Tendon friction rubs
  Arthritis
  Myositis
 Neurologic
  Neuropathy
  Carpal tunnel syndrome
 Serologic
  Antinuclear antibodies
  Systemic sclerosis–specific antibodies (Scl-70, Anticentromere,
   PM-Scl)

---

skin (IL-4, -6, and -8) [14–17]. Specific cytokines such as tumor necrosis factor (TNF) promote fibrosis. Others, such as interferon-γ, are potent suppressors of collagen synthesis (Fig. 1).

 Evidence that endothelial cells are damaged is provided by the elevated levels of factor VIII–related antigen, reduced plasma angiotensin-converting enzyme

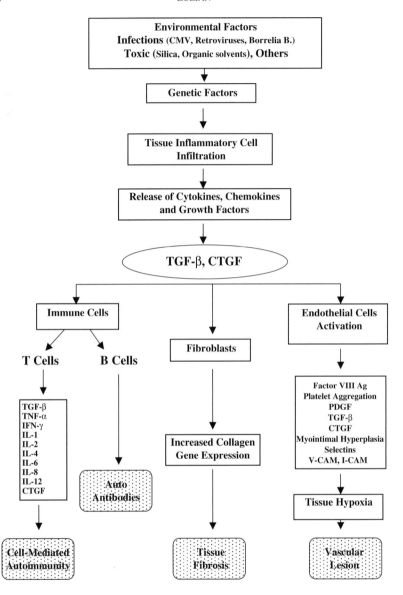

Fig. 1. Sequence of events involved in the onset of juvenile systemic sclerosis. CMV, human cytomegalovirus; CTGF, connective tissue growth factor; ICAM-1, intracellular adhesion molecule-1; IFN-γ, interferon-γ; PDGF, platelet-derived growth factor; VCAM-1, vascular cell adhesion molecule-1. (*Modified from* Jimenez SA, Derk CT. Following the molecular pathways toward an understanding of the pathogenesis of systemic sclerosis. Ann Intern Med 2004;160:37–50; with permission.)

(ACE) activity, and accelerated endothelial cell apoptosis [18–20]. The microvascular injury leads to arteriolar intimal fibrosis and narrowing of the vascular lumen, which results in ischemic damage.

Microchimerism, the presence in an individual of a very low level of cells derived from different individuals, was postulated as a possible cause of scleroderma. This hypothesis was considered because of the frequent occurrence of sclerodermatous skin involvement in patients with graft-versus-host disease. Although microchimerism can be identified in normal persons, chimeric cells are increased in number in patients with scleroderma and are more similar to the maternal cells than in normal persons [21,22]. These studies concluded that fetal antimaternal graft-versus-host reactions may play an important role in the pathogenesis of scleroderma [23].

Clinical features

Early signs and symptoms

The presenting signs and symptoms of juvenile systemic scleroderma are shown in Table 1. The onset is often characterized by the development of Raynaud's phenomenon and tightening, thinning, and atrophy of the skin of the hands and face [24–26]. There is often a diagnostic delay of years because of the subtle nature of this presentation and the insidious onset of cutaneous abnormalities [8,26–28].

Cutaneous changes characteristically evolve in a sequence beginning with edema, followed by induration and sclerosis resulting in marked tightening and contracture, and finally leading to atrophy. During the sclerotic phase, the skin becomes waxy in texture, tight, hard, and bound to subcutaneous structures. This phenomenon is particularly noticeable in skin of the digits and face; the characteristic expressionless appearance of the skin may be the first clue to diagnosis.

The long-term consequence of edema and sclerosis is atrophy of skin and adnexa accompanied by areas of hypopigmentation or hyperpigmentation and, often, by deposition of calcium salts in the subcutaneous tissues [29].

Table 1
Presenting signs and symptoms in children with systemic sclerosis

Signs and symptoms	% patients[a] (N = 164)
Skin tightening	84.4
Raynaud's phenomenon	72.4
Arthralgia	32.2
Muscle weakness and pain	17.1
Subcutaneous calcification	10.2
Dysphagia	15.5
Dyspnea	14.1

[a] Percentage calculated only on those series in which detailed information was provided.
Data from refs [8,24–29].

Telangiectases, characteristic signs of juvenile systemic sclerosis, are fine, macular dilatations of cutaneous or mucous-membrane blood vessels. The periungual nailfold is often the most obvious early location and on examination with an ophthalmoscope demonstrates capillary dropout, tortuous dilated loops, and, occasionally, distorted capillary architecture [30]. Digital pitting, sometimes with ulceration, occurs in the pulp of the fingertips as a result of ischemia.

Raynaud's phenomenon occurs in 80% to 90% of children and is often the initial symptom of the disorder, in some instances preceding other manifestations by years [31]. Raynaud's phenomenon is much more common in the fingers than elsewhere, but it can be observed in toes and, occasionally, ears, tip of the nose, lips, or tongue.

Musculoskeletal symptoms are common in juvenile systemic sclerosis and characteristically occur at or near the onset of the disease. Among the 127 children with juvenile systemic sclerosis included in the Padua International database of PRES, 36% had musculoskeletal symptoms during the course of the disease [8]. Arthralgia is usually mild and transient; joint contractures are most common at the proximal interphalangeal joints and elbows, but other joints are also affected. Muscle inflammation can occur in up to 38% of children and seems to be the characteristic feature of the overlapping presentation of the disease in children [32].

Upper gastrointestinal involvement is present in almost 40% of the patients during the course of the disease, and dysphagia may be one of the presenting signs in 14% of children [8]. Typically, dysphagia is caused by esophageal dysmotility and gastroesophageal reflux. Small bowel involvement develops in up to 50% of children, usually in association with esophageal or colonic disease [33]. Radiologic and functional studies of the gastrointestinal tract often demonstrate characteristic abnormalities even in the absence of symptoms. Manometry and intra-esophageal 24-hour pH monitoring provide more sensitive indicators of diminished lower sphincter tone and presence of reflux [34].

Cardiopulmonary disease, although uncommon at presentation, is a primary cause of morbidity among children with juvenile systemic sclerosis [26,35]. Cardiac fibrosis causes conduction defects, arrhythmias, and impaired ventricular function. Pericardial effusions are quite common but usually are not hemodynamically significant. Severe cardiomyopathy, although rare, can be one of the causes of early death in these patients and requires prompt and aggressive immunosuppressive treatment [35]. Cardiorespiratory complications are probably the greatest cause of juvenile systemic sclerosis–related death. Pulmonary involvement, although frequently asymptomatic, can manifest as dry, hacking cough or dyspnea on exertion [36]. Interstitial pulmonary fibrosis is a devastating complication but, unlike in adults, is rarely reported in children [8]. Pulmonary vascular disease can occur secondary to pulmonary fibrosis, but it is the isolated form of this complication, typically occurring in the limited variety of juvenile systemic sclerosis, that seems to have a much worse prognosis. High-resolution CT (HRCT) may reveal pulmonary disease even in the presence of a normal chest radiograph. In children, the most frequent HRCT findings are ground-glass opacification, subpleural micronodules, linear opacities, and honey combing [37,38]. Pulmonary diffusion (DLCO) and spirometry are sensitive measures of involvement of the respiratory tract. Echocardiography is important in confirming early pulmonary hypertension by documenting a dilated right ventricle and blood pressure in the pulmonary artery.

Few data on the prevalence of renal involvement in children are available, although children seem to have less kidney involvement than adults [25,26]. Among children included in the International Padua database, 9.4% had renal involvement, and only one developed renal crisis [6]. Although renal involvement can be indolent, the abrupt onset of accelerated hypertension with acute renal failure (scleroderma renal crisis) is the most feared complication.

The most frequently described central nervous system (CNS) abnormality is cranial nerve involvement. Peripheral neuropathies are uncommon ($\leq 1.6\%$). Clinical involvement of the CNS is usually secondary to renal or pulmonary disease [39].

Table 2 summarizes the prevalence of the involvement of organ systems during the course of the disease.

Laboratory findings

Anemia, although not common, is present in approximately one fourth of patients and is characteristic of the anemia of chronic disease. Less commonly, in case of chronic malabsorption, macrocytic anemia, reflecting vitamin B_{12} or folate deficiency, may occur. Microangiopathic hemolysis or bleeding from mu-

Table 2
Organ system involvement during the course of disease in children with systemic sclerosis

Organ system	No. observed[a]	Percentage
Skin		
Subcutaneous calcification	28/135	21
Ulcerations	57/133	43
Raynaud's phenomenon	115/141	82
Musculoskeletal system		
Arthritis/arthralgia	46/127	36
Muscle weakness	34/137	25
Gastrointestinal tract		
Abnormal oesophageal motility	51/135	38
Lungs		
Abnormal diffusion	47/89	53
Abnormal vital capacity	66/109	61
Heart		
Electrocardiographic abnormalities	9/139	7
Congestive heart failure	10/139	7

[a] Cumulative series from Martini G, Foeldvari I, Russo R, et al. Systematic scleroderma syndromes in children: clinical and immunological characteristics of 181 patients. Arthritis Rheum 2003:48(9):S512; and Cassidy JT, Sullivan DB, Dabich L, et al. Scleroderma in children. Arthritis Rheum 1977;20:351–4.

cosal telangiectases may also occur. Leukocytosis is not prominent but when present may correlate with advanced visceral or muscle disease. Synovial fluid contains increased protein content and polymorphonuclear leukocytosis. Pericardial fluid has the characteristics of an exudate.

Antinuclear antibodies (ANA) are frequently demonstrated in the sera of children with juvenile systemic sclerosis. The prevalence of ANA positivity in the Padua database was 80.8%, a frequency lower than reported in adults [8]. The prevalence of Scl-70 (anti-topoisomerase I) ranges from 20% to 30%, whereas anticentromere antibodies are much less common than in adults (approximately 7%) [8,32]. In adults, Scl-70 antibodies occur most frequently in patients with diffuse systemic sclerosis, in whom it is associated with peripheral vascular disease and pulmonary interstitial fibrosis [40]. Anticentromere antibodies occur almost exclusively in adult patients with limited systemic sclerosis in association with calcinosis, telangiectases, and the late development of pulmonary hypertension.

Management

The management of patients with juvenile systemic sclerosis presents one of the most difficult and frustrating challenges in pediatric rheumatology. None of the agents currently used as disease-modifying treatments for juvenile systemic sclerosis have undergone rigorous placebo-controlled evaluation.

Methotrexate, a proven effective drug for juvenile idiopathic arthritis, showed clinical benefit in adult systemic sclerosis as documented by skin score and pulmonary function [42]. Unfortunately, a substantially larger study from North America was negative [43]. Mycophenolate mofetil has recently been used for scleroderma. The apparent safety and tolerability of this drug makes it a potential choice as an immunodulatory drug for maintenance [44], but its role needs to be defined by controlled clinical trials.

Glucocorticoids are generally ineffective except during the early inflammatory stage of muscle involvement or in the edematous phase of the cutaneous disease [45]. Because higher doses seem to be associated with an increased frequency of renal crisis [46], their use should be accompanied by vigilant monitoring of the renal function.

Because TNFα antagonizes a number of profibrotic cytokines, including TGF-β1, it was postulated that its blockade would be beneficial in systemic sclerosis. A pilot study treating 10 patients with early diffuse systemic sclerosis suggests that treatment with soluble TNFα receptor (etanercept) is well tolerated, although conclusions about efficacy would be premature [47].

Autologous hemopoietic stem cell transplantation (HSCT) represents one of the most aggressive recent approaches to therapy for juvenile systemic sclerosis [48]. The rationale for this therapy is that ablation of self-reactive lymphocyte clones responsible of the autoimmune process may block pathogenesis of the disease. A multicenter study in adults reported that HSCT improved skin score in nearly 70% of patients, did not affect lung function, and halted pulmonary hypertension. Disease progression occurred in 19% of patients, however, and 17% died of complications related to the procedure [49]. The European Bone Marrow Transplantation/European League Against Rheumatism (EBMT/EULAR) registry has recently reported similar results. In this study, a durable clinical response was observed in two thirds of the patients. Treatment-related mortality was 9% [50]. Because of this mortality rate, HSCT must be considered carefully for systemic sclerosis patients, especially children.

During the last few years, the use of D-penicillamine has decreased. Several studies examining its effect in systemic sclerosis were either retrospective [51,52] or poorly controlled [53]. A carefully executed, double-blind RCT showed no difference between high-dose (750–1000 mg daily) and low-dose (125 mg on alternate days) regimens, certainly providing no justification for using high doses [54]. Although there are no controlled studies on the use of D-penicillamine in juvenile systemic sclerosis, it is a well-known antifibrotic agent and may still have a place in the treatment of this disease in combination with other anti-inflammatory or immunosuppressive agents.

Therapy of specific complications

Raynaud's phenomenon is difficult complication to treat. The most widely used vasodilator agents are the calcium channel blockers. Nifedipine is most widely recommended, although this priority may change as new agents are developed. In several controlled trials, nifedipine has been well tolerated, has reduced the frequency and severity of Raynaud's phenomenon, and promoted healing of cutaneous ischemic ulcers [55–57]. Intermittent infusions of prostacyclin or its analogues have been reported to be safe and effective in treatment of Raynaud's phenomenon and ischemic digits of children with juvenile systemic sclerosis and other connective tissue diseases [58]. Orally active formulations of prostacyclin or its analogues are an attractive alternative, but unfortunately two large studies from Europe and North America have failed to demonstrate efficacy [59,60].

In the past, renal involvement was the leading cause of mortality in patients with systemic sclerosis. ACE inhibitors (eg, captopril, quinapril) are useful in preventing vascular damage, providing effective long-term control of blood pressure, and stabilizing renal function [61–63].

Cyclophosphamide is used in treatment of scleroderma-associated pulmonary fibrosis. A number of retrospective series have suggested its efficacy and have delineated factors associated with responsiveness [41]. As in other disorders, the toxic side effects of cyclophosphamide, such as premature ovarian failure, opportunistic infections, and the possibility of late secondary malignancies, should be carefully balanced against efficacy. Following the experience in adults, it is common practice to combine cyclophosphamide (monthly intravenous infusions of 500–750 mg/m^2) with prednisone (0.3–0.5 mg/kg/day). Treatment is generally recommended for at least 6 to 9 months. Controlled trials comparing cyclophosphamide treatment with placebo are underway, and a recently reported open study was encouraging [64].

Continuous infusion of prostacyclin (or analogues such as epoprostenol) has been used with good results to treat pulmonary hypertension occurring in the context of established interstitial lung fibrosis or in limited systemic sclerosis [65,66]. Recently an endothelin-1 receptor antagonist, bosentan, was demonstrated to be safe and effective in the treatment of pulmonary hypertension [67]. The oral formulation and the potential use for other vascular complications are important factors for its use in juvenile systemic sclerosis.

Course of the disease and prognosis

Generally, the prognosis of juvenile systemic sclerosis is poor. Skin tightness and joint contractures inevitably lead to severe disability [68]. It has been reported that the skin may eventually soften years after onset of the disease. The most common causes of death in children are related to involvement of the cardiac, renal, and pulmonary systems. Arrhythmias may develop during the course of the disease secondary to myocardial fibrosis. Cardiomyopathy, although rare, can be one of the causes of early death, especially in children [35]. Interstitial lung disease and renal failure or acute hypertensive encephalopathy lead to potentially fatal outcomes in a few children and seem more likely to occur early in the course of the disease.

Survivorship has not been determined in any large series of children; because of the rarity of this disease, few retrospective data are available [6,69]. The mortality rate in adults, particularly under the age of 35 years, is significantly increased, and the extent of sclerosis of the skin seems to be an important determining factor in prognosis [70].

Juvenile localized scleroderma

Definition and classification

Juvenile localized scleroderma is a distinct entity from juvenile systemic sclerosis because of its almost exclusive cutaneous involvement and, with some exceptions, internal organs are not involved. The most widely used classification divides juvenile localized scleroderma into five general types: plaque morphea, generalized morphea, bullous morphea, linear scleroderma, and deep morphea (Box 2) [71]. Some conditions, such as atrophoderma of Pasini and Pierini, eosinophilic fasciitis, or lichen sclerosus and atrophicus, are classified among the subtypes of juvenile localized scleroderma, but their inclusion is still controversial. Indeed, this classification does not include the mixed forms of juvenile localized scleroderma in which different types of lesions occur in the same individual and which are probably more common than previously recognized. A multiphase project considering all these issues and sponsored by the PRES is developing new classification criteria for juvenile localized scleroderma [2].

Box 2. The Mayo Clinic classification of localized scleroderma

Plaque morphea
   Morphea en plaque
   Guttate morphea
   Atrophoderma of Pasini and Perini
   Keloid morphea
   [Lichen sclerosus et atrophicus]
Generalized morphea
Bullous morphea
Linear scleroderma
   Linear morphea
   En coup de sabre scleroderma
   Progressive hemifacial atrophy
Deep morphea
   Subcutaneous morphea
   Eosinophilic fasciitis
   Morphea profunda
   Disabling pansclerotic morphea

Epidemiology

Although localized scleroderma is relatively uncommon, it is far more common than systemic sclerosis in childhood, by a ratio of at least 10:1 [72,73]. Few adequate studies have addressed the incidence or prevalence of this disorder, which is believed to occur only in up to 1 per 100.000 of the population [73]. It has been reported that in pediatric rheumatology practice around 2% of the patients have localized scleroderma, that is approximately one case of localized scleroderma for every 20 cases of juvenile rheumatoid arthritis [74]. Many patients seen by dermatologists are never referred to rheumatologists because of the mild nature of their disease, however.

Etiology and pathogenesis

The causes and pathogenesis of the localized sclerodermas are unknown. As in systemic sclerosis, the focus of much investigation is on abnormalities of regulation of fibroblasts, production of collagen, and immunologic abnormalities. Autoimmunity, environmental factors, infection, and trauma have all been associated with localized disease. It seems certain that autoimmunity is an important etiologic factor, given the presence of abnormal serum antibodies in patients with localized scleroderma.

A number of drugs and environmental toxins, including bleomycin, ergot, bromocriptine, pentazocine, carbidopa, and vitamin K_1, have resulted in scleroderma-like reactions [75]. Although some studies have documented evidence of *Borrelia Burgdorferi* infection in patients with morphea [76], serologic testing for Lyme disease is not likely to be helpful in the evaluation of patients with juvenile localized scleroderma unless they have been in an endemic area [77].

Trauma has been implicated in initiation of lesions in 2.6% to 12.7% of the patients [78,79,116]. The mechanism by which a physical trauma may contribute to the development of scleroderma is unclear. Some authors have suggested a role for cytokines and neuropeptides such as endothelin-1 that normally are involved in the process of wound healing [78,80], but further studies are needed to elucidate the pathogenetic process fully.

A positive family history for rheumatic or autoimmune diseases was reported in approximately 12% of patients in two series [78,81].

Clinical features and subtypes of localized scleroderma

Plaque morphea is characterized by oval or round circumscribed areas of induration with a central waxy, ivory area surrounded by a violaceous halo (Fig. 2). It is confined to the dermis with only occasional involvement of the superficial panniculus. Depending on the shape and size of the lesions, various subtypes of plaque morphea have been described (guttate, keloid morphea, atrophoderma of Pasini and Pierini). The plaques may be of different sizes and evolve from an erythematous inflammatory stage through a sclerotic indurated phase with surrounding inflammation and subsequently to softening and dermal atrophy with associated hypopigmentation or hyperpigmentation. Atrophoderma of Pasini and Pierini, characterized by hyperpigmented atrophic patches with well-demarcated borders, may coexist with other sclerotic lesions or represent the involutionary phase of plaque morphea.

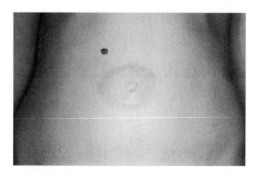

Fig. 2. Plaque morphea.

When individual plaques become confluent or multiply and affect three or more anatomic sites, the condition is called generalized morphea.

In the rare subtype of bullous morphea, lesions are probably related to lymphatic obstruction secondary to the sclerodermatous process [82].

Linear scleroderma is the most common subtype in children and adolescents [73]. It is characterized by one or more linear streaks that typically involve an upper or lower extremity (Fig. 3). With time, the streaks can extend through the dermis, subcutaneous tissue, and muscle to the underlying bone causing significant deformities.

When a linear lesion involves the face or scalp, it is referred to as en coup de sabre scleroderma because the lesion is reminiscent of the depression caused by a dueling stroke from a sword (Fig. 4).

Parry–Romberg syndrome (PRS) is characterized by hemifacial atrophy of the skin and tissue below the forehead, with greater involvement of the lower face than in en coup de saber scleroderma and relatively minor involvement of the superficial skin. PRS probably represents the severe end of the spectrum of en coup de saber scleroderma, because some cases of PRS have definite localized scleroderma lesions on the face and in the other parts of the body [83]. Also, much like PRS, some typical localized scleroderma lesions present no evidence of inflammation and sclerosis preceding the severe atrophy on the limbs [84,85].

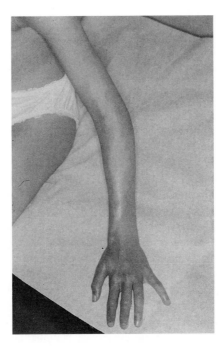

Fig. 3. Linear scleroderma.

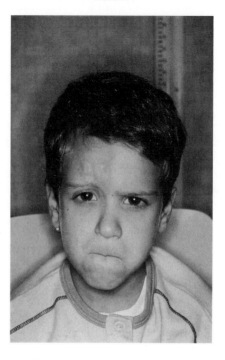

Fig. 4. En coup de sabre scleroderma.

A number of associated disorders, including seizures, uveitis, and dental and ocular abnormalities, have been reported in both conditions,.

Deep morphea is the least common but most disabling variant and includes subcutaneous morphea, eosinophilic fasciitis, morphea profunda, and disabling pansclerotic morphea of children.

In subcutaneous morphea, the primary site of involvement is the panniculus or subcutaneous tissue [86]. The plaques are hyperpigmented, symmetric, and somewhat ill defined.

In morphea profunda, the entire skin feels thickened, taut, and bound down, sometimes with the appearance of a solitary, indurated plaque [87,88]. Disabling pansclerotic morphea, an extremely rare but severe disorder, is characterized by generalized full-thickness involvement of the skin of the trunk, extremities, face, and scalp with sparing of the fingertips and toes (Fig. 5) [89]. In eosinophilic fasciitis, lesions typically involve the extremities but spare the hands and feet and have a peau d'orange appearance [90,91]. Reports of combined syndrome of fasciitis and morphea and histologic changes similar to eosinophilic fasciitis found in some subtypes of localized scleroderma seem to strength the hypothesis that this disorder may be a subtype of juvenile localized scleroderma [92]. Conversely, the characteristic cutaneous features such as pitting edema, diffuse painful areas with peau d'orange appearance, increased serum acute-phase

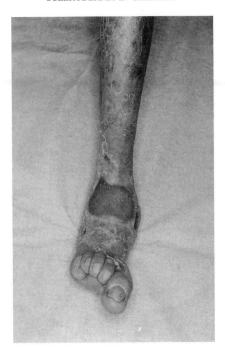

Fig. 5. Pansclerotic morphea.

reactants, peripheral blood eosinophilia, and hypergammaglobulinemia may suggest a separate nosologic classification.

Extracutaneous involvement

During the last decade, the publication of some case reports on possible transition from localized to systemic scleroderma and of case series of patients with localized scleroderma and internal organ involvement [93,94] have raised suspicions that systemic sclerosis and localized scleroderma are not always clearly distinct.

Approximately one fourth of patients with juvenile localized scleroderma have been reported as having one or more extracutaneous manifestations during the course of the disease [93–95]. Articular involvement is the most frequently reported complication of juvenile localized scleroderma, accounting for almost one half of the reported extracutaneous manifestations especially in the linear subtype [95]. Sometimes arthritis is completely unrelated to the site of the skin lesion.

Epilepsy and recent-onset headache are the most frequent reported neurologic involvements [88–99], but behavioral changes and learning disabilities have also been described [100,101]. Other abnormalities on MRI such as calcifications and white matter changes, vascular malformations, and even CNS vasculitis have been reported [102–105].

Ocular changes are almost exclusively reported in linear scleroderma involving the face. They include eyelid or eyelash abnormalities, inflammatory changes such as uveitis, episcleritis, keratitis, glaucoma, and xerophthalmia, and motility disorders [105–110].

Gastroesophageal reflux has been reported in adults and children with localized scleroderma [93,95,111,112]. Respiratory involvement, consisting of restrictive changes with mildly decreased respiratory volume and impaired DLCO, was reported [94,95,113].

Systemic manifestations are rarely observed in localized scleroderma, although internal organ involvement is frequently found when searched for systematically. These extracutaneous manifestations, usually mild, may suggest that localized scleroderma and systemic sclerosis represent two ends of a continuous spectrum of disease.

Single-case reports have reported a transition from localized scleroderma to systemic sclerosis in children [114,115]. In adults this evolution has been reported in 0.9% and 1.3% of the patients [94,116]; it is reported more rarely in children (0.13%) [95].

Considering this low prevalence of transition to systemic sclerosis and the lack of prospective follow-up studies, a practical suggestion could be to investigate for eye and CNS complications in patients with head involvement (en coup de saber scleroderma or PRS) and to look for internal organ involvement in other patients with juvenile localized scleroderma only if they are symptomatic.

Laboratory results

The diagnosis of localized scleroderma is established by the clinical picture, sometimes aided by biopsy of skin or subcutaneous tissues. The erythrocyte sedimentation rate may be increased in the subtypes of the disease with active inflammation, such as eosinophilic fasciitis. Eosinophilia and hypergamma-globulinemia are hallmarks of this disorder but also may occur in linear scleroderma and the other deep subtypes. Rheumatoid factor is present in 25% to 40% of patients [81,117,118], and higher titers are usually associated with more severe cutaneous and articular involvement [114].

ANA can be present in any of the morphea subtypes with a frequency ranging from 23% to 73% [81,119]. ANAs were found in 34% to 50% of patients with plaque morphea, 31% to 100% of those with generalized morphea, and 47% to 67% of those with linear scleroderma [81,120]. Anti-Scl70 antibodies, a marker of systemic sclerosis in adults, were positive in 2% to 3% patients. [81,121,122]

Anticardiolipin antibodies have recently been shown to be present in adults with localized scleroderma with an overall prevalence of 46% that increases to 70% in patients with generalized forms [123]. In children this prevalence falls

Table 3
Role of thermography in juvenile localized scleroderma

Advantages	Disadvantages
Noninvasive	Expensive to set up
Well tolerated	False positivity
Easy interpretation	Atrophy, old lesions, site (ie, scalp)
Possible computerized quantitation	
Rapid results, helpful in decision-making	
Prediction of progress (?)	

to 13%, and, in contrast to adults, the presence of anticardiolipin antibodies is not associated with thromboembolic events or clotting abnormalities [81].

Antihistone antibodies seem to be associated with more extensive localized disease [123]. Serum concentrations of soluble IL-2 receptor have been noted to be increased in localized scleroderma and may differentiate active from inactive disease [124], although this finding is not supported by all studies [78].

Thermography shows promise when associated with clinical examination in discriminating disease activity. Table 3 summarizes the advantages and disadvantages of this methodology. This technique has high reproducibility, but it remains to be seen whether it truly will predict outcome and subclinical areas likely to progress to serious disease [125,126].

The application of newer imaging techniques such as MRI and ultrasound also shows promise in supporting clinical management and greater understanding of disease characteristics. MRI is most useful when CNS or eye involvement is suspected but can demonstrate the true depth of soft tissue lesions and the degree to which different tissues are involved in other sites. In addition, early in lesion development MRI may provide supporting evidence that true inflammation is occurring in tissue thought to be undergoing spontaneous atrophy [127]. High-frequency ultrasound has shown similar promise [128,129]. Table 4 summarizes the advantages and disadvantages of the two different ultrasound modalities, 13- and 20-Mhz probes, used in the management of localized scleroderma.

Table 4
Comparison of 20- and 13-MHz ultrasound probes in the management of localized scleroderma

13-MHz ultrasound		20-MHz ultrasound	
Advantages	Disadvantages	Advantages	Disadvantages
Noninvasive	Difficult in overweight patients	Noninvasive	Penetration depth 7 mm
Good sensitivity and specificity	Worse image definition	Higher resolution = better quality images	
Cost-effective		Clear identification of pathological skin structures	
Penetration depth 60 mm		Useful to evaluate the evolution of sclerotic plaques	

Treatment

Therapy for juvenile localized scleroderma is as challenging as therapy for juvenile systemic sclerosis. The literature contains many case reports or case series, but few controlled trials have been published. Indeed, management decisions must be based on the understanding that these disorders are benign in the many patients and often spontaneously enter remission after 3 to 5 years [116,130].

Morphea en plaque generally is of cosmetic concern only, and therefore treatments with potentially significant toxicity are not justified. In general, these lesions remit spontaneously with residual pigmentation as the only abnormality. Therefore, treatment should be directed mainly at topical therapies such as moisturizing agents, topical glucocorticoids, or calcipotriene [131].

When there is a significant risk for disability, such as in linear scleroderma and the deep subtypes, systemic treatment should be considered. Methotrexate has been used successfully in children with localized scleroderma [132,133]. Unfortunately, these studies were not controlled trials, and the series of treated patients were very small. In adults, a recent well-conducted multicenter randomized, controlled trial in patients with early diffuse systemic sclerosis confirmed that methotrexate is effective in reducing the skin involvement, especially during the first 6 months of treatment [134].

During the last few years, the use of D-penicillamine, a proven antifibrotic agent [135,136], has decreased without clear evidence of lack of efficacy. D-penicillamine has been used successfully for the treatment of localized scleroderma in adults [137]. Although there are no controlled studies on the use of D-penicillamine in the treatment of children with localized scleroderma, it is a well-known antifibrotic agent and may still have a place in the treatment of this disease.

In a well-designed randomized, controlled drug trial, use of the intralesional cytokine interferon-γ proved no better than placebo for established lesions; however, it may prevent the appearance of new lesions [138]. The use of UV light therapy, with or without chemical agents such as psoralen, has been reported in a number of recent studies with suggestions of clinical benefit. It may be much more effective for localized or superficial lesions [139,140]. Extracorporeal photochemotherapy (with UVA and psoralen) has been reported in localized scleroderma, but the evidence to support its usefulness is still relatively weak [141–143]. Topical or systemic use of vitamin D or its analogue has been reported in several case series, again with encouraging results [144–146]; in the only controlled trial, however, it was no more effective than placebo [147].

It is clear that multicenter randomized, controlled trials are needed to evaluate the efficacy of these or other new agents for the treatment of juvenile localized scleroderma by using uniform diagnostic criteria and validated outcome measures.

Physical and occupational therapy usually have a major role in the management of juvenile localized scleroderma, particularly when joint structures are involved. Surgical reconstruction may be considered, usually after the active phase of the disease has abated, and the child's growth is complete [148,149].

References

[1] The American Rheumatism Association Diagnostic and Therapeutic Criteria Committee, Subcommittee for Scleroderma Criteria. Preliminary criteria for the classification of systemic sclerosis (scleroderma). Arthritis Rheum 1980;23:581–90.

[2] Zulian F, Ruperto N, editors. Proceedings of the Second Workshop on Juvenile Scleroderma Syndrome. Padua, Italy, June 3–6, 2004.

[3] Mayes MD. Scleroderma epidemiology. Rheum Dis Clin North Am 2003;29:239–54.

[4] Tuffanelli DL, LaPerriere R. Connective tissue diseases. Pediatr Clin North Am 1971;18: 925–51.

[5] Kornreich HK, King KK, Bernstein BH, et al. Scleroderma in childhood. Arthritis Rheum 1977;20:343–50.

[6] Medsger Jr TA. Epidemiology of systemic sclerosis. Clin Dermatol 1994;12:207–16.

[7] Black CM. Scleroderma in children. Adv Exp Med Biol 1999;455:35–48.

[8] Martini G, Foeldvari I, Russo R, et al. Systemic scleroderma syndromes in children: clinical and immunological characteristics of 181 patients. Arthritis Rheum 2003;48(9):S512.

[9] Jimenez SA, Derk CT. Following the molecular pathways toward an understanding of the pathogenesis of systemic sclerosis. Ann Intern Med 2004;140:37–50.

[10] Abraham DJ, Shiwen X, Black CM, et al. Tumor necrosis factor alpha suppresses the induction of connective tissue growth factor by transforming growth factor-beta in normal and scleroderma fibroblasts. J Biol Chem 2000;275:15220–5.

[11] Varga J, Rosenbloom J, Jimenez SA. Transforming growth factor beta (TGF beta) causes a persistent increase in steady-state amounts of type I and type III collagen and fibronectin mRNAs in normal human dermal fibroblasts. Biochem J 1987;247:597–604.

[12] Stratton R, Shiwen X, Martini G, et al. Iloprost suppresses connective tissue growth factor production in fibroblasts and in the skin of scleroderma patients. J Clin Invest 2001; 108:241–50.

[13] Gore-Hyer E, Pannu J, Smith EA, et al. Selective stimulation of collagen synthesis in the presence of costimulatory insulin signaling by connective tissue growth factor in scleroderma fibroblasts. Arthritis Rheum 2003;48:798–806.

[14] Needleman BW, Wigley FM, Stair RW. Interleukin-1, interleukin-2, interleukin-4, interleukin-6, tumor necrosis factor alpha, and interferon-gamma levels in sera from patients with scleroderma. Arthritis Rheum 1992;35:67–72.

[15] Hasegawa M, Sato S, Ihn H, et al. Enhanced production of interleukin-6 (IL-6), oncostatin M and soluble IL-6 receptor by cultured peripheral blood mononuclear cells from patients with systemic sclerosis. Rheumatology (Oxford) 1999;38:612–7.

[16] Atamas SP, Yurovsky VV, Wise R, et al. Production of type 2 cytokines by CD8 + lung cells is associated with greater decline in pulmonary function in patients with systemic sclerosis. Arthritis Rheum 1999;42:1168–78.

[17] Sato S, Hanakawa H, Hasegawa M, et al. Levels of interleukin 12, a cytokine of type 1 helper T cells, are elevated in sera from patients with systemic sclerosis. J Rheumatol 2000;27: 2838–42.

[18] Matucci-Cerinic M, Pignone A, Lotti T, et al. Reduced angiotensin converting enzyme plasma activity in scleroderma. A marker of endothelial injury? J Rheumatol 1990;17:328–30.

[19] Kahaleh MB, Osborn I, LeRoy EC. Increased factor VIII/von Willebrand factor antigen and von Willebrand factor activity in scleroderma and in Raynaud's phenomenon. Ann Intern Med 1981;94:482–4.

[20] Sgonc R, Gruschwitz MS, Dietrich H, et al. Endothelial cell apoptosis is a primary pathogenetic event underlying skin lesions in avian and human scleroderma. J Clin Invest 1996;98:785–92.

[21] Ohtsuka T, Miyamoto Y, Yamakage A, et al. Quantitative analysis of microchimerism in systemic sclerosis skin tissue. Arch Dermatol Res 2001;293:387–91.

[22] Nelson JL, Furst DE, Maloney S, et al. Microchimerism and HLA-compatible relationships of pregnancy in scleroderma. Lancet 1998;351:559–62.

[23] Artlett CM, Smith JB, Jimenez SA. Identification of fetal DNA and cells in skin lesions from women with systemic sclerosis. N Engl J Med 1998;338:1186–91.

[24] Goel KM, Shanks RA. Scleroderma in childhood. Report of 5 cases. Arch Dis Child 1974; 49:861–6.

[25] Jaffe MO, Winkelmann RK. Generalized scleroderma in children. Acrosclerotic type. Arch Dermatol 1961;83:402.

[26] Cassidy JT, Sullivan DB, Dabich L, et al. Scleroderma in children. Arthritis Rheum 1977; 20:351–4.

[27] Suarez-Almazor ME, Catoggio LJ, Maldonado-Cocco JA, et al. Juvenile progressive systemic sclerosis: Clinical and serologic findings. Arthritis Rheum 1985;28:699–702.

[28] Hanson V. Dermatomyositis, scleroderma, and polyarteritis nodosa. Clin Rheumat Dis 1976; 2:445.

[29] Lababidi HM, Nasr FW, Khatib Z. Juvenile progressive systemic sclerosis: report of five cases. J Rheumatol 1991;18:885–8.

[30] Spencer-Green G, Schlesinger M, Bove KE, et al. Nailfold capillary abnormalities in childhood rheumatic diseases. J Pediatr 1983;102:341–6.

[31] Duffy CM, Laxer RM, Lee P, et al. Raynaud syndrome in childhood. J Pediatr 1989;114:73–8.

[32] Arkachaisri T, Scalapini T, Fertig N, et al. Comparison of clinical and serological findings in childhood and adult onset systemic sclerosis. Arthritis Rheum 2004;50(9):S686–7.

[33] D'Angelo WA, Fries JF, Masi AT, et al. Pathologic observations in systemic sclerosis (scleroderma). A study of fifty-eight autopsy cases and fifty-eight matched controls. Am J Med 1969; 46:428–40.

[34] Weber P, Ganser G, Frosch M, et al. Twenty-four hour intraesophageal pH monitoring in children and adolescents with scleroderma and mixed connective tissue disease. J Rheumatol 2000;27:2692–5.

[35] Quartier P, Bonnet D, Fournet JC, et al. Severe cardiac involvement in children with systemic sclerosis and myositis. J Rheumatol 2002;29:1767–73.

[36] Eid NS, Buchino JJ, Schikler KN. Pulmonary manifestations of rheumatic diseases. Pediatr Pulmonol Suppl 1999;18:91–2.

[37] Koh DM, Hansell DM. Computed tomography of diffuse interstitial lung disease in children. Clin Radiol 2000;55:659–67.

[38] Seely JM, Jones LT, Wallace C, et al. Systemic sclerosis: using high-resolution CT to detect lung disease in children. Am J Roentgenol 1998;170(3):691–7.

[39] Lee P, Bruni J, Sukenik S. Neurological manifestations in systemic sclerosis (scleroderma). J Rheumatol 1984;11:480–3.

[40] Sato S, Hamaguchi Y, Hasegawa M, et al. Clinical significance of anti-topoisomerase I antibody levels determined by ELISA in systemic sclerosis. Rheumatology (Oxford) 2001;40:1135–40.

[41] Steen VD, Lanz Jr JK, Conte C, et al. Therapy for severe interstitial lung disease in systemic sclerosis. A retrospective study. Arthritis Rheum 1994;37:1290–6.

[42] van den Hoogen FH, Boerbooms AM, Swaak AJ, et al. Comparison of methotrexate with placebo in the treatment of systemic sclerosis: a 24 week randomized double-blind trial, followed by a 24 week observational trial. Br J Rheumatol 1996;35:364–72.

[43] Pope JE, Bellamy N, Seibold JR, et al. A randomized, controlled trial of methotrexate versus placebo in early diffuse scleroderma. Arthritis Rheum 2001;44:1351–8.

[44] Stratton RJ, Wilson H, Black CM. Pilot study of anti-thymocyte globulin plus mycophenolate mofetil in recent-onset diffuse scleroderma. Rheumatology (Oxford) 2001;40:84–8.

[45] Clements PJ, Furst DE, Campion DS, et al. Muscle disease in progressive systemic sclerosis: Diagnostic and therapeutic considerations. Arthritis Rheum 1978;21:62–71.

[46] Steen VD, Medsger Jr TA. Case-control study of corticosteroids and other drugs that either precipitate or protect from the development of scleroderma renal crisis. Arthritis Rheum 1998;41:1613–9.

[47] Ellman MH, MacDonald PA, Hayes FA. Etanercept as treatment for diffuse scleroderma: a pilot study [abstract]. Arthritis Rheum 2000;43:S392.

[48] Wulffraat NM, Sanders LA, Kuis W. Autologous hemopoietic stem-cell transplantation for children with refractory autoimmune disease. Curr Rheumatol Rep 2000;2:316–23.

[49] Binks M, Passweg JR, Furst D, et al. Phase I/II trial of autologous stem cell transplantation in systemic sclerosis: procedure related mortality and impact on skin disease. Ann Rheum Dis 2001;60:577–84.

[50] Farge D, Passweg J, van Laar J, et al. Autologous stem cell transplantation in the treatment of systemic sclerosis: report from the EBMT/EULAR Registry. Ann Rheum Dis 2004;63(8): 974–81.

[51] Jayson MIV, Lovell C, Black CM, et al. Penicillamine therapy in systemic sclerosis. Proc R Soc Med 1977;70(Suppl 3):82–8.

[52] Steen VD, Medsger Jr TA, Rodnan GP. D-penicillamine therapy in progressive systemic sclerosis: a retrospective analysis. Ann Intern Med 1982;97:652–9.

[53] Jimenez SA, Sigal SH. A 15-year prospective study of treatment of rapidly progressive systemic sclerosis with D-penicillamine. J Rheumatol 1991;18:1496–503.

[54] Clements PJ, Furst DE, Wong WK, et al. High-dose versus low-dose D-penicillamine in early diffuse systemic sclerosis: analysis of a two-year, double blind, randomized, controlled clinical trial. Arthritis Rheum 1999;42:1194–203.

[55] Smith CD, McKendry RJ. Controlled trial of nifedipine in the treatment of Raynaud's phenomenon. Lancet 1982;2:1299–301.

[56] Rodeheffer RJ, Rommer JA, Wigley F, et al. Controlled double-blind trial of nifedipine in the treatment of Raynaud's phenomenon. N Engl J Med 1983;308:880–3.

[57] Sauza J, Kraus A, Gonzalez-Amaro R, et al. Effect of the calcium channel blocker nifedipine on Raynaud's phenomenon. A controlled double blind trial. J Rheumatol 1984;11:362–4.

[58] Zulian F, Corona F, Gerloni V, et al. Safety and efficacy of iloprost for the treatment of ischaemic digits in paediatric connective tissue diseases. Rheumatology (Oxford) 2004;43: 229–33.

[59] Black CM, Halkier-Sorensen L, Belch JJ, et al. Oral iloprost in Raynaud's phenomenon secondary to systemic sclerosis: a multicentre, placebo-controlled, dose-comparison study. Br J Rheumatol 1998;37:952–60.

[60] Wigley FM, Korn JH, Csuka ME, et al. Oral iloprost treatment in patients with Raynaud's phenomenon secondary to systemic sclerosis: a multicenter, placebo-controlled, double-blind study. Arthritis Rheum 1998;41:670–7.

[61] Beckett VL, Donadio Jr JV, Brennan Jr LA, et al. Use of captopril as early therapy for renal scleroderma: a prospective study. Mayo Clin Proc 1985;60:763–71.

[62] Steen VD, Costantino JP, Shapiro AP, et al. Outcome of renal crisis in systemic sclerosis: relation to availability of angiotensin converting enzyme (ACE) inhibitors. Ann Intern Med 1990;113:352–7.

[63] Moddison P. Prevention of vascular damage in scleroderma with angiotensin-converting enzyme (ACE) inhibition. Rheumatology (Oxford) 2002;41:965–71.

[64] White B, Moore WC, Wigley FM, et al. Cyclophosphamide is associated with pulmonary function and survival benefit in patients with scleroderma and alveolitis. Ann Intern Med 2000;132:947–54.

[65] Kuhn KP, Byrne DW, Arbogast PG, et al. Outcome in 91 consecutive patients with pulmonary arterial hypertension receiving epoprostenol. Am J Respir Crit Care Med 2003;167:580–6.

[66] Badesch DB, Tapson VF, McGoon MD, et al. Continuous intravenous epoprostenol for pulmonary hypertension due to the scleroderma spectrum of disease. A randomized, controlled trial. Ann Intern Med 2000;132:425–34.

[67] Rubin LJ, Badesch DB, Barst RJ, et al. Bosentan therapy for pulmonary arterial hypertension. N Engl J Med 2002;346:896–903.

[68] Bottoni CR, Reinker KA, Gardner RD, et al. Scleroderma in childhood: a 35-year history of cases and review of the literature. J Pediatr Orthop 2000;20:442–9.

[69] Foeldvari I, Zhavania M, Birdi N, et al. Favourable outcome in 135 children with juvenile systemic sclerosis: results of a multi-national survey. Rheumatology (Oxford) 2000;39:556–9.

[70] Jacobsen S, Halberg P, Ullman S. Mortality and causes of death of 344 Danish patients with systemic sclerosis. Br J Rheumatol 1998;37:750–5.

[71] Peterson LS, Nelson AM, Su WPD. Subspecialty clinics: rheumatology and dermatology. Classification of morphea (localized scleroderma). Mayo Clin Proc 1995;70:1068–76.

[72] Bodemer C, Belon M, et al. Scleroderma in children: a retrospective study of 70 cases. Ann Dermatol Venereol 1999;126:691–4.

[73] Peterson LS, Nelson AM, Su WP, et al. The epidemiology of morphea (localized scleroderma) in Olmsted County 1960–1993. J Rheumatol 1997;24:73–80.

[74] Levinson JE, Bove KE. Scleroderma. In: Gershwin ME, Robbins DE, editors. Musculoskeletal diseases of children. Orlando (FL): Grune & Stratton; 1983. p. 195–208.

[75] Haustein UF, Haupt B. Drug-induced scleroderma and sclerodermiform conditions. Clin Dermatol 1998;16:353–66.

[76] Aberer E, Neumann R, Stanek G. Is localised scleroderma a Borrelia infection? Lancet 1985; 2:278.

[77] Fan W, Leonardi CL, Penneys NS. Absence of Borrelia burgdorferi in patients with localized scleroderma (morphea). J Am Acad Dermatol 1995;33:682–4.

[78] Vancheeswaran R, Black CM, David J, et al. Childhood onset scleroderma: is it different from adult onset disease? Arthritis Rheum 1996;39:1041–9.

[79] Falanga V, Medsger TA, Reichlin M, et al. Linear scleroderma: clinical spectrum, prognosis and laboratory abnormalities. Ann Intern Med 1986;104:849–57.

[80] Kanzler MH, Gorsulowsky DC, Swanson NA. Basic mechanisms in the healing of cutaneous wound. J Dermatol Surg Oncol 1986;12:1156–64.

[81] Zulian F, De Oliveira SKF, Lehman TH, et al. Juvenile localized scleroderma: clinical epidemiological features of 688 patients [abstract]. Arthritis Rheum 2003;48(9):512.

[82] Daoud MS, Su WP, Leiferman KM, et al. Bullous morphea: clinical, pathologic, and immunopathologic evaluation of thirteen cases. J Am Acad Dermatol 1994;30:937–43.

[83] Menni S, Marzano AV, Passoni E. Neurologic abnormalities in two patients with facial hemiathrophy and sclerosis coexisting with morphea. Pediatr Dermatol 1997;14:113–6.

[84] Blaszczyk M, Jablonska S. Linear scleroderma en coup de sabre: relationship with progressive facial hemiatrophy. Adv Exp Med Biol 1999;455:101–4.

[85] Lehman TJ. The Parry Romberg syndrome of progressive facial herniathrophy and linear scleroderma en cop de sabre: mistaken diagnosis or overlapping conditions? J Rheumatol 1992; 19:844–5.

[86] Person JR, Su WP. Subcutaneous morphoea: a clinical study of sixteen cases. Br J Dermatol 1979;100:371–80.

[87] Su WP, Person JR. Morphea profunda: a new concept and a histopathologic study of 23 cases. Am J Dermatopathol 1981;3:251–60.

[88] Whittaker SJ, Smith NP, Jones RR. Solitary morphoea profunda. Br J Dermatol 1989;120: 431–40.

[89] Diaz-Perez JL, Connolly SM, Winkelmann RK. Disabling pansclerotic morphea in children. Arch Dermatol 1980;116:169–73.

[90] Shulman LE. Diffuse fasciitis with eosinophilia: a new syndrome? Trans Assoc Am Physicians 1975;88:70–86.

[91] Rodnan GP, Di Bartolomeo A, Medsgar Jr TA. Eosinophilic fasciitis. Report of six cases of a newly recognized scleroderma-like syndrome. Arthritis Rheum 1975;18:525.

[92] Miller III JJ. The fasciitis-morphea complex in children. Am J Dis Child 1992;146:733–6.

[93] Lunderschmidt C, König G, Leisner B, et al. Zirkumskripte sklerodermie: interne manifestationen und signifikante correlation zu HLA-DR1 und –DR5. Hautarzt 1985;36:516–21.

[94] Dehen L, Roujeau JC, Cosnes A, et al. Internal involvement in localized scleroderma. Medicine 1994;73:241–5.

[95] Zulian F, Russo R, Laxer R, et al. Is juvenile localized scleroderma really "localized"? [abstract]. Arthritis Rheum 2003;48(9):512.

[96] Heron E, Hernigou A, Fornes P, et al. Central nervous system involvement in scleroderma. Ann Med Interne (Paris) 2002;153(3):179–82.

[97] Blaszczyk M, Krolicki L, Krasu M, et al. Progressive facial hemiatrophy: central nervous system involvement and relationship with scleroderma *en coup de sabre*. J Rheumatol 2003; 30:1997–2004.

[98] Grosso S, Fioravanti A, Biasi G, et al. Linear scleroderma associated with progressive brain atrophy. Brain Dev 2003;25:57–61.

[99] Woolfenden AR, Tong DC, Norbash AM, et al. Progressive facial hemiatrophy: abnormality of intracranial vasculature. Neurology 1998;50(6):1915–7.

[100] David J, Wilson J, Woo P. Scleroderma *"en coup de saber"*. Ann Rheum Dis 1991;50:260–2.

[101] Goldberg-Stern H, deGrauw T, Passo M, et al. Parry-Romberg syndrome: follow-up imaging during suppressive therapy. Neuroradiology 1997;39(12):873–6.

[102] Flores-Alvarado DE, Esquivel-Valerio JA, Garza-Elizondo M, et al. Linear scleroderma *en coup de sabre* and brain calcifications: is there a pathogenic relationship? J Rheumatol 2003;30: 193–5.

[103] Higashi Y, Kanekura T, Fukumaru K, et al. Scleroderma *en coup de sabre* with central nervous system involvement. J Dermatol 2000;27(7):486–8.

[104] Luer W, Jockel D, Henze T, et al. Progressive inflammatory lesions of the brain parenchyma in localized scleroderma of the head. J Neurol 1990;237:379–81.

[105] Miedziak AI, Stefanyszyn M, Flamagan J, et al. Parry-Romberg syndrome associated with intracranial vascular malformations. Arch Ophthalmol 1998;116:1235–7.

[106] Goldenstein-Schainberg C, Pereira RM, Gusukuma MC, et al. Childhood linear scleroderma "en coup de sabre" with uveitis. J Pediatr 1990;117:581–4.

[107] Serup J, Alsbirk PH. Localized scleroderma "en coup de sabre" and iridopalpebral atrophy at the same line. Acta Derm Venereol 1983;63:75–7.

[108] Campbell WW, Bajandas FJ. Restrictive ophthalmopathy associated with linear scleroderma. J Neuroophthalmol 1995;15:95–7.

[109] Tang RA, Mewis-Christmann L, Wolf J, et al. Pseudo-oculomotor palsy as the presenting sign of linear scleroderma. J Pediatr Ophthalmol Strabismus 1986;23:236–8.

[110] Suttorp-Schulten MS, Koornneef L. Linear scleroderma associated with ptosis and motility disorders. Br J Ophthalmol 1990;74:694–5.

[111] Zaninotto G, Peserico A, Costantini M, et al. Oesophageal motility and lower oesophageal sphincter competence in progressive systemic sclerosis and localized scleroderma. Scand J Gastroenterol 1989;24:95–102.

[112] Weber P, Ganser G, Frosh M, et al. Twenty-four hour intraesophageal pH monitoring in children and adolescents with scleroderma and mixed connective tissue disease. J Rheumatol 2000; 27:2692–5.

[113] Bourgeois-Droin C, Touraine R. Sclérodermie en plaque: Perturbations immunologique et viscérales. Ann Med Interne (Paris) 1978;129:107–12.

[114] Birdi N, Laxer RM, Thorner P, et al. Localized scleroderma progressing to systemic disease. Case report and review of the literature. Arthritis Rheum 1993;36:410–5.

[115] Mayorquin FJ, McCurley TL, Levernier JE, et al. Progression of childhood linear scleroderma to fatal systemic sclerosis. J Rheumatol 1994;21:1955–7.

[116] Christianson HB, Dorsey CS, O'Leary PA, et al. Localized scleroderma. A clinical study of two hundred thirty-five cases. Arch Dermatol 1956;74:629–39.

[117] Kornreich HK, King KK, Bernstein BH, et al. Scleroderma in childhood. Arthritis Rheum 1977;20(Suppl 2):343–50.

[118] Torok E, Ablonczy E. Morphoea in children. Clin Exp Dermatol 1986;11:607–12.

[119] Uziel Y, Krafchik BR, Silverman ED, et al. Localized scleroderma in childhood: a report of 30 cases. Semin Arthritis Rheum 1994;23:328–40.

[120] Takehara K, Moroi Y, Nakabayashi Y, et al. Antinuclear antibodies in localized scleroderma. Arthritis Rheum 1983;26:612–6.

[121] Blaszczyk M, Jarzabek-Chorleska M, Jablonska S. Relationship between cutaneous and systemic scleroderma. Are immunopathological studies helpful in evaluating transition of cutaneous to systemic scleroderma? Przegl Dermatol 2000;2:119–25.

[122] Marzano AV, Menni S, et al. Localized scleroderma in adults and children. Clinical and laborator investigations on 239 cases. Eur J Dermatol 2003;13:171–6.

[123] Sato S, Fujimoto M, Hasegawa M, et al. Antiphospholipid antibody in localized scleroderma. Ann Rheum Dis 2003;62:771–4.

[124] Uziel Y, Krafchik BR, Feldman B, et al. Serum levels of soluble interleukin-2 receptor. A marker of disease activity in localized scleroderma. Arthritis Rheum 1994;37:898–901.

[125] Martini G, Murray KJ, Howell KJ, et al. Juvenile-onset localized scleroderma activity detection by infrared thermography. Rheumatology (Oxford) 2002;41(10):1178–82.

[126] Birdi N, Shore A, Rush P, et al. Childhood linear scleroderma: a possible role of thermography for evaluation. J Rheumatol 1992;19:968–73.

[127] Liu P, Uziel Y, Chuang S, et al. Localized scleroderma: imaging features. Pediatr Radiol 1994; 24:207–9.

[128] Seidenari S, Conti A, Pepe P, et al. Quantitative description of echographic images of morphea plaques as assessed by computerized image analysis on 20 MHz B-scan recordings. Acta Derm Venereol 1995;75:442–5.

[129] Cosnes A, Anglade MC, Revux J, et al. Thirteen-megahertz ultrasound probe: its role in diagnosing localized scleroderma Br. J Dermatol 2003;148:724–9.

[130] Chazen EM, Cook CD, Cohen J. Focal scleroderma. J Pediatr 1962;60:385–93.

[131] Cunningham BB, Landells ID, Langman C, et al. Topical calcipotriene for morphea/linear scleroderma. J Am Acad Dermatol 1998;39:211–5.

[132] Uziel Y, Feldman BM, Krafchik BR, Yeung RS, Laxer RH. Methotrexate and corticosteroid therapy for pediatric localized scleroderma. J Pediatr 2000;136:91–5.

[133] Walsh J, Martini G, Murray KJ, et al. Evaluation and treatment of childhood onset localized scleroderma [abstract]. Arthritis Rheum 1999;42(9):231.

[134] Pope JE, Bellamy N, Seibold JR, et al. A randomized controlled trial of methotrexate versus placebo in early diffuse scleroderma. Arthritis Rheum 2001;44(6):1351–8.

[135] Herbert CM, Lindberg KA, Jayson MIV, et al. Biosynthesis and maturation of skin collagen in scleroderma and effect of D-penicillamine. Lancet 1974;1:187–92.

[136] Uitto J, Helin P, Rasmussen O, et al. Skin collagen in patients with scleroderma: biosynthesis and maturation in vitro, and the effect of D-penicillamine. Ann Clin Res 1970;2:228–34.

[137] Falanga V, Medsger Jr TA. D-penicillamine in the treatment of localised scleroderma. Arch Dermatol 1990;126:609–12.

[138] Hunzelmann N, Anders S, Fierlbeck G, et al. Double-blind, placebo-controlled study of intra-lesional interferon gamma for the treatment of localized scleroderma. J Am Acad Dermatol 1997;36(3 Pt 1):433–5.

[139] De Rie MA, Bos JD. Photochemotherapy for systemic and localized scleroderma. J Am Acad Dermatol 2000;43:725–6.

[140] Kerscher M, Volkenandt M, Gruss C, et al. Low dose UVA phototherapy for treatment of localized scleroderma. J Am Acad Dermatol 1998;38:21–6.

[141] Camacho NR, Sanchez JE, Martin RF, et al. Medium dose UVA phototherapy in localized scleroderma and its effect in CD34-positive dendritic cells. J Am Acad Dermatol 2001;45:697–9.

[142] Cribier B, Faradij T, Le Coz C, et al. Extracorporeal photochemotherapy in systemic sclerosis and severe morphea. Dermatology 1995;191:25–31.

[143] Grundmann-Kollmann M, Ochsendorf F, Zollner TM, et al. PUVA cream photochemotherapy for the treatment of localized scleroderma. J Am Acad Dermatol 2000;43:675–8.

[144] Caca-Biljanovska NG, Vlckova-Laskoska MT, Dervendi DV, et al. Treatment of generalized morphea with oral 1,25-dihydroxyvitamin D3. Adv Exp Med Biol 1999;455:299–304.

[145] Cunningham BB, Landells ID, Langman C, et al. Topical calcipotriene for morphea/linear scleroderma. J Am Acad Dermatol 1998;39(2 Pt 1):211–5.

[146] Hulshof MM, Pavel S, Breedveld FC, et al. Oral calcitriol as a new therapeutic modality for generalized morphea. Arch Dermatol 1994;130:1290–3.

[147] Hulshof MM, Bouwes BJN, Bergman W, et al. Double-blind, placebo-controlled study of oral calcitriol for the treatment of localized scleroderma and systemic scleroderma. J Am Acad Dermatol 2000;43:1017–23.

[148] Sengezer M, Deveci M, Selmanpakoglu N. Repair of "coup de sabre," a linear form of scleroderma. Ann Plast Surg 1996;37:428–32.

[149] Lapiere J, Aasi S, Cook B, et al. Successful correction of depressed scars of the forehead secondary to trauma and morphea en coup do sabre by en bloc autologous dermal fat graft. Dermatol Surg 2000;26:793–7.

PEDIATRIC CLINICS
OF NORTH AMERICA

Pediatr Clin N Am 52 (2005) 547–575

Vasculitis in Children

Fatma Dedeoglu, MD[a,b], Robert P. Sundel, MD[a,b],*

[a]*Program in Rheumatology, Division of Immunology, Department of Medicine, Children's Hospital, Boston, MA 02115, USA*
[b]*Department of Pediatrics, Harvard Medical School, 25 Shattuck Street, Boston, MA 02115, USA*

Vasculitis implies a straightforward process, inflammation of blood vessels. The conditions included in this category are anything but straightforward, however, because of the variability of vessels that may be involved and the multitude of ways in which they may be affected. Thus, damage to mural structures can lead to anything from numbness to pain, thrombosis to bleeding, aneurysm formation to necrosis.

Further confounding the study of vasculitides in children are the large gaps in the understanding of the nosology, etiology, and pathogenesis of these entities. This lack of understanding, in turn, complicates attempts at classification, hamstrings clinicians' ability to quantify prognosis, and thwarts rationalization of therapy. This article begins with a general overview of vasculitis, situations in which the diagnosis should be considered, diagnostic methods, and therapeutic considerations. Details and treatments unique to specific vasculitides are then reviewed.

Diagnosis

Early in the course of a vasculitis, findings are generally nonspecific, primarily reflecting systemic inflammation (fever, malaise, fatigue, failure to thrive, elevated acute-phase reactants). As vessel damage progresses, more characteristic abnormalities, including evidence of vascular compromise on physical examina-

This article was supported in part by the Samara Jan Turkel Center for Pediatric Autoimmune Disease.

* Corresponding author. Children's Hospital Rheumatology Program, 300 Longwood Avenue, Boston, MA 02115.

E-mail address: robert.sundel@childrens.harvard.edu (R.P. Sundel).

tion, elevation of markers of vascular injury (eg, von Willebrand's factor antigen, pentraxin 3), and distinctive autoantibodies (especially antineutrophil cytoplasmic antibodies [ANCA] or anti-endothelial antibodies) may be detected. Although these findings are often specific for vasculitis, they are seldom part of a routine screening evaluation, so a physician often must consider the diagnosis of vasculitis before its manifestations are pathognomonic. Should the diagnosis be delayed beyond this stage, irreversible tissue damage may occur; it is important that therapy be initiated while the findings remain subtle. Thus a "Catch-22" exists: little information specifically suggestive of vasculitis may be apparent when the diagnosis needs to be made; the condition tends to become more evident only after severe and irreversible morbidity is present.

Despite the inherent variability of the manifestations of vasculitis, certain specific symptoms are particularly suggestive of vascular inflammation. Involvement of large- or medium-sized muscular arteries, as may be seen in Takayasu arteritis (TA) or polyarteritis nodosa (PAN), initially causes symptoms related to the severity of the inflammatory response. As vascular compromise progresses, symptoms of arterial insufficiency begin to dominate. Involvement of large vessels to the extremities, such as the subclavian or femoral arteries, typically leads to claudication, whereas involvement of visceral vessels causes hypertension (renal arteries), abdominal pain (mesenteric and celiac axes), chest pain (aortic or coronary artery involvement), or neurologic symptoms (focal neurologic deficits or neuropathic pain).

Inflammation of smaller arteries and arterioles leads to symptoms in richly vascularized organs. Skin involvement—livedo reticularis, purpuric (generally palpable) or nonblanching lesions, and palmar or plantar rashes—is most suggestive of vascular inflammation. Pulmonary, renal, and gastrointestinal arterial beds are often involved as well. Consequently, hemoptysis, hematuria, hypertension, abdominal pain, or melena may signify the development of vessel damage. Capillary and venous inflammation typically involves the same organs, although the lower volume of blood flow through these vessels tends to make capillaritis and venulitis less of an acute emergency than arteritis.

Whenever vasculitis is considered as a diagnosis, a thorough history and careful general physical examination should be augmented by focus on clinical features of vascular disease. History should include recent illnesses, in particular infections, other exposures (including prescription and over-the-counter drugs), travel, and family history. All pulses must be palpated carefully, and bilateral Allen's tests should be performed to confirm patency of the radial and ulnar arteries and volar arch. The neck, abdomen, and proximal extremities should be auscultated for bruits, and blood pressures in all four extremities should be compared for asymmetry. The skin should be examined carefully for lesions that are nodular or do not blanch, and the two other windows on small vessel abnormalities—ocular fundi and nailbed capillaries—should be assessed as well.

Laboratory studies specific for the diagnosis of vasculitis are not yet available. When vasculitis is being considered, laboratory investigation should include a complete blood cell count and acute-phase reactants (especially erythrocyte sedimentation rate [ESR] and C-reactive protein [CRP]) for evidence of systemic inflammation. Ongoing immune activation leads to hypergammaglobulinemia in many cases of systemic vasculitis. Certain small-vessel diseases are characterized by ANCA. Von Willebrand factor antigen is released by damaged vascular endothelium, so it is elevated in small-vessel vasculitides but also in other conditions that cause vessel damage, including stroke, trauma, and severe infections [1]. New assays currently under development, including measurement of PTX3, a pentraxin expressed by endothelial cells and monocytes [2], hold promise as more sensitive and specific markers of diffuse vascular inflammation, but they are not yet routinely available.

Imaging procedures should be used to confirm a clinical suspicion of vasculitis, not to hunt blindly for a diagnosis. When pulmonary involvement is suspected, pulmonary function tests and imaging of the lungs with radiographs or CT are often useful. Vascular imaging must be interpreted in light of clinical and laboratory data unique to the individual case. Doppler ultrasound studies and CT or MRI angiograms are adequate for resolving abnormalities in large- or medium-sized vessels, but conditions involving smaller vessels often can be visualized only by use of focused angiograms. Even in the hands of interventional radiologists experienced in pediatric angiography, these procedures are potentially morbid, so careful attention to history and physical examination should be relied upon to minimize the number of unnecessary studies.

The reference standard for diagnosing a vasculitis remains histopathologic demonstration of vascular inflammation, although tissue specimens may not be available in many cases because of the inaccessibility of lesions or patchiness of the vascular involvement. When skin lesions are present, deciding to obtain a biopsy is relatively easy; when inaccessible structures such as the brain are involved, calculating the risks and benefits of a biopsy is significantly more complicated.

Classification

Primary vasculitides may be classified according to their clinical manifestations, the size of blood vessels involved, the histology of vascular damage, or the presumed disease pathogenesis. An etiologic classification system would be ideal, especially because it could potentially shed light on anticipated responsiveness to treatment. For example, in adults, inhibition of tumor necrosis factor (TNF) seems to be effective in TA [3] but apparently is less so in Wegener's granulomatosis [4]. On the other hand, using rituximab to target B cells seems to be uniquely safe and effective in ANCA-associated vasculitides [5]. This information might warrant empiric use of rituximab in other vasculitides associated with autoantibodies (eg, anti-endothelial antibodies) but perhaps not in cases of vascular damage caused by cell-mediated mechanisms.

Most current classification systems are based on a combination of histologic and clinical features of the vasculitides [6]. Unfortunately, as new data emerge, conditions previously thought to be similar turn out to differ in fundamental

Box 1. Classification of pediatric vasculitides

Primary vasculitides
  Large vessel diseases
    Takayasu arteritis
    Giant cell (temporal) arteritis
  Medium vessel disease
    Polyarteritis nodosa
      Cutaneous
      Systemic
      Cogan's syndrome
    Kawasaki disease
  Small-vessel disease
    Henoch-Schönlein purpura
    Hypersensitivity vasculitis
    Primary angiitis of the central nervous system
  ANCA-positive vasculitis
    Wegener's granulomatosis
    Microscopic periarteritis
    Churg–Strauss syndrome
Secondary vasculitides
  Infection-related vasculitis
    Hepatitis viruses
    Herpes viruses (EBV, CMV, varicella)
  Vasculitis secondary to connective tissue disease
    Dermatomyositis,
    Systemic lupus erythematosus,
    Rheumatoid arthritis
    Hypocomplementemic uticarial vasculitis
  Drug hypersensitivity –related vasculitis
  Malignancy-related vasculitis
  Post–organ transplant vasculitis
  Pseudovasculitic syndromes
    Myxoma
    Endocarditis
    Sneddon syndrome
  Vasculitides with strong genetic component
    Periodic fever syndromes
    Behçet's disease

Modified from Hunder GG, Wilking AP. Classification of the vasculitides in children. UpToDate, 2005. Available at: http://www.utdol.com/application/search.asp. Accessed February 14, 2005.

ways. Thus, PAN, first described pathologically by Rokitansky in 1852 [7], classically refers to a medium-sized muscular arteritis. Although most cases involve both visceral and cutaneous vessels, some show a particular predilection for the skin (cutaneous PAN), or involve the eyes and ears (Cogan's syndrome). Most recently, with the discovery that some patients with PAN demonstrate antibodies to myeloperoxidase, ANCA-positive microscopic PAN was added to the nomenclature. The result is that today the name PAN might refer to a bewildering array of conditions, some of which are limited, others systemic, some benign, others life-threatening. Clearly, such a classification system requires modification, but the tools for doing so in a coherent manner remain elusive [8].

No classification system is infallible, and a certain degree of overlap is unavoidable. Recently, for example, a young patient of the authors was diagnosed as having primary angiitis of the central nervous system (CNS) on the basis of a brain biopsy. Three years later, he was found to have Hodgkin's lymphoma, a condition associated with vasculitis of the CNS in adults. Should his condition retrospectively be reclassified as a vasculitis secondary to a malignancy? Because this form of vasculitis generally remits when the underlying tumor is treated, this reclassification would be reasonable from a therapeutic perspective. Nonetheless, both tumor-associated vasculitis and primary angiitis of the CNS accurately describe his condition, according to the knowledge available at the time of classification. Allowing for such ambiguities, the authors include a working scheme for classifying pediatric vasculitides, attempting to include current knowledge of disease pathogenesis but leaving open the possibility of reclassification as new data emerge (Box 1) [104].

Epidemiology

Vasculitis is rare in children of all backgrounds, although the incidence of particular diseases varies by location, ethnicity, gender, and underlying conditions. The most complete survey was performed by Gardner-Medwin et al [9] in West Midlands, UK, in 2002. The overall estimated annual incidence of primary vasculitis among children under 17 years of age was 20.4/100 000, with Henoch-Schönlein purpura (HSP) the most prevalent. The Pediatric Rheumatology Database Group reported that 3.3% of children followed at 26 pediatric rheumatology referral centers in the United States carried a diagnosis of vasculitis between 1992 and 1995 [10]. This percentage probably represents an underestimate, because children with HSP or Kawasaki disease (KD) are often treated by pediatricians and not referred to specialty care centers.

Pathogenesis

Despite extensive research, mechanisms underlying the onset and perpetuation of vascular inflammation are generally not understood. Epidemiology, animal models, basic experiments, and responses to directed therapy are shedding light on the processes involved in a variety of vasculitides, and these studies are mentioned in discussions of specific conditions. More generally, theories of pathogenesis may be divided into the following categories:

1. Humoral factors: Vascular damage secondary to specific antibodies is best demonstrated in the ANCA-associated vasculitides [11]. These antibodies may activate neutrophils, causing vascular inflammation, although the lack of a direct correlation between antibody titers and disease activity suggests that additional factors are important in mediating the vessel damage. Anti-endothelial antibodies are also present in a variety of vasculitides, but whether they are markers or mediators of vascular pathology remains unclear [12].
2. Immune complexes: The size, charge, and immunoreactivity of immune complexes help explain aspects of the pathogenesis of HSP and cryo-globulinemic vasculitis [13]. Similarly, PAN associated with hepatitis B or C seems to be triggered by inflammation incited by immune complexes deposited upon vessel walls [14].
3. T lymphocytes attracted to damaged or infected endothelium may contribute to vascular inflammation through direct cytotoxicity or release of inflammatory cytokines. Evidence of restricted expression of T-cell receptors supports a role for selection of antigen-specific lymphocytes in some types of vasculitis [15]. In addition, suppression of autoreactive lymphocytes may be dependent upon populations of T-regulatory cells. When these cells fail to restrict lymphocyte reactivity with autoantigens, the result may be breaking of tolerance and development of autoimmunity. Once the cycle of immune targeting against blood vessels begins, damage may continue through activation of the complement cascade and recruitment of effector cells such as natural killer cells or phagocytes [16]. Indeed, biopsy samples from different types of vasculitis demonstrate different populations of cells invading vessel walls (eg, macrophages in KD and eosinophils in Churg–Strauss syndrome [CSS]) [17].
4. The characteristic predilection of different vasculitides for different anatomic sites remains unexplained, although it seems to depend on a variety of factors, including specificity of the triggering antigen, regional variations in cell surface receptors, and unidentified contributions of surrounding tissues.

Henoch-Schönlein purpura

The most common pediatric vasculitis is HSP, IgA immune complex–mediated small-vessel leukocytoclastic vasculitis that classically presents with the triad of nonthrombocytopenic palpable purpura, colicky abdominal pain, and arthritis. The major cause of morbidity is renal involvement: although HSP is mild in most children, it may progress to chronic renal failure in up to 1% of cases. HSP is significantly more prevalent in young children, but cases in older children and adults seem to have a higher propensity for causing significant renal damage [18]. Symptomatic involvement of other organs is not common, although one study found that a large percentage of children with HSP had abnormalities of pulmonary diffusion capacity despite having no respiratory symptoms [19]. In rare cases, CNS or respiratory lesions may lead to hemorrhage with serious sequelae [20].

A wide variety of infections may trigger HSP. Group A streptococcus is the most common precipitant, demonstrable in up to one third of cases, but exposure to *Bartonella*, *Haemophilus parainfluenza*, and numerous vaccines and drugs may precede the development of HSP [21]. Consistent with the contribution of infectious triggers in children, HSP seems to be slightly more common in boys than in girls, and it occurs more commonly during winter and spring than during warmer months. In adults, however, HSP is reported most frequently in the summer, suggesting different predisposing factors in these cases.

Skin involvement in HSP may begin as urticaria, but in most cases it progresses to dramatic purple, nonblanching lesions (Fig. 1). The disease seems to be mediated by activation of the alternate pathway of complement by large IgA-containing immune complexes [22]. This association may explain the predilection of skin lesions for the lower legs and buttocks in ambulatory children and the sacrum, ears, and buttocks in infants, because gravity causes immune complexes to deposit and incite inflammation in dependent areas.

The arthritis of HSP is usually transient, and it does not cause chronic joint changes or permanent sequelae. Gastrointestinal involvement ranges from colicky abdominal pain to profuse bleeding, intussusception (typically ilio-ilial, unlike intussusceptions associated with infections) and perforation [23]. Pancreatitis, cholecystitis, and protein-losing enteropathy may also occur [24]. Frequently, gastrointestinal symptoms follow the rash; when they occur first, distinguishing appendicitis or other abdominal catastrophes from HSP may be quite challenging [25].

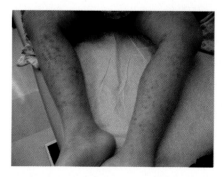

Fig. 1. Typical lower extremity palpable purpura seen in HSP.

In most cases, renal disease is observed early in the disease course, during the first days or weeks. One series found that nephritis occurred within the first 3 months of the illness in 97% of patients [26]. In this study, risk factors for renal involvement included age over 47 years, gastrointestinal bleeding, purpura of more than 1 month's duration, factor XIII activity less than 80% of normal, and factor XIII concentrate treatment. HSP recurs in about one third of patients, especially those with nephritis. It usually recurs during the first 4 to 6 months of the disease. Recurrent episodes resemble the initial presentation, although they are generally less severe, and they do not adversely impact prognosis.

In general, long-term outcomes in HSP are quite good. The major exception is patients with significant kidney involvement, although some female patients with milder renal involvement nonetheless seem to develop hypertension and proteinuria during pregnancy [27]. More generally, there is a correlation between the severity of urinary abnormalities and the chances of developing chronic renal disease, with patients demonstrating both nephritic and nephrotic changes at greatest risk. Renal biopsy is useful for confirming the extent and severity of nephritis and planning treatment: the higher the percentage of glomeruli with crescents, the more likely is development of end-stage renal disease [28]. In a research setting, high serum levels of nitric oxide and urinary nitrate excretion [29], and increased urinary excretion of the tubular proteins N-acetyl b-D-glucoseaminidase and α-1-microglobulin also proved useful in identifying patients at higher risk of long-term renal disease [30]. Overall, about 1% to 5% of HSP patients develop some degree of chronic renal disease. Another study found that nailfold capillary abnormalities may be detected well after clinical symptoms remit, suggesting that subclinical vasculitis persists longer than may be readily apparent [31].

HSP most commonly must be distinguished from two other purpuric conditions of childhood: acute hemorrhagic edema of infancy and hypersensitivity vasculitis. Acute hemorrhagic edema of infancy characteristically presents with fever, large purpuric lesions, and edema [32] (Fig. 2). It is a self-limited condition, but clinicians must exclude infectious and noninfectious causes of pur-

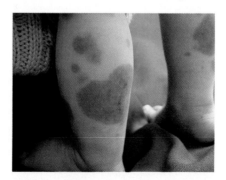

Fig. 2. Purpuric rash of acute hemorrhagic edema of childhood. The lesions are larger and more macular than those seen in HSP.

pura before reassuring parents that the rash is likely to resolve within weeks. Hypersensitivity vasculitis is an inflammatory condition of small vessels that occurs after exposure to drugs or infections or may be idiopathic [33]. Histologic evaluation shows leukocytoclastic vasculitis, primarily involving postcapillary venules. Immune complexes are usually present, and mononuclear or poly-morphonuclear cells may be present as well. Clinical features include fever, urticaria, lymphadenopathy, arthralgias, low serum complement levels, and ele-vated ESR. Low serum concentrations of C3 and C4 and the absence of IgA deposition in vessel walls help to distinguish this entity from HSP, in which serum complement levels are normal.

Therapy of HSP is primarily supportive, aiming for symptomatic relief of arthritis and abdominal pain. Acetaminophen or nonsteroidal anti-inflammatory drugs (NSAIDs) seem to be effective in most cases; there is no evidence that these agents increase the likelihood of gastrointestinal hemorrhage in HSP. Use of steroids in children who do not respond to NSAIDs or in those thought to be at highest risk of developing renal compromise continues to be controversial. Prednisone, at a dose of 2 mg/kg/day, seems to relieve symptoms rapidly in most cases, but caregivers must avoid excessively rapid tapering of the steroids, be-cause precipitate tapers commonly trigger a flare of symptoms [34]. More potent immunosuppressive agents, such as cyclophosphamide or azathioprine, are re-served for children with biopsy-proven crescentic glomerulonephritis or other life-threatening complications such as cerebral or pulmonary hemorrhage [35].

Kawasaki disease

Etiology and epidemiology

Although KD or mucocutaneous lymph node syndrome is classified as a vasculitis, it is unique in several respects. Unlike other inflammatory conditions of blood vessels, it is a self-limited condition, with fever and manifestations of acute inflammation lasting for an average of 12 days without therapy [36]. It is diagnosed by clinical criteria (Box 2) [105], not histology or angiography. It is almost entirely a disease of children, with 80% to 90% of cases occurring before the fifth birthday. For all of its similarities to infectious exanthema of childhood, however, KD is not necessarily a benign disease: historically, up to 1.5% of untreated children died from KD.

More than 100,000 cases of KD have been registered in Japan since its ini-tial description in 1967 [37]. Genetic factors seem to account for the varying susceptibility of different ethnic groups to KD, with polymorphisms of che-mokines and TNF receptors and variations in HLA haplotypes all possibly contributing. Overall, Asians are affected 5 to 10 times as frequently as whites; blacks and Hispanics have an intermediate risk [38].

The cause of KD remains unknown. As in other vasculitides, blood vessel damage seems to result from an aberrant immune response leading to endothe-

---

Box 2. Criteria for diagnosis of Kawasaki disease

Fever lasting 5 days or more (4 days if treatment with IVIG eradicates fever) plus at least four of the following clinical signs not explained by another disease process (numbers in parentheses indicate the approximate percentage of children with KD who display the criterion):

1. Bilateral conjunctival injection (80%–90%)
2. Changes in the oropharyngeal mucous membranes (including one or more of the following symptoms: injected or fissured lips, strawberry tongue, injected pharynx) (80%–90%)
3. Changes in the peripheral extremities, including erythema or edema of the hands and feet (acute phase) or periungual desquamation (convalescent phase) (80%)
4. Polymorphous rash, primarily truncal; nonvesicular (> 90%)
5. Cervical lymphadenopathy: anterior cervical lymph note at least 1.5 cm in diameter (50%)

Modified from Centers for Disease Control. Revised diagnostic criteria for Kawasaki disease. MMWR Morb Mortal Wkly Rpt 1990; 39(No. 44-13):27–8.

---

lial cell injury and vessel wall damage. Pathologically, however, KD seems to be unique: macrophages [17] and IgA-producing plasma cells [39] have been described in the vessel walls, features recognized in no other conditions.

Many aspects of KD suggest that it is caused by a transmissible agent. A synthetic monoclonal IgA antibody was found to bind to an unidentified cytoplasmic component of macrophages within the coronary arteries of 9 of 12 fatal cases of KD but in none of 10 controls [40]. Similar binding to the respiratory epithelium of proximal bronchi was noted in 77% of fatal cases, never in controls. The significance of these findings is unclear, but one interpretation is that a particular respiratory pathogen may be associated with KD.

Many epidemiologic data also support the theory that KD is triggered by a transmissible agent or agents. Boys are affected 50% more commonly than girls, a feature typical of infectious diseases. The average age of children with KD is about 2 years, and occurrence beyond late childhood is extremely rare [41], suggesting a ubiquitous agent to which most people are exposed and become immune by late childhood. Epidemics occurred regularly in the 1980s, and during these outbreaks the average age of patients dropped while the percentage of girls increased, again typical of infections. Nonetheless, suggestions that certain viruses (eg, Epstein–Barr virus, parvovirus, HIV-2) or bacterial toxins (eg, streptococcal erythrogenic toxin, staphylococcal toxic shock toxin) account for the majority of cases have not been substantiated [42]. Thus, many researchers now believe that KD represents a final common pathway of immune-mediated vascular inflammation following a variety of inciting infections.

Clinical manifestations

Guidelines for the diagnosis of KD were established by Tomisaku Kawasaki in 1967. Diagnosis requires the presence of fever lasting 5 days or more without any other explanation, combined with at least four of five manifestations of mucocutaneous inflammation (Box 2) [34,43]. As with all clinical criteria, these guidelines are imperfect, with less than 100% sensitivity and specificity. Children who do not meet the criteria may have an incomplete or atypical form of KD. In addition, some patients who manifest five or six signs may have other conditions. For example, one study of patients referred for possible KD found that the standard clinical diagnostic criteria for KD were fulfilled in 18 of 39 patients (46%) in whom other diagnoses were established [44].

Kawasaki published his diagnostic guidelines before cardiac involvement was recognized in this disease. Thus, the criteria were never intended to identify children at risk for developing coronary artery abnormalities. Indeed, at least 10% of children who develop coronary artery aneurysms never meet criteria for KD [45]. In an attempt to improve clinicians' ability to diagnose KD in all cases at risk of developing coronary artery changes, an American Heart Association working group has recommended modifications of the criteria [38]. These recommendations have yet to be validated prospectively.

Fever is probably the most consistent manifestation of KD. It reflects elevated levels of proinflammatory cytokines such as TNF and interleukin (IL)-1 that are also thought to mediate the underlying vascular inflammation [46]. The fever is typically hectic, minimally responsive to antipyretic agents, and remains above 38.5°C during most of the illness. Because KD may be so pleomorphic, it should always be considered in a child with prolonged, unexplained fever, irritability, and laboratory signs of inflammation, especially in the presence of other manifestations of mucocutaneous inflammation. Conversely, the diagnosis must be suspect in the absence of fever.

Bilateral nonexudative conjunctivitis is present in as many as 90% of cases of KD. The predominantly bulbar injection typically begins within days of the onset of fever, and the eyes have a brilliant erythema that spares the limbus. Children are also frequently photophobic, and anterior uveitis may develop [47]. Slit-lamp examination may be helpful in ambiguous cases; the presence of uveitis provides further evidence for the diagnosis of KD because it is seen more commonly in KD than in mimics of the vasculitis.

As KD progresses, mucositis often becomes evident. Cracked, red lips and a strawberry tongue are characteristic; the latter is caused by sloughing of filiform papillae and denuding of the inflamed glossal tissue. Discrete oral lesions, such as vesicles or ulcers, as well as tonsillar exudate, suggest a viral or bacterial infection rather than KD.

The cutaneous manifestations of KD are polymorphous. The rash typically begins as perineal erythema and desquamation, followed by macular, morbilliform, or targetoid lesions of the trunk and extremities. Vesicular or bullous lesions are rare.

Changes in the extremities are generally the last manifestation of KD to develop. Children demonstrate an indurated edema of the dorsum of the hands and feet and a diffuse erythema of the palms and soles. The convalescent phase of KD may be characterized by sheetlike desquamation that begins in the periungual region of the hands and feet (Fig. 3) and by linear nail creases (Beau's lines). In addition, one third of children have arthritis. The arthritis is typically a small joint polyarthritis during the first week of illness, followed by a large joint pauciarthritis. It never persists beyond 1 to 2 months, nor is it erosive.

Cervical lymphadenopathy is the least consistent of the cardinal features of KD, absent in as many as 50% of children with the disease. When present, lymphadenopathy tends to involve primarily the anterior cervical nodes overlying the sternocleidomastoid muscle [48]. Diffuse lymphadenopathy or other signs of reticuloendothelial involvement (eg, splenomegaly) should prompt a search for alternative diagnoses.

Children suspected of having KD who have fewer than four signs of mucocutaneous inflammation may have incomplete or atypical KD. Clinical manifestations of KD tend to be most incomplete and atypical in the youngest patients, and a particularly high level of suspicion is needed in infants younger than 1 year of age. In a retrospective review of 45 cases of KD, for example, 5 of 11 infants (45%) had atypical disease, compared with 4 of 33 older children (12%) [49]. Magnifying the gravity of the situation is the fact that infants are the group with the highest risk of developing coronary artery aneurysms. In the study by Joffe et al [49], coronary artery complications occurred in seven infants (64%) compared with three older children (9%) and occurred in all five infants with incomplete disease. Overall, among the 2221 children under 5 years of age analyzed for the Japanese nationwide survey of KD in 1995 and 1996, infants under 1 year of

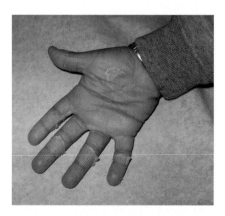

Fig. 3. Periungual desquamation seen during the subacute phase of KD.

age had an odds ratio of 1.54 for developing cardiac sequelae [50]. Similarly, in a recent retrospective survey, the rate of treatment failure was 8.5% in patients under 12 months of age [51], compared with a 1.8% incidence of coronary artery abnormalities in those at least 12 months of age.

Thus, KD should be considered in any infant or young child with prolonged, unexplained fever. Although alternative explanations for the child's symptoms must be carefully excluded before instituting empiric treatment with intravenous immunoglobulin (IVIG), a high index of suspicion should be maintained for the diagnosis of incomplete disease. Consultation with an expert is recommended if the diagnosis is in question. Although no laboratory studies are included among the diagnostic criteria for KD, certain findings may help distinguish KD from mimics in ambiguous cases [44]:

- Systemic inflammation is most characteristic, manifested by elevation of acute-phase reactants (eg, CRP, ESR, and alpha-1 antitrypsin), leukocytosis, and a left shift in the white blood cell count. By the second week of illness, platelet counts generally rise and may reach 1,000,000/mm^3 in the most severe cases.
- Children with KD often present with a normocytic, normochromic anemia; hemoglobin concentrations more than two SD below the mean for age are noted in 50% of patients within the first 2 weeks of illness.
- The urinalysis commonly reveals white blood cells on microscopic examination. The pyuria is of urethral origin and therefore will be missed on urinalyses obtained by bladder tap or catheterization. In addition, the white cells are mononuclear and are not detected by dipstick tests for leukocyte esterase. Renal involvement may occur in KD but is uncommon.
- Measurement of liver enzymes often reveals elevated transaminase levels or mild hyperbilirubinemia caused by intrahepatic congestion. In addition, a minority of children develops obstructive jaundice from hydrops of the gallbladder.
- Other body fluids also demonstrate inflammation: cerebrospinal fluid (CSF) typically displays a mononuclear pleocytosis without hypoglycorrhachia or elevation of CSF protein. A chart review of 46 children with KD found that 39% had elevated CSF white cell counts; the median count was 22.5 cells with 6% neutrophils and 91.5% mononuclear cells, although cell counts as high as 320/mm^3 with up to 79% neutrophils were reported [52]. Similarly, arthrocentesis of involved joints demonstrates 50 to 300,000 white cells/mm^3, primarily consisting of neutrophils.

Differential diagnosis

KD is most commonly confused with infectious exanthems of childhood [53]:

- Measles, echovirus, and adenovirus may share many of the signs of mucocutaneous inflammation, but they typically have less evidence of systemic inflammation and generally lack the extremity changes seen in KD.

- Toxin-mediated illnesses, especially beta-hemolytic streptococcal infection and toxic shock syndrome, lack the ocular and articular involvement typical of KD
- Rocky Mountain spotted fever and leptospirosis are two additional infectious illnesses to be considered in the differential diagnosis of KD. Headache and gastrointestinal complaints typically are prominent features of these infections.
- Drug reactions such as Stevens–Johnson syndrome or serum sickness may mimic KD but with subtle differences in the ocular and mucosal manifestations.
- Systemic-onset juvenile rheumatoid arthritis is marked by prominent rash, fever, and systemic inflammation and may be difficult to distinguish from KD until its chronicity and polyarthritis are evident.
- Mercury hypersensitivity reaction (acrodynia) shares certain clinical features with KD, including fever, rash, swelling of the palms and feet, desquamation, and photophobia. Unless there is a convincing history of exposure to mercury, however, treatment of a child with possible KD should not be delayed while awaiting mercury levels, because acrodynia is rare in the developed world.

Therapy

Patients who fulfill the criteria for KD are hospitalized and treated with IVIG and aspirin. Patients suspected of having incomplete disease may require further testing such as slit-lamp examination and echocardiography to confirm the diagnosis. At times, children are treated for suspected KD when the diagnosis is uncertain but no clear alternative explanation for the clinical findings can be identified. Markers of increased risk of developing coronary artery aneurysms, including age under 1 year, signs of severe systemic inflammation (especially marked anemia and left shift in the white blood cell count), and a consumptive coagulopathy, may shift the balance toward empiric therapy [54].

Aspirin was the first medication used for treatment of KD because of its anti-inflammatory and antithrombotic effects [55]. Although aspirin was useful for management of fever and arthritis, it did not lower the incidence of coronary artery aneurysm development. A reduction in the occurrence of this complication was first reported with IVIG in 1984 [56]. IVIG offers a remarkable combination of efficacy and safety for the treatment of KD. Therapy within the first 10 days of illness reduces the incidence of coronary artery aneurysms by more than 70% [36]. IVIG therapy also largely eliminates the development of giant coronary artery aneurysms (more than 8 mm in diameter), which are associated with the highest risk of morbidity and mortality, and rapidly restores disordered lipid metabolism and depressed myocardial contractility to normal [45].

Aspirin traditionally is given initially in relatively high doses to achieve an anti-inflammatory effect; doses of 30 mg/kg/day to more than 80 mg/kg/day in four divided doses have been used during the acute phase of illness. Subsequently, aspirin is administered in low doses (3 to 5 mg/kg/day) for its antiplatelet action. Alternative anti-inflammatory agents such as ibuprofen may be used for prolonged episodes of arthritis. No study has demonstrated long-term benefit from the use of aspirin, and a recent trial found no differences in outcomes between children treated with IVIG alone and those who also received aspirin [57]. In view of the potential risks and lack of obvious benefits of aspirin, it should be withheld in the presence of any contraindications to its use, including bleeding, exposure to influenza or varicella, or a history of hypersensitivity to salicylates. When used, the initial dose should be no higher than 100 mg/kg/day. Once fever resolves, patients receive a dose of 3 to 5 mg/kg/day. Treatment with aspirin is continued until laboratory studies (eg, platelet count and sedimentation rate) return to normal, unless coronary artery abnormalities are detected by echocardiography. This phase of therapy typically is complete within 2 months of the onset of disease.

Corticosteroids—prednisone and related medications—are mainstays of the therapeutic regimen in other forms of vasculitis, but they have been considered unsafe in KD. This conclusion is based primarily on a single study that demonstrated an extraordinarily high incidence of coronary artery aneurysms (11 of 17 patients) in a group that received oral prednisolone at a dose of 2 to 3 mg/kg/day for at least 2 weeks, followed by 1.5 mg/kg/day for an additional 2 weeks [58]. These data are difficult to interpret, because treatment groups were not stratified according to risk factors for the development of aneurysms, and no information about randomization methods was given. In addition, a smaller group of seven patients in the same study received prednisolone plus aspirin, and none of these patients developed aneurysms.

A detrimental effect of steroids in patients with vasculitis would be unprecedented, and several recent reports have rekindled interest in a possible role for steroids in the management of KD. A retrospective survey of the records of almost 300 children treated with or without steroids between 1982 and 1998 [59] and two open, randomized, prospective trials [60,61] found that patients who received corticosteroids in addition to IVIG had shorter durations of fever and more rapid decrease in inflammatory markers than those in the standard-therapy group. In all reports, corticosteroid therapy has been well tolerated, with no significant adverse effects. At present, most clinicians who specialize in the care of KD use pulsed doses of intravenous methylprednisolone (IVMP) in children whose inflammation persists despite at least two doses of IVIG [51]. A trial supported by the National Institutes of Health comparing outcomes in children who received initial therapy with IVMP plus IVIG versus IVIG alone has completed enrollment. Results of this trial soon should supply definitive information concerning the potential role of steroids in the primary treatment of KD.

Re-treatment

Fever persists or returns 48 hours after the start of initial treatment with IVIG in 10% to 15% of patients [62]. Persistent or recrudescent fever is particularly concerning, because it usually indicates ongoing vasculitis with increased risk of developing coronary artery aneurysms (12.2% versus 1.4% in one analysis) [54]. In another study, persistent fever was the only factor that predicted subsequent development of aneurysms [37]. Thus, it is extremely important not to dismiss mild temperature elevations in children with KD; one should assume that these elevations represent incompletely controlled disease unless proved otherwise. Patients who remain febrile after the first dose of IVIG are usually treated with a second and perhaps even a third dose of IVIG, 2 g/kg [51]. This practice is based on the apparent dose–response effect of IVIG [63]. Nonetheless, children are not usually re-treated until at least 48 hours after the start of the initial IVIG infusion, because fever before this time may represent a reaction to the medication.

A subgroup of patients with KD seems to be resistant to IVIG therapy, even after multiple doses. These patients are at greatest risk for development of coronary artery aneurysms and long-term sequelae of the disease. Therapies that are effective in other forms of vasculitis, such as corticosteroids, pentoxyfylline, plasmapheresis, and immunosuppression, have been used in these patients. Prospective studies have not compared these options, but most specialists treat children who have not responded to IVIG and still have active KD with one to three daily doses of pulsed methylprednisolone (30 mg/kg) [51]. If this treatment is ineffective, a single dose of infliximab, 5 mg/kg, may be beneficial [64].

The need for more potent immunosuppressive agents (eg, cyclophosphamide or cyclosporine) in KD is not clear. These medications are relatively toxic, with delayed onsets of action. Because fever generally lasts less than 3 weeks even in the most severe cases of KD, few patients will remain sick enough to consider immunosuppression by the time routine therapies have been exhausted. When symptoms are prolonged beyond 3 to 4 weeks, consideration should be given to an alternative diagnosis, including chronic vasculitides such as PAN.

Additional considerations

An echocardiogram should be obtained early in the acute phase of illness and 6 to 8 weeks after onset to confirm the efficacy of treatment [38]. Patients should also have repeated physical examinations during the first 2 months to detect arrhythmias, heart failure, valvular insufficiency, or myocarditis. Children with coronary artery abnormalities generally receive long-term antithrombotic therapy with aspirin, dipyridamole, or other agents, as well as regular cardiac evaluations.

Coronary artery dilatation of less than 8 mm generally regresses over time, and most smaller aneurysms fully resolve by echocardiogram [65]. Healing is by fibrointimal proliferation, often accompanied by calcification, and vascular reactivity does not return to normal despite grossly normal appearance [66]. Children should thus be followed indefinitely after KD, a point highlighted by a report of the sudden death of a 3.5-year-old child 3 months after dilated coronary arteries had regained a normal echocardiographic appearance [67]. Autopsy revealed obliteration of the lumen of the left anterior descending coronary artery by fibrosis, with evidence of ongoing active inflammation in the epicardial arteries.

Children with severe KD who develop coronary occlusion may experience myocardial infarction, arrhythmias, or sudden death, and those who develop peripheral artery occlusion may experience ischemia or gangrene [68]. Various therapies have been attempted to restore circulation, although control of vascular inflammation with sufficient IVIG or corticosteroids is an essential prerequisite to arterial reperfusion. Thereafter, treatments may include thrombolytic therapy, if arterial thrombosis is present, or vasodilators, if tissue viability is threatened primarily by vasospasm.

At least one report suggests a potential role for abciximab, a monoclonal antibody that inhibits platelet glycoprotein IIb/IIIa receptor [69]. A group from the University of Utah reported increased resolution of aneurysms in patients with KD who received abciximab compared with those who received conventional treatment. Subsequent case reports have been less promising, however.

Overall, with modern treatment and cardiologic follow-up, the prognosis of children with KD is excellent. Long-term follow-up of children without persistent coronary artery abnormalities in Japan has demonstrated no increase in morbidity or mortality after 25 years [70]. In fact, studies suggest that fear of a cardiac event is more disabling than actual medical problems in most children who have had KD [71]. Thus, caregivers should be particularly careful to reassure families when appropriate.

Polyarteritis nodosa

PAN is a systemic necrotizing vasculitis with aneurysm formation affecting medium or small arteries. This condition is important historically as the first noninfectious cause of vascular damage to be identified. In 1866, Kussmaul and Maier's extensive report described a 27-year old tailor with diffuse visceral involvement as well as features of systemic inflammation (fever, fatigue, weight loss). At least one third of children with PAN, however, have a more limited form, restricted largely to the skin and joints.

Worldwide, PAN is most commonly associated with hepatitis B or C infections [72]. Perhaps because of the relative infrequency of these infections in children, pediatric PAN is quite rare, especially in North America. When it does occur before adulthood, PAN incidence peaks at 9 to 10 years of age, and it may be slightly more common in boys than in girls [14]. No clear genetic association has been identified, although several reports suggest an association with familial Mediterranean fever (FMF). Up to 1% of FMF patients develop PAN, but in these patients it seems to be milder than idiopathic disease and is associated with a better prognosis [73].

Cutaneous PAN is usually limited to skin and the musculoskeletal system. It commonly occurs after a sore throat or streptococcal pharyngitis. Livedo reticularis, maculopapular rash, painful skin nodules, panniculitis, brawny edema, and arthritis mostly affect the knees and ankles [74]. Acute-phase reactants may be normal or elevated, at least partially reflecting the severity of the inciting infection [75,76] Constitutional symptoms are generally mild. Even though systemic involvement is quite rare, these patients should be observed closely for development of systemic disease. Symptoms are more troubling than disabling, and treatment generally consists of NSAIDs and steroids. The disease does tend to persist or relapse, so many patients require steroid-sparing agents for long-term management. These drugs may include methotrexate or other immunosuppressive agents; TNF inhibitors have been reported to be effective, as well [77]. Penicillin prophylaxis may prevent disease flares caused by recurrent streptococcal infections.

Systemic PAN may involve virtually any muscular artery. Consequently, in addition to constitutional symptoms, it may cause a vast array of organ dysfunction. Palpable purpura, livedo, necrotic dermal lesions (Fig. 4), abdominal pain, arthritis/arthralgia, myositis/myalgia, renovascular hypertension, neurologic deficits, pulmonary disease, and coronary arteritis may be seen at presentation or during the course of the disease, so PAN should be considered in the differential diagnosis of any undiagnosed systemic inflammatory condition [78]. Because of its pleomorphism, PAN may be confused with systemic-onset juvenile rheumatoid arthritis, KD, or dermatomyositis. Small vessels are spared in classical PAN, however, so glomerulonephritis typically is not a feature of this condition.

Laboratory evaluation usually reflects the ongoing systemic inflammation including anemia, leukocytosis, thrombocytosis, and elevated ESR, CRP, and immunoglobulins. A positive ANCA generally indicates pauci-immune glomerulonephritidies rather than PAN. Proteinuria, hematuria, and increases in serum urea nitrogen and creatinine levels are also common findings. Complement levels are normal. The diagnosis usually requires tissue biopsy or radiologic documentation of vasculitis. Imaging studies demonstrate the typical beading of vessels caused by alternating areas of vascular narrowing and dilatation that give PAN its name. Pathologically this manifestation corresponds to segmental vascular involvement with nodule and aneurysm formation resulting from panmural fibrinoid necrosis. No overt complement or immunoglobulin deposition is seen.

Treatment usually aims at decreasing systemic vascular inflammation, mainly with high-dose steroids. Other immunosuppressive agents, primarily daily oral

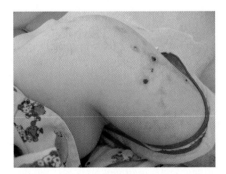

Fig. 4. Ulcerating livedo reticularis characteristic of polyarteritis nodosa.

or monthly intravenous doses of cyclophosphamide, seem to be beneficial in improving outcome. Azathioprine, methotrexate, IVIG, and, more recently biologic response modifiers such as TNF-inhibitors, have been used in a number of patients. Randomized, controlled trials are needed to determine the most effective remittive and maintenance therapies as well as predictors of individual patients' responses. Nonetheless, recent reviews of PAN in children suggest an excellent overall prognosis, with a 4-year mortality rate under 5% [14].

Takayasu arteritis

TA is the third most common form of childhood vasculitis [79]. The cause of TA remains unknown, although histopathology and immunohistochemistry of biopsy and autopsy samples from adults with TA suggest a primarily T-cell–mediated mechanism [80]. Pathologically TA lesions consist of granulomatous changes progressing from the vascular adventitia to the media, indistinguishable from those seen in giant cell arteritis and temporal arteritis [81]. The diagnosis of TA is based on the distribution of involvement—primarily the aorta and its branches—and the young age of patients, typically under 40 years. TA is more common in the Far East and West Africa than in Europe and North America. Certain HLA associations have been found in Japan, but these have not been confirmed in other populations [82].

Onset of TA is most commonly during the third decade of life, but childhood disease has been reported as early as the first year of life [75] As in adults, there is a significant preponderance of female patients in children with TA, and the distribution of vessel involvement parallels that in adults as well, with diffuse aortic involvement predominating. In a recent review of childhood TA, the mean age of onset was 11.4 years, and two thirds of the patients were female [83]. Signs and symptoms included hypertension, cardiomegaly, elevated ESR, fever, fatigue, palpitations, vomiting, nodules, abdominal pain, arthralgia, claudication, weight loss, and chest pain. The delay in diagnosis in children was 19 months, notably longer than that reported in most adult series [84]. Possibly because of delayed diagnosis, mortality was 33%, also significantly higher than reported in adult series.

Once TA is suspected, angiography has been the standard method used for diagnosis. The size of the vessels involved and the spotty nature of the vascular inflammation make biopsies impractical. In recent years, CT and MR angiograms have proven to be as useful as traditional angiograms and far less invasive. MRI has the added advantage of revealing evidence of ongoing vessel wall inflammation. This information is particularly helpful because of the need to suppress the vasculitis completely to prevent disease progression. Laboratory markers may be entirely normal despite ongoing inflammation, so MRI offers a potentially more sensitive test for residual disease [85].

As with all vasculitides, early diagnosis and aggressive therapy are important in TA to prevent irreversible vessel damage with resulting compromise of vital organs. Steroids and the typical immunosuppressive agents used in other vasculitides (including cyclophosphamide, methotrexate, and azathioprine) have shown variable efficacy in TA. A recent report in adults with TA from the Cleveland Clinic documented a high response rate to TNF-inhibitors [3]. Before starting such treatment, however, it is important to test patients for tuberculosis, because aortitis is associated with mycobacterial infections, especially in less developed countries [86].

Primary angiitis of the central nervous system

Primary angiitis of the central nervous system (PACNS) is potentially one of the most challenging diseases a physician might face, both diagnostically and therapeutically [87]. By definition, systemic manifestations of the disease are usually absent, acute-phase reactants are typically normal, and examination of CSF might be unrevealing as well [88]. Thus, to make the diagnosis before the patient comes to autopsy, clinicians must have a high level of suspicion when children have even scanty suggestion of a vasculitis. A recent review based on 62 patients with childhood PACNS (cPACNS) helps shed light on symptoms that might suggest inclusion of PACNS in a child's differential diagnosis [89]. Headache (80%) and focal neurologic deficits (78%) were the most common presenting complaints, followed by hemiparesis in 62%. When a clearly defined infectious, toxic, or vascular abnormality cannot account for such findings, brain and cerebral vessel imaging are indicated. Normal MRI together with normal CSF have high negative predictive value for cPACNS. Nonetheless in 5% to 10% of cases of cPACNS, only a meningeal and brain biopsy, guided by clinical or MRI abnormalities or performed blindly, reveals diagnostic evidence of the vasculitis.

Although brain biopsy remains the reference standard for the diagnosis of cPACNS, even these results may be falsely negative because of the patchy nature of the disease. Biopsy is also useful in excluding mimics of CNS vasculitis, especially atypical infections that could worsen if immunosuppressive therapy is started empirically. PACNS may be rapidly progressive and neurologically devastating, so the risks of diagnostic procedures must be weighed against the need for prompt diagnosis and initiation of therapy. Treatment invariably includes corticosteroids and a potent immunosuppressive agent, usually cyclophosphamide. Outcomes using these agents to achieve initial disease control, followed by methotrexate or azathioprine for maintenance therapy, are excellent [89].

Anti-neutrophil cytoplasmic antibody-associated vasculitides

Wegener's granulomatosis

Wegener's granulomatosis (WG) is uncommon in children. It is a necrotizing granulomatous inflammation of small- to medium-sized vessels involving the kidneys and upper and lower respiratory tracts. As with other ANCA-associated vasculitides, biopsies of active lesions reveal a microscopic pauci-immune polyangiitis. Serologic testing is positive for cANCA directed against PR-3. Available data suggest that clinical manifestations in children are similar to those in adults [90]. In a recent report of 17 children, nasal and sinus involvement were seen in 100%, respiratory disease in 87%, arthralgias, ocular findings, or skin or renal involvement each in just over 50%, gastrointestinal disease in 41%, and CNS involvement in 12% [91]. In this and other pediatric series, subglottic stenosis has been more frequent than in adults, noted in almost 50% of children with WG.

Although the cause of WG remains unknown, pathogenesis seems to be related to ANCA. ANCA most likely stabilize adherence of rolling neutrophils to endothelium and activate neutrophils and monocytes to undergo an oxidative burst. Activation of phagocytic cells causes increased expression of proinflammatory cytokines (eg, TNF-α and IL-8), with resultant localized endothelial cell cytotoxicity [11].

Most children with WG present with upper respiratory symptoms such as epistaxis, sinusitis, otitis media, or hearing loss. Cough, wheezing, dyspnea, and hemoptysis are among the lower respiratory tract manifestations. Because benign causes of these symptoms are so much more prevalent than WG in children, these patients usually are treated for infections or allergies. Further, despite the potential severity of the glomerulonephritis seen in WG, kidney involvement may initially be asymptomatic. Thus, as with other rare conditions, pediatricians must remember to consider WG in a child with respiratory disease that is unusually persistent or severe. Chest radiographs may be particularly helpful when a diagnosis of WG is suspected, because even in asymptomatic children up to one third have radiographic abnormalities.

Confirmation of a diagnosis of WG relies heavily on biopsy results. Necrotizing granulomatous vascular inflammation is strongly suggestive in a child with consistent clinical features. cANCA targeted against PR-3 is positive in most patients [92]. Although this autoantibody is highly specific, it may be found in other diseases, such as cystic fibrosis, which are more common in children. Accordingly, a positive ANCA titer should not replace a tissue biopsy in confirming the diagnosis of WG, nor should ANCA screening substitute for a careful history and physical examination. The role of monitoring of ANCA titers as a marker of disease activity is also controversial. Some studies have shown a correlation between rising ANCA titers and relapses of WG, whereas others found no correlation [93]. Currently, intra- and interpatient variability in antibody titers means that treatment of anticipated relapses based on rising ANCA titers alone is not generally recommended.

Without effective immunosuppressive therapy, WG is commonly rapidly progressive and even fatal. Current therapeutic practices reflect this potential, relying on potent combination therapies including steroids, cyclophosphamide, azathioprine, methotrexate, and, more recently, mycophenolate mofetil and TNF-α blockers. Preliminary data showed that the anti-TNF agent etanercept did not prove effective in adults with WG, but infliximab apparently was effective [4]. It is not clear whether this finding represents a fundamental difference in the agents or simply different potencies, but it does highlight the need for cooperative studies of new agents in the treatment of rare diseases, rather than haphazard experimentation by individual practitioners.

Despite progress in the management of WG, the disease continues to cause significant morbidity and mortality from relapses and treatment-related toxicity. Subglottic stenosis does not respond to systemic therapy but requires surgical dilatation and local steroid injections. In patients with limited upper respiratory disease, trimethoprim/sulfamethoxazole has been shown to be beneficial [94], perhaps by suppressing upper respiratory infections that might activate vascular inflammation.

Microscopic polyangiitis

Microscopic polyangiitis is a necrotizing vasculitis of the small vessels without granuloma formation. Clinical manifestations typically center around kidney and pulmonary involvement, especially focal segmental glomerulonephritis and pulmonary hemorrhage. The disease is characterized by a positive pANCA with reactivity to myeloperoxidase (MPO) by immunoblotting. In fact, these auto-antibodies seem to be integral to disease pathogenesis, activating neutrophils whose cytotoxic granules cause local vascular damage [95]. Thus, one must be cautious about making the diagnosis of microscopic polyangiitis in the absence of a positive ANCA. Biopsy or radiographic confirmation of vascular inflammation is also necessary to confirm the diagnosis, however, because nonspecific ANCA may be seen in a variety of other conditions, including inflammatory bowel disease, primary sclerosing cholangitis, and silicosis.

A diagnosis of microscopic polyangiitis seems to identify a disease with a severe and chronic course and significant risk of chronic renal failure. Most patients seem to require cyclophosphamide to achieve disease control. Milder agents may be adequate for maintaining remissions [96]. Most recently, a small, uncontrolled series suggested that a single 4-week course of rituximab might replace both cyclophosphamide and long-term steroids [5]. Larger studies aimed at confirming this finding will begin enrolling patients shortly.

Churg–Strauss syndrome

CSS is extremely rare in children. The first report of this small-vessel disease of the lungs, skin, peripheral nerves, heart, and gastrointestinal tract occurring in a preteen-aged child was made only in the past decade. The prodromal phase of CSS is manifested only as allergic rhinitis and asthma, and it may persist for many years. The second phase is characterized by worsening asthma, peripheral eosinophilia, and pulmonary infiltrates. Only during the third or vasculitic phase do manifestations of systemic vasculitis become evident, with weight loss, fever, arthralgia, myalgia, nodular rash, and neuropathy. Asthma symptoms usually subside during the vasculitic phase. In some cases, it may be difficult to differentiate CSS from PAN, although in CSS renal hypertension and nephritis are uncommon, and peripheral eosinophilia is quite striking. Tissue biopsy is generally diagnostic, with significant perivascular eosinophilic infiltrates and occasional extravascular granulomas. ANCA directed against both PR-3 and MPO may be seen in CSS.

The optimal regimen for treating CSS is not clear, although an initial aggressive remittive therapy, followed by milder maintenance treatment, may offer the best combination of safety and efficacy [96]. Disease control is necessary because untreated CSS is usually progressive. Most deaths are caused by cardiac involvement, followed by severe gastrointestinal and CNS disease. Fortunately, because CSS is exquisitely sensitive to corticosteroids, they offer a good bridging therapy until effects of remittive agents become evident.

Secondary vasculitides

Vasculitis may occur in the setting of a wide variety of infections, medications, and systemic diseases. These settings seem to represent a heightened susceptibility to vascular inflammation, because most people exposed to these viruses (parvovirus B19, HIV, varicella), Rickettsia, bacteria, fungi, mycobacteria, systemic inflammatory conditions (systemic lupus erythematosus, juvenile dermatomyositis [JDMS], juvenile rheumatoid arthritis, sarcoidosis, inflammatory bowel syndrome, tumors) and drugs (including leflunomide, TNF inhibitors, and anti-thyroid agents) do not develop vasculitis. Both leukocytoclastic and necrotizing vasculitis have been reported [97]. In most cases, removal of the trigger or control of the inciting condition leads to remission of the vasculitis.

Behçet's disease

Behçet's disease (BD) is a multisystem inflammatory disorder with manifestations similar to those of spondyloarthropathies. BD is characterized by the triad of recurrent oral ulcers, genital ulcers, and uveitis, but any organ system may be involved including skin, joints [98], CNS, or gastrointestinal tract, and vascular inflammation is often a prominent feature. Both arteries and veins may be affected, but there seems to be a particular predilection for the venules. Also characteristic of BD is a propensity for development of thromboses, including deep vein thrombosis and thrombophlebitis. Arterial aneurysms may also occur, and pulmonary aneurysms are a significant cause of mortality [99].

BD is thought to occur when an infectious agent triggers an amplified inflammatory response in a genetically susceptible host. In the Japanese and Turkish populations, in whom the disease is most prevalent, HLA-B51 is a marker for BD [100], and the aberrant cellular immune response seems to involve γδ-T cells. Antibody-mediated immune mechanisms may also play a role, given the cases of transient neonatal BD apparently caused by transplacental passage of antibodies from affected mothers. Various immunomodulatory agents, including IFN-α, thalidomide, and dapsone, are effective in some cases of BD, as are a variety of immunosuppressive agents, such as steroids, cyclophosphamide, and azathioprine [101]. The prognosis of BD seems to be worse in young males. Overall, the disease is less severe in Western countries.

Periodic fever syndromes

During the past 5 years, novel autoinflammatory conditions caused by mutations in regulators of inflammation have been described. As these periodic fever syndromes have been further characterized, an association with vasculitis has come to light. The gene defect responsible for FMF, a dysfunctional mutation of the protein pyrin, predisposes carriers to the development of HSP and PAN [102]. A group from Germany recently reported a small-vessel vasculitis in a patient who was found to have another periodic fever syndrome caused by the TNF receptor–associated periodic syndrome mutation [103]. They hypothesize that abnormal metabolism of TNF in this patient led to premature leukocyte activation and endothelial damage. The extent to which similar abnormalities in regulators of inflammation may account for other cases of vasculitis remains unknown, but these discoveries have opened new avenues of investigation into the pathogenesis of systemic vascular diseases.

Summary

Vasculitis is rare in children, and, apart from HSP and perhaps KD, most practicing pediatricians will never encounter a case. Nonetheless, progress in the diagnosis and treatment of these conditions has afforded most children with vasculitis a reasonably good prognosis. Accordingly, it is important to consider vasculitis as a potential cause of unexplained inflammation, perplexing rashes, or strange combinations of symptoms. Although evaluation and management of suspected vasculitis are difficult in the best of situations, they are impossible if the diagnosis is not considered.

References

[1] Bowyer SL, Ragsdale CG, Sullivan DB. Factor VIII related antigen and childhood rheumatic diseases. J Rheumatol 1989;16:1093–7.

[2] Fazzini F, Peri G, Doni A, et al. PTX3 in small-vessel vasculitides: an independent indicator of disease activity produced at sites of inflammation. Arthritis Rheum 2001;44:2841.

[3] Hoffman GS, Merkel PA, Brasington RD, et al. Anti-tumor necrosis factor therapy in patients with difficult to treat Takayasu arteritis. Arthritis Rheum 2004;50:2296.

[4] Wegener's Granulomatosis Etanercept Trial (WGET) Research Group. Etanercept plus standard therapy for Wegener's granulomatosis. N Engl J Med 2005;352:351–61.

[5] Keogh KA, Wylam ME, Stone JH, Specks U. Induction of remission by B lymphocyte depletion in 11 patients with refractory antineutrophil cytoplasmic antibody-associated vasculitis. Arthritis Rheum 2005;52:262–8.

[6] Jennette JC, Falk RJ. Do vasculitis categorization systems really matter? Curr Rheumatol Rep 2000;2:430.

[7] Tesar V, Kazderova M, Hlavackova L. Rokitansky and his first description of polyarteritis nodosa. J Nephrol 2004;17:172.

[8] Ozen S, Besbas N, Saatci U, et al. Diagnostic criteria for polyarteritis nodosa in childhood. J Pediatr 1992;120:206.

[9] Gardner-Medwin JM, Dolezalova P, Cummins C, et al. Incidence of Henoch-Schonlein purpura, Kawasaki disease, and rare vasculitides in children of different ethnic origins. Lancet 2002;360:1197.

[10] Bowyer S, Roettcher P. Pediatric rheumatology clinic populations in the United States: results of a 3 year survey. Pediatric Rheumatology Database Research Group. J Rheumatol 1996; 23:1968.

[11] Huugen D, Tervaert JW, Heeringa P. Antineutrophil cytoplasmic autoantibodies and pathophysiology: new insights from animal models. Curr Opin Rheumatol 2004;16:4.

[12] Praprotnik S, Rozman B, Blank M, et al. Pathogenic role of anti-endothelial cell antibodies in systemic vasculitis. Wien Klin Wochenschr 2000;112:660.

[13] Yoshinoya S. [Immune complex and vasculitis]. Nippon Rinsho 1994;52:1992–9 [in Japanese].

[14] Ozen S, Anton J, Arisoy N, et al. Juvenile polyarteritis: results of a multicenter survey of 110 children. J Pediatr 2004;145:517.

[15] Brogan PA, Shah V, Bagga A, et al. T cell Vbeta repertoires in childhood vasculitides. Clin Exp Immunol 2003;131:517.

[16] Kallenberg CG, Heeringa P. Pathogenesis of vasculitis. Lupus 1998;7:280.

[17] Jennette JC. Implications for pathogenesis of patterns of injury in small- and medium-sized-vessel vasculitis. Cleve Clin J Med 2002;69(Suppl 2):SII33.

[18] Blanco R, Martinez-Taboada VM, Rodriguez-Valverde V, et al. Henoch-Schonlein purpura in adulthood and childhood: two different expressions of the same syndrome. Arthritis Rheum 1997;40:859.

[19] Chaussain M, De Boissai D, Kalifa G, et al. Impairment of lung diffusion capacity in HSP. J Pediatr 1992;121:12.

[20] Dengler LD, Capparelli EV, Bastian JF, et al. Cerebrospinal fluid profile in patients with acute Kawasaki disease. Pediatr Infect Dis J 1998;17:478.

[21] Coppo R, Amore A, Gianoglio B. Clinical features of Henoch-Schonlein purpura. Italian Group of Renal Immunopathology. Ann Med Interne (Paris) 1999;150:143.

[22] Robson WL, Leung AK. Henoch-Schonlein purpura. Adv Pediatr 1994;41:163.

[23] Saulsbury FT. Henoch-Schonlein purpura in children. Report of 100 patients and review of the literature. Medicine (Baltimore) 1999;78:395.

[24] Chang WL, Yang YH, Lin YT, et al. Gastrointestinal manifestations in Henoch-Schonlein purpura: a review of 261 patients. Acta Paediatr 2004;93:1427.

[25] Gunasekaran TS, Berman J, Gonzalez M. Duodenojejunitis: is it idiopathic or is it Henoch-Schonlein purpura without the purpura? J Pediatr Gastroenterol Nutr 2000;30:22.

[26] Sano H, Izumida M, Shimizu H, et al. Risk factors of renal involvement and significant proteinuria in Henoch-Schonlein purpura. Eur J Pediatr 2002;161:196.

[27] Ronkainen J, Nuutinen M, Koskimies O. The adult kidney 24 years after childhood Henoch-Schonlein purpura: a retrospective cohort study. Lancet 2002;360:666.

[28] Kawasaki Y, Suzuki J, Sakai N, et al. Clinical and pathological features of children with Henoch-Schoenlein purpura nephritis: risk factors associated with poor prognosis. Clin Nephrol 2003;60:153.

[29] Soylemezoglu O, Ozkaya O, Erbas D, et al. Nitric oxide in Henoch-Schonlein purpura. Scand J Rheumatol 2002;31:271.

[30] Muller D, Greve D, Eggert P. Early tubular proteinuria and the development of nephritis in Henoch-Schonlein purpura. Pediatr Nephrol 2000;15:85.

[31] Martino F, Agolini D, Tsalikova E, et al. Nailfold capillaroscopy in Henoch-Schonlein purpura: a follow-up study of 31 cases. J Pediatr 2002;141:145.

[32] Saraclar Y, Tinaztepe K, Adalioglu G, et al. Acute hemorrhagic edema of infancy (AHEI)– a variant of Henoch-Schonlein purpura or a distinct clinical entity? J Allergy Clin Immunol 1990;86:473.

[33] Calabrese LH, Michel BA, Bloch DA, et al. The American College of Rheumatology 1990 criteria for the classification of hypersensitivity vasculitis. Arthritis Rheum 1990;33:1108.

[34] Sundel R, Szer I. Vasculitis in childhood. Rheum Dis Clin North Am 2002;28:625.

[35] Flynn JT, Smoyer WE, Bunchman TE, et al. Treatment of Henoch-Schonlein purpura glo- merulonephritis in children with high-dose corticosteroids plus oral cyclophosphamide. Am J Nephrol 2001;21:128.

[36] Newburger JW, Takahashi M, Burns JC, et al. The treatment of Kawasaki syndrome with intravenous gamma globulin. N Engl J Med 1986;315:341.

[37] Newburger JW, Taubert KA, Shulman ST, et al. Summary and abstracts of the Seventh International Kawasaki Disease Symposium: December 4–7, 2001, Hakone, Japan. Pediatr Res 2003;53:153.

[38] Newburger JW, Takahashi M, Gerber MA, et al. Diagnosis, treatment, and long-term management of Kawasaki disease: a statement for health professionals from the Committee on Rheumatic Fever, Endocarditis, and Kawasaki Disease, Council on Cardiovascular Disease in the Young, American Heart Association. Pediatrics 2004;114:1708.

[39] Rowley AH, Shulman ST, Spike BT, et al. Oligoclonal IgA response in the vascular wall in acute Kawasaki disease. J Immunol 2001;166:1334.

[40] Rowley AH, Baker SC, Shulman ST, et al. Detection of antigen in bronchial epithelium and macrophages in acute Kawasaki disease by use of synthetic antibody. J Infect Dis 2004; 190:856.

[41] Yanagawa H, Yashiro M, Nakamura Y, et al. Nationwide surveillance of Kawasaki disease in Japan, 1984 to 1993. Pediatr Infect Dis J 1995;14:69.

[42] Rowley AH, Wolinsky SM, Relman DA, et al. Search for highly conserved viral and bacterial nucleic acid sequences corresponding to an etiologic agent of Kawasaki disease. Pediatr Res 1994;36:567.

[43] Kawasaki T. [Acute febrile mucocutaneous syndrome with lymphoid involvement with spe- cific desquamation of the fingers and toes in children]. Arerugi 1967;16:178 [in Japanese].

[44] Burns JC, Mason WH, Glode MP, et al. Clinical and epidemiologic characteristics of patients referred for evaluation of possible Kawasaki disease. United States Multicenter Kawasaki Disease Study Group. J Pediatr 1991;118:680.

[45] Sundel RP. Update on the treatment of Kawasaki disease in childhood. Curr Rheumatol Rep 2002;4:474.

[46] Leung DY. The potential role of cytokine-mediated vascular endothelial activation in the pathogenesis of Kawasaki disease. Acta Paediatr Jpn 1991;33:739.

[47] Smith LB, Newburger JW, Burns JC. Kawasaki syndrome and the eye. Pediatr Infect Dis J 1989;8:116.

[48] April MM, Burns JC, Newburger JW, et al. Kawasaki disease and cervical adenopathy. Arch Otolaryngol Head Neck Surg 1989;115:512.

[49] Joffe A, Kabani A, Jadavji T. Atypical and complicated Kawasaki disease in infants. Do we need criteria? West J Med 1995;162:322.

[50] Yanagawa H, Tuohong Z, Oki I, et al. Effects of gamma-globulin on the cardiac sequelae of Kawasaki disease. Pediatr Cardiol 1999;20:248.

[51] Burns JC, Capparelli EV, Brown JA, et al. Intravenous gamma-globulin treatment and retreatment in Kawasaki disease. US/Canadian Kawasaki Syndrome Study Group. Pediatr Infect Dis J 1998;17:1144.

[52] Wen YK, Yang Y, Chang CC. Cerebral vasculitis and intracerebral hemorrhage in Henoch-Schonlein purpura treated with plasmapheresis. Pediatr Nephrol 2005;20:223–5.

[53] Yanagihara R, Todd JK. Acute febrile mucocutaneous lymph node syndrome. Am J Dis Child 1980;134:603.

[54] Beiser AS, Takahashi M, Baker AL, et al. A predictive instrument for coronary artery aneurysms in Kawasaki disease. US Multicenter Kawasaki Disease Study Group. Am J Cardiol 1998;81:1116.

[55] Kusakawa S, Tatara K. Efficacies and risks of aspirin in the treatment of the Kawasaki disease. Prog Clin Biol Res 1987;250:401.

[56] Furusho K, Kamiya T, Nakano H, et al. High-dose intravenous gammaglobulin for Kawasaki disease. Lancet 1984;2:1055.

[57] Hsieh KS, Weng KP, Lin CC, et al. Treatment of acute Kawasaki disease: aspirin's role in the febrile stage revisited. Pediatrics 2004;114:e689.

[58] Kato H, Koike S, Tanaka C, et al. Coronary heart disease in children with Kawasaki disease. Jpn Circ J 1979;43:469.

[59] Shinohara M, Sone K, Tomomasa T, et al. Corticosteroids in the treatment of the acute phase of Kawasaki disease. J Pediatr 1999;135:465.

[60] Okada Y, Shinohara M, Kobayashi T, et al. Effect of corticosteroids in addition to intravenous gamma globulin therapy on serum cytokine levels in the acute phase of Kawasaki disease in children. J Pediatr 2003;143:363.

[61] Sundel RP, Baker AL, Fulton DR, et al. Corticosteroids in the initial treatment of Kawasaki disease: report of a randomized trial. J Pediatr 2003;142:611.

[62] Burns JC, Glode MP. Kawasaki syndrome. Lancet 2004;364:533.

[63] Newburger JW, Takahashi M, Beiser AS, et al. A single intravenous infusion of gamma globulin as compared with four infusions in the treatment of acute Kawasaki syndrome. N Engl J Med 1991;324:1633.

[64] Weiss JE, Eberhard BA, Chowdhury D, et al. Infliximab as a novel therapy for refractory Kawasaki disease. J Rheumatol 2004;31:808.

[65] Fukushige J, Takahashi N, Ueda K, et al. Long-term outcome of coronary abnormalities in patients after Kawasaki disease. Pediatr Cardiol 1996;17:71.

[66] Dhillon R, Clarkson P, Donald AE, et al. Endothelial dysfunction late after Kawasaki disease. Circulation 1996;94:2103.

[67] McConnell ME, Hannon DW, Steed RD, et al. Fatal obliterative coronary vasculitis in Kawasaki disease. J Pediatr 1998;133:259.

[68] Tomita S, Chung K, Mas M, et al. Peripheral gangrene associated with Kawasaki disease. Clin Infect Dis 1992;14:121.

[69] Williams RV, Wilke VM, Tani LY, et al. Does abciximab enhance regression of coronary aneurysms resulting from Kawasaki disease? Pediatrics 2002;109:E4.

[70] Nakamura Y, Yanagawa H, Harada K, et al. Mortality among persons with a history of Kawasaki disease in Japan: the fifth look. Arch Pediatr Adolesc Med 2002;156:162.

[71] Baker AL, Gauvreau K, Newburger JW, et al. Physical and psychosocial health in children who have had Kawasaki disease. Pediatrics 2003;111:579.

[72] Blanco R, Martinez-Taboada VM, Rodriguez-Valverde V, et al. Cutaneous vasculitis in children and adults. Associated diseases and etiologic factors in 303 patients. Medicine (Baltimore) 1998;77:403.

[73] Ozen S, Saatci U, Balkanci F, et al. Familial Mediterranean fever and polyarteritis nodosa. Scand J Rheumatol 1992;21:312.

[74] Fink CW. Vasculitis. Pediatr Clin North Am 1986;33:1203.

[75] David J, Ansell BM, Woo P. Polyarteritis nodosa associated with streptococcus. Arch Dis Child 1993;69:685.

[76] Sheth AP, Olson JC, Esterly NB. Cutaneous polyarteritis nodosa of childhood. J Am Acad Dermatol 1994;31:561.

[77] Garcia-Porrua C, Gonzalez-Gay MA. Successful response to infliximab in a patient with undifferentiated spondyloarthropathy coexisting with polyarteritis nodosa-like cutaneous vasculitis. Clin Exp Rheumatol 2003;21:S138.

[78] Mouthon L, Le Toumelin P, Andre MH, et al. Polyarteritis nodosa and Churg-Strauss angiitis: characteristics and outcome in 38 patients over 65 years. Medicine (Baltimore) 2002;81:27.

[79] Brogan PA, Dillon MJ. Vasculitis from the pediatric perspective. Curr Rheumatol Rep 2000; 2:411.

[80] Noris M. Pathogenesis of Takayasu's arteritis. J Nephrol 2001;14:506.

[81] Seo P, Stone JH. Large-vessel vasculitis. Arthritis Rheum 2004;51:128.

[82] Kimura A, Ota M, Katsuyama Y, et al. Mapping of the HLA-linked genes controlling the susceptibility to Takayasu's arteritis. Int J Cardiol 2000;75(Suppl 1):S105.

[83] Yalcindag A, Sundel R. Vasculitis in childhood. Curr Opin Rheumatol 2001;13:422.

[84] Kerr GS, Hallahan CW, Giordano J, et al. Takayasu arteritis. Ann Intern Med 1994;120:919.

[85] Tso E, Flamm SD, White RD, et al. Takayasu arteritis: utility and limitations of magnetic resonance imaging in diagnosis and treatment. Arthritis Rheum 2002;46:1634.

[86] Seo JW, Park IA, Yoon DH, et al. Thoracic aortic aneurysm associated with aortitis–case reports and histological review. J Korean Med Sci 1991;6:75.

[87] Calabrese L. Primary angiitis of the central nervous system: the penumbra of vasculitis. J Rheumatol 2001;28:465.

[88] Gallagher KT, Shaham B, Reiff A, et al. Primary angiitis of the central nervous system in children: 5 cases. J Rheumatol 2001;28:616.

[89] Benseler S, Schneider R. Central nervous system vasculitis in children. Curr Opin Rheumatol 2004;16:43.

[90] Rottem M, Fauci AS, Hallahan CW, et al. Wegener granulomatosis in children and adolescents: clinical presentation and outcome. J Pediatr 1993;122:26.

[91] Langford CA, Sneller MC, Hallahan CW, et al. Clinical features and therapeutic management of subglottic stenosis in patients with Wegener's granulomatosis. Arthritis Rheum 1996;39:1754.

[92] Yu F, Zhao MH, Huang JP, et al. [Clinical and pathological features of anti-neutrophil cytoplasm antibody associated systemic vasculitis in children]. Zhonghua Er Ke Za Zhi 2003; 41:831 [in Japanese].

[93] Langford CA, Sneller MC. Update on the diagnosis and treatment of Wegener's granulomatosis. Adv Intern Med 2001;46:177.

[94] Langford CA, Talar-Williams C, Barron KS, et al. A staged approach to the treatment of Wegener's granulomatosis: induction of remission with glucocorticoids and daily cyclophosphamide switching to methotrexate for remission maintenance. Arthritis Rheum 1999; 42:2666.

[95] Heeringa P, Tervaert JW. Pathophysiology of ANCA-associated vasculitides: are ANCA really pathogenic? Kidney Int 2004;65:1564.

[96] Sanders JS, Slot MC, Stegeman CA. Maintenance therapy for vasculitis associated with antineutrophil cytoplasmic autoantibodies. N Engl J Med 2003;349:2072.

[97] Weyand CM, Goronzy JJ. Medium- and large-vessel vasculitis. N Engl J Med 2003;349:160.

[98] Eldem B, Onur C, Ozen S. Clinical features of pediatric Behcet's disease. J Pediatr Ophthalmol Strabismus 1998;35:159.

[99] Uziel Y, Brik R, Padeh S, et al. Juvenile Behcet's disease in Israel. The Pediatric Rheumatology Study Group of Israel. Clin Exp Rheumatol 1998;16:502.

[100] Park SH, Park KS, Seo YI, et al. Association of MICA polymorphism with HLA-B51 and disease severity in Korean patients with Behcet's disease. J Korean Med Sci 2002;17:366.

[101] Sakane T, Takeno M. Current therapy in Behcet's disease. Skin Therapy Lett 2000;5:3.

[102] Ozen S. Vasculopathy, Behcet's syndrome, and familial Mediterranean fever. Curr Opin Rheumatol 1999;11:393.

[103] Lamprecht P, Moosig F, Adam-Klages S, et al. Small vessel vasculitis and relapsing panniculitis

in tumour necrosis factor receptor associated periodic syndrome (TRAPS). Ann Rheum Dis 2004;63:1518.

[104] Hunder GG, Wilking AP. Classification of the vasculitides in children. UptoDate, 2005. Available at: http://www.utdol.com/application/search.asp. Accessed February 14, 2005.

[105] Centers for Disease Control. Revised diagnostic criteria for Kawasaki disease. MMWR 1990; 39(No. 44-13):27–8.

ELSEVIER
SAUNDERS

PEDIATRIC CLINICS
OF NORTH AMERICA

Pediatr Clin N Am 52 (2005) 577–609

Periodic Fever Syndromes

Shai Padeh, MD[a,b,*]

[a]Pediatric Rheumatology, Edmond & Lily Safra Children Hospital, The Chaim Sheba Medical Center,
Tel Hashomer 52621, Israel
[b]Sackler School of Medicine, Tel-Aviv University, Tel Aviv, Israel

The term auto-inflammatory disease has been proposed to describe a group of disorders characterized by attacks of seemingly unprovoked inflammation without significant levels of either autoantibodies or autoreactive T cells. The genetic causes of eight hereditary autoinflammatory syndromes have been identified in the last 7 years:

Familial Mediterranean fever (FMF)
Tumor necrosis factor (TNF) receptor–associated periodic syndrome (TRAPS)
Hyperimmunoglobulinemia D and periodic fever syndrome (HIDS)
Familial cold autoinflammatory syndrome (FCAS)/familial cold urticaria syndrome (FCUS)
Muckle-Wells syndrome (MWS)
Neonatal-onset multisystem inflammatory disease (NOMID)/chronic infantile neurologic cutaneous and articular (CINCA) syndrome
Blau syndrome
PAPA (Pyogenic sterile Arthritis, Pyoderma gangrenosum and Acne) syndrome

This article discusses those syndromes that are associated with recurrent fevers. Members of a recently described family of genes, the pyrin family, account for several hereditary periodic fever syndromes. The study of autoinflammatory disease has progressed from clinical characterization to genetic analysis and to definition of the functional defects, linking pyrin genes or domains to apoptotic proteins and signal transduction pathways. As a result, the periodic fever syn-

* Pediatric Rheumatology, Edmond & Lily Safra Children Hospital, The Chaim Sheba Medical Center, Tel Hashomer 52621, Israel.
E-mail address: padeh@012.net.il

0031-3955/05/$ – see front matter © 2005 Elsevier Inc. All rights reserved.
doi:10.1016/j.pcl.2005.01.005

pediatric.theclinics.com

dromes have been associated with the field of innate immunology, and the classification of these disorders has been changed to autoimmune hereditary fevers. Most patients with hereditary periodic fevers have mutations in either the pyrin or the tumor-necrosis factor (TNF) receptor superfamily of molecules, both of which are intimately involved in innate immunity.

Both pyrin and a related gene, cryopyrin, contain an N-terminal domain that encodes a death domain–related structure, now known as the pyrin domain, or PyD. The PyD is a conserved sequence motif identified in more than 20 human proteins with putative functions in apoptotic and inflammatory signaling pathways [1]. Both pyrin and cryopyrin interact through their PyDs with a common adaptor protein, apoptotic speck protein (ASC). ASC itself participates in apoptosis, recruitment, and activation of pro-caspase-1 (with associated processing and secretion of interleukin [IL]-1 beta), and nuclear factor (NF)-kappa B,

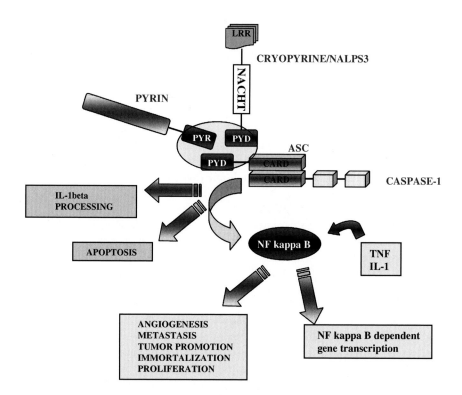

Fig. 1. Proteins containing PyD domain regulate inflammation through their interaction with apoptotic speck protein (ASC). The assembly of cryopyrin and ASC induces IL-1 processing through caspase-1, whereas pyrin may act as an inhibitor. Loss of function by mutations in the pyrin could potentially lead to autoinflammation by reducing the pyrin inhibitory role. Alternatively, gain-of-function mutations in cryopyrin, as found in MWS/FCU/NOMID patients, could activate this pathway. ASC participates in apoptosis and activation of NF-kappa B, a transcription factor involved in both initiation and resolution of the inflammatory response. IL-1, interleukin-1; LRR, LLR, leucine-rich repeats; TNF, tumor necrosis factor.

a transcription factor involved in both initiation and resolution of the inflammatory response (Fig. 1). Pyrin protein associates with tubulin and actin, leading to speculation that pyrin might regulate cytoskeletal organization in leukocytes. Hereditary pyrin mutants do not show altered cellular distribution and still colocalize with ASC. In contrast, cryopyrin displays granular cytoplasmic localization [2]. Expression of some PyD-containing proteins, including pyrin, and of ASC is controlled by interferons (IFNs). Inflammatory mediators such as lipopolysaccharide (LPS) and TNF increase the expression of cryopyrin, and its expression is also increased at sites of inflammation [2]. Likewise, pyrin is induced as an immediate early gene by proinflammatory molecules (eg, TNF, LPS, and IFNs), but inducibility is inhibited by anti-inflammatory cytokines (eg, IL-4, IL-10, and transforming growth factor-beta) [2]. In summary, pyrin and cryopyrin, through PyD:PyD interactions, seem to modulate the activity of apoptotic proteins and signal transduction pathways, playing a crucial role in the inflammatory pathways of the innate immune system [3–5].

Familial Mediterranean fever

FMF is an autosomal recessive disease mainly affecting ethnic groups living around the Mediterranean basin: Sephardic and Ashkenazi Jews, Armenians, Turks, Arabs, and Druze [6]. Scattered cases of FMF have been reported throughout the world, however, and cases are increasingly reported from other ethnicities, such as Greeks, Italians, Japanese, and others [7–9]. Although FMF existed in early Biblical times, it was first described as a separate nosologic entity in 1945 [10]. In the early 1950s, French investigators [11] described the disease in Jews of Sephardic extraction in North Africa and first reported nephropathy as part of the disease. In the same period, the disease was described in Armenian families [12]. Following the waves of emigration of Jews from North Africa, Iraq, and Turkey to the newly formed state of Israel in the 1950s, Sohar et al [13] and Heller et al [14] established a detailed clinical description of the condition. This description included recessive inheritance, arthritis, the nature of amyloid nephropathy, and the name familial Mediterranean fever. The benefit of prophylactic treatment with colchicine was first suggested by Goldfinger [15] and was later assessed by double-blind studies [16].

The gene responsible for FMF, *MEFV*, has been mapped to the short arm of chromosome 16 [17]. The protein encoded by this gene, termed pyrin/Marenostrin, is present almost exclusively in neutrophils and their precursors [18,19]. The role of pyrin is believed be to decrease inflammation, specifically in neutrophils.

Clinical features

Painful febrile episodes constitute the hallmark of the disease. The febrile episodes are characterized by elevated temperatures of 38.5° to 40°C and in most cases accompanied by signs of peritonitis, pleuritis, or acute synovitis, mainly of the knee, ankle, or hip. The attacks are short-lived, lasting for 1 to 3 days, and resolve without treatment. Between attacks, patients are perfectly well. Children commonly complain of headache and general malaise accompanying the elevated temperature. Recurrent oral aphthae are often reported, unassociated with attacks. Repeated attacks at irregular intervals and in an unpredicted sequence, rather than truly periodic attacks, are typical of the disease. The frequency of attacks may vary from once per week to periods of remissions of weeks or months with no apparent explanation. Over the course of the illness, a patient will probably experience several forms of attacks, but the recurrence of one type over many years is common [6]. In children, febrile attacks alone could be the first manifestation of the disease, occurring years before other forms of attacks appear. The age of onset in the cohort of 704 FMF patients followed in the Pediatric National Clinic in the Sheba Medical Center in Tel Hahsomer, Israel, is depicted in Fig. 2. About half of the cases had symptoms before the age of 4 years, and 80% had symptoms before the age of 10 years. The delay in diagnosis was in direct correlation to the age of patients at the onset, probably representing the difficulties in diagnosing very young patients (Fig. 3).

Abdominal attacks

Other than fever, the most frequent manifestation of FMF is the abdominal attack, experienced by 90% of patients. This attack is marked by the sudden onset of fever and generalized abdominal pain, guarding of the abdominal muscles, rebound tenderness, and abdominal distention, mimicking acute appendicitis. After 6 to 20 hours, the signs and symptoms recede, and within 24 to 48 hours the attack is usually over [6]. Often vomiting or diarrhea accompanies the abdominal pain. Many patients note that diarrhea terminates the attack. In severe cases, analgesics or intravenous rehydration is required. Organization of the exudate,

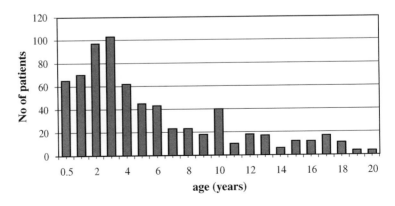

Fig. 2. The age at onset in a cohort of 704 FMF patients followed in the Pediatric National Clinic in the Sheba Medical Center in Tel Hahsomer, Israel.

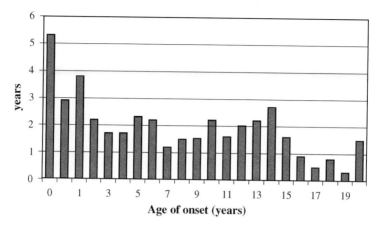

Fig. 3. The delay in diagnosis in a cohort of 704 FMF patients followed in the Pediatric National Clinic in the Sheba Medical Center in Tel Hahsomer, Israel.

which is formed in the peritoneum during the acute inflammation, may result in fibrous adhesions that in rare cases may give rise to mechanical ileus [20]. The adhesions are probably the cause of sterility in some women affected by FMF [21]. In the author's cohort of pediatric FMF patients, 65 (9%) underwent emergent appendectomy, but only 35 patients (5%) had acute appendicitis. Prophylactic appendectomy is not recommended, because in most cases both children and their parents can clearly distinguish between an abdominal attack of FMF and abdominal pain from other causes.

Acute scrotum

In males, inflammation of the tunica vaginalis testis may mimic episodes of torsion of the testis. Unilateral, erythematous, and tender swelling of the scrotum occurs in scrotal attacks. Fever and pain are present in all cases. The episodes are self-limiting and last from a few hours to 4 days [22].

Pleural attacks

Pleural attacks occur in 15% to 30% of patients [23]. Attacks present an acute one-sided febrile pleuritis resembling the peritoneal attacks in their abrupt onset, unpredictable recurrence, and rapid resolution. Breathing is painful, and breath sounds may be diminished in severe cases. There may be radiologic evidence of a small pleural effusion or mild pleural thickening.

Pericarditis attacks

Pericarditis is a rare feature of FMF. The author and colleagues observed clinical attacks of pericarditis in only six children with FMF (0.8%) [24]. This type of attack also resolves within 1 to 3 days. Four of the children also had other forms of FMF attacks, but two had only pericarditis.

Articular attacks

Articular involvement is the second-most common form of FMF. The acute arthritis of FMF is abrupt and accompanied by high fever in the first 24 hours. In most cases, it is monoarticular and affects one of the large joints of the lower extremities (ie, the ankle, knee, or hip, in that order). The arthritis lasts longer than other FMF manifestations, usually peaking within 24 to 48 hours and then gradually subsiding, leaving no residua. Attacks often are precipitated by minor trauma or effort, such as prolonged walking. The arthritis of FMF differs significantly from juvenile idiopathic arthritis in many respects: the affected joint is hot, tender, and often red, resembling septic arthritis. The synovial fluid is sterile, but varies in appearance from cloudy to purulent and contains large numbers of neutrophils [6,14]. Nonsteroidal anti-inflammatory drugs (NSAIDs) are generally effective in FMF arthritis, and naproxen is used successfully during the attack. Rarely, FMF patients experience protracted arthritic attacks that may persist for more than a month (reported in 6% of adult patients [25]). These attacks usually occur in the hip or knee. Although not described in children, joint damage (mostly in the hip) can be severe and cause permanent deformity that may require joint replacement in some adult cases [25,26].

Myalgia

Muscle pain occurs in about 10% of children with FMF. The pain is usually mild, occurs mainly in the lower extremities after physical exertion or prolonged standing, lasts a few hours to 1 day, and subsides with rest or NSAIDs. In 1994 Langevitz et al [27] first described FMF patients with a syndrome of protracted febrile myalgia. This syndrome is characterized by severe debilitating myalgia, prolonged fever, abdominal pain without peritoneal irritation, a higher sedimentation rate than commonly found in FMF (around 100 mm in the first hour), leukocytosis, and hyperglobulinemia. In patients treated with NSAIDs the attacks lasted for 6 to 8 weeks but subsided promptly after treatment with prednisone, 1 mg/kg [27]. Because on rare occasions colchicine can induce neuropathy, it is important to differentiate colchicine-induced myopathy from protracted febrile myalgia.

Skin manifestations

Attacks of erysipelas-like erythema (ELE) (Fig. 4) are characteristic of FMF and sometimes are combined with arthritis. ELE occurred in 28.3% of the author's cohort of 704 pediatric FMF patients. Tender, hot, swollen, sharply bordered red lesions appear on the skin of the lower extremities. Usually located

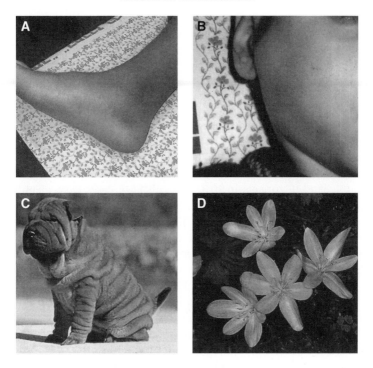

Fig. 4. (*A*) Erysipelas-like erythema of FMF and arthritis of the ankle. (*B*) Temporomandibular arthritis in FMF. (*C*) Familial Shar-Pei fever is a periodic disease occurring in Shar-Pei dogs. Clinically, the disease resembles FMF: febrile attacks are accompanied by arthritis, peritonitis, pleuritis, and amyloidosis. The *MEFV* gene is not found in the dog. (*D*) *Colchicum automnale*, the flower from which colchicine is made.

between the knee and ankle, on the dorsum of the foot, or in ankle region, the dermatitis is often accompanied by abrupt elevation of body temperature and lasts 24 to 48 hours [6,28]. An erroneous diagnosis of cellulitis is often made and an antibiotic prescribed. Histologic examination of the lesions reveals edema of the superficial dermis and sparse perivascular infiltrate without vasculitis. In all cases, direct immunofluorescence shows deposits of C3 in the wall of the small vessels of the superficial vascular plexus [29].

Isolated febrile attacks

Isolated, short-lived elevation of temperature to 40°C without pain or signs of localized inflammation occurs mainly in young children and lasts a few hours. This phenomenon of FMF is often attributed falsely to viral infection [6]. The result is a delay in diagnosis and initiation of prophylactic colchicine therapy. In the author's cohort, in 50 children who first exhibited fever as the only manifestation of FMF, other manifestations of FMF developed 4.5 ± 2.2 years after the onset of fevers (unpublished data). Once additional forms of attacks are present, the fever-only attacks subside, and the recognized pattern of FMF disease continues.

Vasculitis in familial Mediterranean fever

Vasculitides are found in FMF patients at a higher incidence than in the unaffected population. Henoch-Schonlein purpura (HSP) have been reported in 3% to 11% of FMF patients [6,30,31]. Occult FMF cases were identified in a series of children with HSP from Israel. Polyarteritis nodosa (PAN) also occurs more commonly in patients with FMF [32], with a younger age of onset [32]. Although abdominal pain and fever occur in both FMF attacks and PAN, hypertension, nephritis, and the persistence of symptoms are more likely to occur in PAN. Hematuria, sometimes only microscopic, has been observed in some patients during and between attacks of FMF.

Various types of glomerulonephritis have also been reported in FMF [33], but data are insufficient to determine whether these disorders are more common in FMF patients than in the general population. In the author's pediatric cohort, two patients had poststreptococcal glomerulonephritis, and five had Berger nephropathy. Transient microscopic hematuria is a common finding.

Amyloidosis of familial Mediterranean fever

Amyloidosis occurs frequently in untreated patients with FMF, and is of the AA type. It usually presents in FMF patients with persistent heavy proteinuria leading to nephrotic syndrome. The prevalence of amyloidosis in children in the colchicine era is unknown. In the cohort of 704 children seen by the author and colleagues, only 1 child developed end-stage renal disease, probably as a result of poor compliance with colchicine treatment. Amyloidosis is more common in other populations, however, and amyloidosis of different magnitude has been reported in children in Turkey [34]. Amyloid nephropathy has been reported in a child as young as 5 years of age [34]. In a study of 425 Turkish children with FMF from a registry of 20 years in a main referral center, 180 children developed amyloidosis. In the presence of a family history of amyloidosis plus consanguinity in FMF, patients had a 6.04-fold increased risk of amyloidosis [23].

Laboratory investigation

In all forms of attack, leukocytosis and elevated acute-phase reactants, including an accelerated erythrocyte sedimentation rate (ESR) and elevated levels of

C-reactive protein (CRP), fibrinogen, haptoglobin, C3, C4, and serum amyloid A are characteristic. Markers of inflammation often distinguish FMF attacks from common viral illnesses, functional abdominal pain, and irritable bowel syndrome. According to the reports of Gillmore et al [35], the increase in CRP was found to correlate better with FMF attacks, with levels much higher than in other inflammatory conditions. The mean ESR levels found during the attacks in the author's cohort of pediatric FMF patients was 52 ± 25 mm for the first hour. A very prolonged ESR (80–120 mm for the first hour) was indicative, in many cases, of other causes such as pneumonia or vasculitis. Proteinuria, as an indication of amyloidosis, will develop over the years if FMF is not treated. A yearly urinalysis to detect microalbuminuria is recommended in all patients.

Diagnosis and differential diagnosis

Until 1998, the diagnosis of FMF was based on clinical grounds alone. The presence of short-lived febrile episodes accompanied by inflammation of one of the serous membranes, the development of nephropathic amyloidosis, and the response to colchicine treatment were the grounds for the diagnosis. The ethnic origin of the patients and a family history of FMF may help direct the physician to a correct diagnosis but are not crucial for establishing a diagnosis of FMF. The most common differential diagnosis of FMF is functional abdominal pain, irritable bowel syndrome, and recurrent (intercurrent) infections in young children, and these symptoms are responsible for most referrals to FMF centers. The differential diagnosis includes diseases characterized by recurrent fever, such as hyper-IgD immunoglobulinemia (HIDS), TRAPS, and the periodic fever, adenopathy, pharyngitis, aphthae (PFAPA) syndrome.

Treatment

Until 1973, the treatment of FMF was restricted to alleviating pain. Daily prophylactic treatment with colchicine was suggested by Goldfinger [15] and assessed by double-blind studies [16]. Treatment is started with 1 mg colchicine per day (or 1.2 mg in the United States, where tablets of 0.6 mg are available), regardless of age or body weight. This dose is increased to 1.5 or 2 mg until remission is achieved. Doses higher than 1.5 mg must be divided and given twice a day. Some authors recommended adjusting the doses according to body weight or surface area. In one study, mean colchicine doses according to the body weight and surface area were 0.03 ± 0.02 mg/kg/day and 1.16 ± 0.45 mg/m^2/day, respectively. Children younger than 5 years of age needed colchicine doses as high as 0.07 mg/kg/day or 1.9 mg/m^2/day. These dosages were approximately 2.5 to three times higher than the mean colchicine dose for persons aged 16 to 20 years [36]. Omission of only one daily dose may result in an attack. The author and colleagues found that 65% of FMF patients enjoy complete remission of attacks if they adhere to the daily dose of colchicine. An additional 30% of patients experience partial remission, defined as a significant decrease in the frequency and severity of attacks. In 5% of treated patients, the attack rate remains unchanged [16]. Nevertheless, these patients are maintained on 2 mg colchicine per day to prevent amyloidosis. The author's experience showed that continuous prophylactic treatment with colchicine in FMF patients inhibits the development of nephropathic amyloidosis. None of the patients without proteinuria who began treatment and adhered to the treatment regime developed amyloidosis during the 30-year follow-up. Side effects of colchicine are rare and generally mild, with diarrhea and nausea being the most common. These side effects are controlled easily by diet and gastrointestinal antispasmodic medications [16]. The author and colleagues prescribe colchicine to children as young as 1 year (at a dose of 0.5 mg/day), increased to an adult dose at the age of 2 years and have seen no serious toxicity. Diarrhea is often more severe at this age. Colchicine induces significant lactose malabsorption in FMF patients, and this malabsorption is partially responsible for the gastrointestinal side effects of the drug. [37]. The safety of colchicine is even more convincing, as evidenced by its continuing use during pregnancy without any complications [21,38]. In patients who do not respond to colchicine, the use of intravenous colchicine or IFN-alfa should be considered [39,40].

Genetic analysis and pathophysiology

The MEFV gene

In 1992, the gene responsible for FMF, *MEFV*, was found to reside on the short arm of chromosome 16 [17]. Five years later, the *MEFV* gene locus was discovered [18,19]. The International FMF Consortium has named the protein pyrin, from the Greek word for fire and fever, whereas the French FMF Consortium prefers to call it marenostrin, which is Latin for "our sea." Pyrin plays a role in mitigating an inflammatory response [19,41]. To date, more than 40 missense mutations are noted in association with FMF. One specific mutation, *M694V*, has been implicated as a risk factor for amyloidosis.

Pyrin is found in large quantities in neutrophils and is released in response to inflammatory stimuli. Additionally, a recently discovered pyrin-like domain was found to exist at the amino-terminal of several proteins involved in cell-signaling pathways inherent to inflammation. The pyrin protein encoded by the *MEFV* gene belongs to a larger class of the PyD family and is involved in the NF-kappa B cell-signaling pathway. NF-kappa B is an important transcription factor involved in inflammation through induction of proinflammatory gene products. In individuals with the wild-type *MEFV* gene, pyrin serves a key role in regulating the intensity of the inflammatory response. In contrast, individuals with one or more missense mutations at the *MEFV* locus produce a pyrin protein with altered or absent function. Consequently, the ability to regulate the inflammatory response is reduced, and the resultant dysregulated inflammatory response often exceeds physiologic parameters and is disproportionate to the insult that initially triggered the neutrophil activation [4,42–45]. The exclusive expression of *MEFV* in neutrophils supports the clinical observations that neutrophils accumulate in large numbers at sites of inflammation during FMF attacks.

The recent cloning of *MEFV* and its putative role in white blood cells suggest that the gene may provide an advantage over an infectious agent prevalent in the region. Failure to control inflammation might give heterozygotes an advantage in dealing with some infections and may have given rise to the proliferation of the mutated gene. On the other hand, it has been shown that other inflammatory diseases (such as multiple sclerosis) progress rapidly in patients carrying one mutated *MEFV* gene, particularly *M694V*, because of the increased inflammatory damage inflicted by autoimmune responses [46].

Genotype–phenotype correlation

The cloning of the FMF gene *MEFV* and the identification of the mutations causing the disease raised hopes for a more rapid and accurate diagnostic test for FMF [18]. Molecular diagnosis is still not sensitive enough, however, because it fails to confirm the diagnosis of FMF in a large number of patients with typical presentation, even after the entire gene has been sequenced. In an analysis of 216 children with FMF, the author and colleagues found one of the three common *MEFV* mutations in 56% of the studied alleles, but only 38% of the children had two mutated alleles [47]. In another center in Israel [48], molecular testing for the common mutations identified two mutations in 48 of 67 patients (71.6%) of Jewish and Arab extraction (46.3% were Arab children). Divergent results reported from different centers may stem from differences in patient population, patient selection for genetic testing, and diagnostic criteria. Nevertheless, a significant proportion of patients with a typical clinical presentation of FMF and a favorable response to colchicine had only one mutation or none. With respect to genotyping, comparable findings were reported in adults [49] and children [48,50], showing that patients homozygous for the *M694V* mutation had an earlier onset, a more severe course, more joint involvement [51], higher temperature during attacks, higher prevalence of pleuritis, splenomegaly, ELE [50], and amyloidosis [52,53]. Since the identification of the *MEFV* gene, 40 point mutations have been reported. Most laboratories providing routine genetic testing of FMF screen for at least the five most frequent mutations *(M694V, V726A, V680I, E148Q,* and *M694I)*, because the other mutations were found in fewer than 1% of FMF alleles. Genetic analysis does add valuable information, supporting the clinical diagnosis and reassuring the patients of the necessity of lifelong colchicine prophylaxis. Because FMF carries a high risk for the development of amyloidosis, leading to chronic renal failure if untreated [6,16], colchicine treatment should not be withheld because of a nonsupportive mutation analysis. Individuals who meet the clinical criteria for FMF but who have only

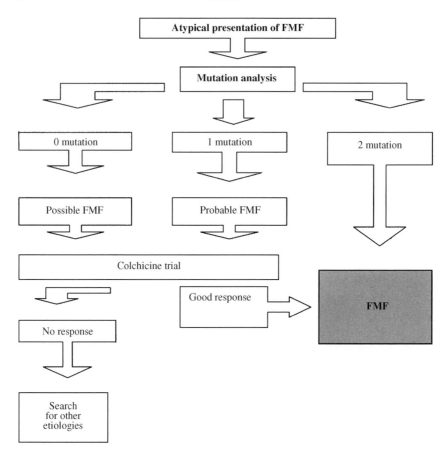

Fig. 5. An algorithm for the diagnosis of atypical clinical presentation of FMF. Patients with two mutations should be diagnosed with FMF and prescribed prophylactic colchicine therapy. Patients with one mutation should be considered as probably having FMF, and patients with no mutations should be considered as possibly having FMF. The last two groups of patients should undergo a colchicine trial consisting of 6 months of treatment followed by drug discontinuation. Those who have a favorable response are diagnosed as having FMF and should continue prophylactic colchicine treatment. Other causes for their symptomatology should be sought for those with no response.

one demonstrable mutation in the FMF gene may still harbor an unknown mutation (Fig. 5) [54,55].

Periodic fever accompanied by aphthous stomatitis, pharyngitis, and cervical adenitis syndrome

PFAPA syndrome is a chronic disease of unknown cause characterized by periodic episodes of high fever accompanied by aphthous stomatitis, pharyngitis, and cervical adenitis, often associated with headache or abdominal or joint pain [56–58]. This syndrome belongs to the group of recurrent fever syndromes, which includes systemic-onset juvenile rheumatoid arthritis, cyclic neutropenia, and the group of hereditary fevers [59]. Unlike hereditary autoimmune fevers, however, PFAPA is a sporadic syndrome, and second cases in siblings are not found.

Clinical features

The earliest report of the syndrome was by Miller et al [60] who described 29 patients with febrile episodes occurring every 21.6 days for an average of 4.6 days. In 1987 Marshall et al [61] described a syndrome of periodic fever in 12 children, lasting 3 to 6 days and recurring every 3 to 8 weeks, accompanied by aphthous stomatitis, pharyngitis, and cervical adenitis. In 1989 they coined the acronym PFAPA to describe this entity [62]. They later described a larger series of 94 children identified with PFAPA and provided the long-term follow-up on 83 [56]. The author and colleagues have reported their experience with 28 cases [57]. PFAPA episodes last 4 to 5 days and resolve spontaneously. Attacks recur every 4 to 6 weeks, with temperatures up to 40.5°C. The affected children had no long-term sequelae. Episodes of fevers begin at the age of 4.2 ± 2.7 years. Fever, chills, sweats, headache, and muscle and bone pain are common. General malaise, resembling streptococcal pharyngitis, tonsillitis with negative throat cultures, and cervical adenopathy are typical of the syndrome. Less common are aphthae, abdominal pain, and arthralgia. Mild hepatosplenomegaly is observed in some patients. There is complete resolution between episodes; appetite and energy return to normal, and lost weight is regained. Affected children grew and developed normally, had no associated diseases, and experienced no long-term sequelae. The clinical presentation of patients with PFAPA in two large series [56,57] is summarized in Table 1. The differences between the two series probably derive from the differences in the diagnostic criteria of the two centers (Table 2). Except for the prevalence of aphthae, these figures have not changed in the current series of 220 children with PFAPA followed in the Sheba Medical Center.

Laboratory investigation

Laboratory investigation at onset of the fever showed a normal hemoglobin level, mild leukocytosis of $13 \times 10^{-9}/mm^3$, moderate elevation of the ESR (41–56 mm for the first hour), and normal platelet count [56,57]. Serum IgD levels were elevated in 12 of the 18 patients (66%) in whom they were measured [57]. The levels were higher than 100 U/mL, which is the cut-off level for HIDS. The serum IgD levels (140.2 ± 62.4 U/mL) were significantly higher than those found in healthy children in an age-matched control group (16.5 ± 15.8 U/mL) or children with juvenile rheumatoid arthritis (85.9 ± 47.4 U/mL). Serum IgD levels were normal in the reports from Europe and the United States [56]. Immunologic

Table 1
Clinical presentation of patients with periodic fever, adenopathy, pharyngitis, aphthae syndrome

Symptom	Thomas et al (%)	Padeh et al (%)
Fever	100	100
Exudative tonsillitis	72[a]	100
Malaise	NA	100
Cervical adenopathy	88	100
Aphthae	70	68
Headache	60	18
Abdominal pain	49	18
Arthralgia	79	11
Chills	80	NA
Cough	13	NA
Nausea	32	NA
Diarrhea	16	NA
Rash	9	NA

Abbreviations: NA, not available.
  [a] Pharyngitis rather than exudative tonsillitis.
Data from Thomas KT, Feder Jr HM, Lawton AR, et al. Periodic fever syndrome in children. J Pediatr 1999;135:15–21; Padeh S, Brezniak N, Zemer D, et al. Periodic fever, apthous stomatitis, pharyngitis, and adenopathy syndrome: clinical characteristics and outcome. J Pediatr 1999;135: 98–101.

and serologic studies were uniformly nondiagnostic [56]. Distributions of T-lymphocyte subsets were normal in all 12 patients studied [56]. IgE levels were elevated in 8 of 16 patients. Imaging studies included chest films, sinus films, gastrointestinal series, CT scans of the head and abdomen, gallium scans, and bone scans, all of which were negative [56].

Table 2
Differences in the diagnostic criteria of two centers for PFAPA syndrome

Thomas et al	Padeh
Regularly recurring fevers with an early age of onset (<5 years of age)	Monthly fevers – cyclic fever at any age groups
Constitutional symptoms in the absence of upper respiratory infection with at least 1 of the following clinical signs: Aprhthous stomatitis Cervical lymphadenitis Pharyngitis	Possibly aphthous stomatitis Cervical lymphadenitis Exudative tonsilitis + negative throat culture Completely asymptomatic interval between episodes
Exclusion of cyclic neutropenia	Rapid response to a single dose of corticosteroids
Completely asymptomatic interval between episodes	
Normal growth and development	

Abbreviations: PFAPA, periodic fever, adenopathy, pharyngitis, apthae syndrome.
Data from Thomas KT, Feder Jr HM , Lawton AR, et al. Periodic fever syndrome in children. J Pediatr 1999;135:15–21; Padeh S, Brezniak N, Zemer D, et al. Periodic fever, apthous stomatitis, pharyngitis, and adenopathy syndrome: clinical characteristics and outcome. J Pediatr 1999;135:98–101.

Differential diagnosis

Periodic fever without other systemic manifestations or sites of disease has a short list of differential diagnoses. An infectious disease or malignancy is rarely diagnosed in an individual with predictable periodic fever [58,63]. Unexplained episodic fever can be the early manifestation that precedes frank Crohn's disease by months to years. Young age, normal growth, sustained sense of well-being, normal hemoglobin level, normal ESR between febrile episodes, and absence of recurring, even mild, pathologic signs or symptoms related to the bowel help distinguish patients with the PFAPA syndrome. Recurrent fever can be associated with congenital or acquired immunodeficiency disorders [64,65], such as deficiency of total immunoglobulins, IgG, or its subclasses; hyperimmunoglobulinemia M (mutations of CD40 ligand) [66] and E [67]; dysfunction/deficiency of T lymphocytes, phagocytic cells, or complement; cyclic neutropenia [68]; and HIV infection. Recurrent unusual or severe infections do not follow in PFAPA syndrome, however. Oral lesions are not distinctively different from the common, recurrent aphthous ulcers seen in individuals without systemic illness, although those ulcers tend to be singular or few, large, deep, and painful, and they frequently follow an identifiable insult. The prevalence of aphthae has dropped since the author and colleagues' first report of 28 patients and is now only 22% among the 220 patients with PFAPA followed in their clinic. Other manifestations of Behçet's disease, such as arthritis, genital ulcers, uveitis, erythema nodosum–like skin lesions, evidence of systemic vasculitis, and pathergy, are not seen in PFAPA patients. Systemic-onset juvenile idiopathic arthritis has hectic spiking fevers, generalized adenopathy, hepatosplenomegaly, and arthritis. Fever may persist for months without remission. Other than complicating infections and neutropenia, the clinical manifestations of cyclic neutropenia and PFAPA are remarkably similar. Although hereditary periodic fever syndromes share features of PFAPA, paroxysmal serosal or synovial inflammation is their dominant feature, with fever less consistent or cyclic. In HIDS, patients are predominantly (but not exclusively) of Dutch ancestry and have onset of fevers with predictable periodicity in infancy. Unlike PFAPA, abdominal symptoms, especially vomiting (56%) and diarrhea (82%), were dominant features in HIDS,, and 80% of patients had polyarthralgia; aphthous stomatitis was not a manifestation [69]. Modestly elevated serum concentrations of IgD [57] and minimally to modestly elevated IgE levels [56] have been reported in PFAPA syndrome. Whether findings reflect normal variations in immunoglobulins, are results or markers of another abnormality, or represent one or more immunologic dysregulations as the cause of PFAPA syndrome remains unclear.

Treatment

Glucocorticoids are highly effective in controlling symptoms. Most of the patients given one dose of corticosteroid (2 mg/kg/day prednisone or prednisolone or, preferably, 0.3 mg/kg of bethamethasone, which has a longer half-life), report a dramatic resolution of fever within 2 to 4 hours after the ingestion of the corticosteroid. In many cases, lower doses of corticosteroids successfully aborted the attacks, and the parents adjusted the doses individually. In addition, most of the associated symptoms resolved, with aphthous stomatitis being the slowest manifestation to respond. Although corticosteroid therapy did not prevent subsequent attacks, patients continued to respond on subsequent cycles. In the report by Thomas et al [56], some patients defervesced only after a longer course. As a starting point, they recommend a dose of 1 mg/kg prednisone or prednisolone at the beginning of an attack, the same dose on the next morning, and one half of that dose on days 3 and 4. Doses on days 3 and 4 may be omitted in some patients, as determined by trial during subsequent episodes. The author and colleagues usually instruct the patient's parents to administer the medication at the onset of the attack and consult the pediatrician only if the attack does not abort. In many patients, the cycles of fever became more closely spaced after initiation of glucocorticoid treatment, a phenomenon that is worrisome to the parents but always abates with time. The syndrome completely resolves over a period of 8 ± 2.5 years. In the Sheba Medical Center, attacks in most of the patients stopped before the age of 10 years. Two therapies reported to be effective in some patients are cimetidine [56,70] and tonsillectomy, with or without adenoidectomy. Tonsillectomy had been previously associated with resolution of PFAPA recurrences [71]. In the Sheba Medical Center, 12 patients underwent tonsillectomy. Histology and electron microscopy of the specimens were unrevealing, and deep cultures were negative. Attacks continued in patients (a 25% failure rate), and therefore the author and colleagues do not currently recommend tonsillectomy.

Pathophysiology

The cause of PFAPA is unknown. One potential clue is the remarkable similarity of uncomplicated episodes of cyclic neutropenia and febrile attacks in PFAPA [72]. Cyclic neutropenia is caused by an unidentified defect in hemato-poietic precursor cells [73] or by alterations in the regulation of cytokines [74]. Mutations of the gene *ELA2* encoding neutrophil elastase cause a perturbed interaction between neutrophil elastase and serpins or other substrates that regulate the clocklike timing of hematopoiesis [75].

Perhaps PFAPA and cyclic neutropenia share common pathways of im-mune dysregulation. The ability of a single dose of corticosteroid to abort attacks of PFAPA suggests that the symptoms may be caused by inflammatory cytokines rather than by infection. Preliminary studies of cytokines in patients with PFAPA indicate that several cytokines are elevated during febrile episodes, most notably γ-IFN, TNF, and IL-6 [56]. It seems that an abnormal host immune response to yet unidentified commensally microorganisms in the tonsils or the oral mucosae may account for the symptomatology. Long [76] has hypothesized that the periodicity of the PFAPA syndrome derives from intermittent expression or suppression of antigens or epitopes of infectious agents or an alteration in the nature or kinetics of immunologic response. Lack of second cases in siblings or other close contacts, lack of seasonal or geographic clustering, and the progression-free duration of PFAPA for years weigh heavily against an infectious disease.

Tumor necrosis factor receptor–associated periodic syndrome

TRAPS, formerly known as familial Hibernian fever (FHF), was first described in 1982 as an autosomal dominant periodic disease characterized by recurrent attacks of fever, abdominal pain, localized tender skin lesions, and myalgia in persons of Irish-Scottish ancestry. Pleurisy, leukocytosis, and high ESR were other features. The disease has a benign course, but later, secondary amyloidosis has been reported [77]. In patients with FHF, McDermott et al [78] identified germline mutations in the *TNFRSF1A* gene, which had been identified as a candidate gene by linkage studies [78]. The type 1 receptor (the *p55* TNF receptor) is encoded by a gene located on chromosome 12p13.2. [79] Twenty mutations have been identified since the initial discovery of the mutations in TNF receptor superfamily 1A (*TNFRSF1A*). Although originally found in patients of Irish or Scottish ancestry, mutations have been reported from diverse ethnicities, suggesting that the diagnosis of TRAPS should not be excluded based on a patient's ancestry [80].

Clinical features

The median age of onset is 3 years (range, 2 weeks to 53 years). Attacks last 21 days on average and occur every 5 to 6 weeks; however, this occurrence is extremely variable. Attacks are commonly described as beginning with the subtle onset of deep muscle cramping that crescendos over the course of 1 to 3 days and climaxes for a minimum of 3 days but frequently lasts longer. No definite stimulus is recognized, but several patients note that physical or emotional stress or physical trauma may trigger an attack. Fever is invariably seen in pediatric patients but may be absent during some attacks in adults. The temperature is higher than 38°C (maximally 41°C), lasts longer than 3 days, and generally heralds the onset of other inflammatory symptoms. Myalgia, typically affecting only a single area of the body and waxing and waning throughout the course of the attack, is nearly always present in TRAPS. Areas over the involved muscles are warm and tender to palpation. Myalgia migrates centrifugally over the course of several days. When myalgia involves a joint, there is often evidence of synovitis and effusion, as well as transient contracture of the affected limb. Serum creatine kinase and aldolase concentrations are within normal limits. Muscle biopsies suggest that the myalgia of TRAPS results from monocytic fasciitis, not from myositis [81]. The most common and distinctive cutaneous manifestation is a centrifugal, migratory, erythematous patch, most typically overlying a local area of myalgia. These lesions are tender to palpation, warm, and blanch with pressure. They range in size from 1 to 28 cm. Although most occur in a single location, they may occasionally involve two separate areas. Skin biopsy reveals both a superficial and a deep perivascular and interstitial infiltrate of lymphocytes and monocytes without evidence of granuloma formation, vasculitis, or mast cell or eosinophilic infiltration [81]. Other, less distinct rashes, including urticaria-like plaques and generalized erythematous serpiginous patches and plaques, are also commonly observed. Abdominal pain occurs in 92% of TRAPS patients and may reflect inflammation within the peritoneal cavity or the musculature of the abdominal wall. Vomiting and constipation, with or without bowel obstruction, are common. Signs of an acute abdomen often result in laparotomy and appendectomy. In the series reported by Hull et al, 45% of patients had intra-abdominal surgery for acute abdominal pain, and 10% had later presented with necrotic bowel [81]. Eighty-two percent of patients presented with conjunctivitis, periorbital edema, or periorbital pain as a frequent manifestation of their attacks. Chest pain may be either musculoskeletal or pleural in origin and is present in 57% of patients. Testicular and scrotal pain has been reported during attacks. Prominent lymphadenopathy is not a universal feature of TRAPS; when observed, it is generally limited to a single anatomic location.

Laboratory investigation

All laboratory investigations measuring the acute-phase response show abnormalities during an attack including elevation of the ESR, CRP, haptoglobin, fibrinogen, and ferritin. Most patients demonstrate a polyclonal gammopathy that probably reflects IL-6–induced immunoglobulin production during attacks. The acute-phase reactants are often elevated between attacks, although not as significantly as during the attacks.

Diagnosis and differential diagnosis

A wide variability in clinical presentation has been reported [81]. The diagnosis of TRAPS should be considered when

1. A combination of the inflammatory symptoms, as described previously, recurs in episodes lasting more than 5 days.
2. Myalgia is associated with an overlying erythematous rash that together display a centrifugal migratory pattern over the course of days and occur on the limbs or trunk.
3. There is ocular involvement with attacks.
4. Symptoms respond to glucocorticosteroids but not to colchicine.
5. Symptoms segregate in the patient's family in an autosomal dominant pattern.

Clinically, the differential diagnosis includes all other periodic fevers, and the final diagnosis relies on mutation analysis.

Treatment

NSAIDs have some beneficial effect in TRAPS, mostly in relieving symptoms of fever, but are generally unable to resolve musculoskeletal and abdominal symptoms. Unlike in FMF, glucocorticoids are able to decrease the severity of symptoms but do not alter the frequency of attacks. Prednisone, 1 mg/kg/day taken in a single dose in the morning and tapered over the course of 7 to 10 days as tolerated, is recommended. Colchicine, azathioprine, cyclosporine, thalidomide, cyclophosphamide, chlorambucil, intravenous immunoglobulin, dapsone, and methotrexate have been tried empirically but have not been found to be beneficial [80]. In a pilot study involving nine TRAPS patients with various mutations in *TNFRSF1A* treated with etanercept over 6 months, an overall 66% response rate (as determined by decreased number of attacks) was observed [80,81].

Mutation analysis and pathophysiology

There does not seem to be a distinct correlation between patients' genotypes and their phenotypic presentations, with two notable exceptions: patients with the *R92Q* mutation seem to have a more heterogeneous clinical presentation than do other TRAPS patients, and patients with *TNFRSF1A* mutations involving cysteine residues seem to be at a greater risk of developing life-threatening AA amyloidosis. When TNF binds to its membrane receptor, the TNFRSF1A, it triggers a three-dimensional conformational change in the extracellular domain, which then induces an intracellular signal. Once activated, the extracellular portion of the receptor sheds from the cell membrane, contributing to the pool of soluble receptors that may attenuate the inflammatory response by removing TNF from the circulation and thereby preventing its binding to the cell-bound receptors. In their original description of TRAPS, Hull et al [81] showed that TRAPS patients possess lower serum levels of soluble TNFRSF1A than seen in normal controls. They hypothesized that the *TNFRSF1A* mutations mediated their effect through decreased shedding of TNFRSF1A, thereby decreasing the amount of soluble receptor available to bind soluble TNF-α and quell the inflammatory response. Later data, however, suggested that defective receptor shedding does not account entirely for the pathophysiologic mechanism observed, and that other mechanisms most likely contribute [81]. Although it is not entirely clear how these mutations alter TNFRSF1A receptor signaling, it is clear that the result is an inflammatory phenotype. Amelioration of inflammation in TRAPS by the anti-TNF p75:fusion protein etanercept suggests that the inflammation is dependent on the presence of TNF ligand and not on constitutive signaling by the mutated receptor [80,81].

Hyper-IgD and periodic fever syndrome

HIDS is a syndrome characterized by periodic febrile attacks occurring every 4 to 8 weeks with an intense inflammatory reaction accompanied by lymphadenopathy, abdominal pain, diarrhea, joint pain, hepatosplenomegaly, and cutaneous signs. HIDS was originally described in six patients by Van der Meer [82] in 1984. Subsequently, reports of similar cases have come from United Kingdom, France, and, later, Italy [83–85]. In 1995, by consensus, the acronym of HIDS was selected to designate the hyper-IgD syndrome [86]. Mutations in the gene encoding the enzyme mevalonate kinase (*MVK*) are responsible for this syndrome. The gene is located at chromosome 12q24 and is subjected to autosomal recessive inheritance [87,88]. *MVK* deficit has also been reported in mevalonic aciduria, a rare inherited disorder that is characterized by developmental delay, failure to thrive, hypotonia, ataxia, myopathy, and cataracts and is a completely different disease [87].

The diagnosis of HIDS is based on clinical signs associated with an elevated serum concentration of IgD, low activity of mevalonate kinase, and *MVK* gene mutation analysis. In a large series of 50 patients described by Drenth and van der Meer [89] most patients originated from Europe, namely The Netherlands (28 cases, 56%), France (10 cases, 20%), and Italy (3 cases, 6%). One patient was from Japan.

Clinical features

Patients present at a very early age at onset (median, 0.5 years) and have a life-long persistence of periodic fever. The attacks generally recur every 4 to 6 weeks, but the intervals between attacks can vary substantially in an individual patient and from one patient to another. Febrile attacks continue throughout the patients' lives, although the frequency of attacks is highest in childhood and adolescence. Patients may be free of attacks for months or even years. Attacks can be provoked by vaccination, minor trauma, surgery, or stress [89]. Attacks feature high spiking fever, preceded by chills in 76% of patients. Lymphadenopathy (94% of patients), abdominal pain, (72%), vomiting (56%), diarrhea (82%), headache (52, and skin lesions (82%) are common manifestations of the syndrome. Polyarthralgia was noted in 80% of patients, and a nondestructive arthritis, mainly of the large joints (knee and ankle), was reported in 68% of patients. Serositis is rare, and amyloidosis has not been reported. A minority of patients report painful, aphthous ulcers in the mouth or vagina. After an attack, patients are free of symptoms, although skin and joint symptoms resolve slowly. As a rule, attacks of arthritis do not lead to joint destruction, but there are exceptions [69,82,83,86,89]. Erythematous macules are the most common cutaneous manifestation, followed by erythematous papules, urticarial lesions, and erythematous nodules. Skin biopsy usually shows mild features of vasculitis [89,90].

Laboratory investigation

During an attack, there is a brisk acute-phase response, with leukocytosis, high levels of CRP and serum amyloid A, and activation of the cytokine network. The serum IgD level is persistently elevated (> 100 U/mL) in all except very young patients (< 3 years old). In 82% of cases, the serum IgA is likewise elevated (≥ 2.6 g/L). IgD should be measured on two occasions at least 1 month apart but may be normal in very young patients. More than 80% of patients have high IgA levels in conjunction with high IgD levels. Mevalonate kinase is a key enzyme in the cholesterol metabolic pathway and follows 3-hydroxy-3-methylglutaryl–coenzyme A reductase. In classic HIDS, the activity of mevalonate kinase is reduced to 5% to 15% of normal; as a result, serum cholesterol levels are slightly reduced; urinary excretion of mevalonic acid is slightly elevated during attacks [69,82,83,86,89].

Diagnosis and differential diagnosis

The diagnosis is based on clinical signs associated with an elevated serum concentration of IgD, low activity of mevalonate kinase, and *MVK* gene mutation analysis. None of the other periodic syndromes shares all these features. FMF resembles HIDS in many aspects. Increased IgD levels were found in 13% patients with FMF, significantly lower than the prevalence reported for HIDS [91]. Lymphadenectomy, skin eruption, and symmetrical oligoarthritis are seen only in HIDS, whereas monoarthritis, peritonitis, and pleuritis are more characteristic of FMF and are the main clinical features distinguishing FMF from HIDS. Unlike FMF, colchicine has no preventive effect against febrile episodes in HIDS [91].

Treatment

No effective treatment is known, and many of medications have been tried with limited response [89]. Thalidomide had a limited effect in decreasing the acute-phase protein synthesis without an effect on the attack rate [92]. Simvastatin resulted in a drop in urinary mevalonic acid concentration in six patients and decreased the number of febrile days [93]. Favorable experience with etanercept for the treatment of HIDS in two patients has been reported recently [94].

Genetic analysis and pathophysiology

HIDS is an autosomal recessive disease, and most patients are compound heterozygotes for missense mutations in the *MVK* gene. One mutation, *V377I*, is present in more than 80% of patients; the other mutations are less frequent [87,4]. The *V377I* mutation results in a slight reduction of the stability of recombinant human mevalonate kinase protein and in the catalytic activity of the enzyme. Fewer than 1% of patients have a complete deficiency of, which is associated with mevalonic aciduria, in which disease-associated mutations are mainly clustered within a specific region of the protein [87]. How a deficiency of mevalonate kinase is linked to an inflammatory periodic fever syndrome is not yet known. Mevalonate kinase, a product of *MVK*, catalyzes the conversion of mevalonate to 5-phosphomevalonic acid in the biosynthesis of cholesterol and nonsterol isoprenoid compounds. Decreased mevalonate kinase activity, which is aggravated by fever, leads to accumulation of its substrate, mevalonate. Some clinical features in patients with mevalonic aciduria may result directly from the accumulation of mevalonate. In one report, however, patients with mevalonic aciduria developed severe febrile attacks following treatment with lovastatin [94], despite an initial decrease of mevalonate levels in the serum and urine [95], and it is therefore less likely that increased production of mevalonate itself is directly involved in the pathogenesis of febrile attacks. Decreased *MVK* activity also leads to decreased production of the molecules involved in prenylation, which is the posttranslational modification of proteins with isoprenoids such as farnesyl or geranyl moieties. Impaired prenylation, particularly of proteins providing regulatory control over ligand-induced cellular activation, may lower the threshold for the production of proinflammatory cytokine. An increased IL-1 production by HIDS leukocytes was found in vitro [94], but a direct link between disrupted prenylation and cytokine production or febrile attacks has yet to be elucidated.

CIAS1-related autoinflammatory syndromes

The CIAS1 (named for cold-induced autoinflammatory syndrome) gene, located on chromosome 1p44, encodes a pyrin-like protein, cryopyrin, expressed predominantly in peripheral blood leukocytes. CIAS1-related autoinflammatory syndromes (CRAS) are three different diseases caused by mutation in the CIAS1 gene: CINCA syndrome (also known as NOMID/CINCA syndrome), FCUS, and MWS [59,96,97]. The first clinical signs of severe CRAS occur during childhood, sometimes presenting right after birth, and comprise urticaria, recurrent fever, severe joint inflammation, myalgia, chronic meningitis often resulting in generalized neurologic impairment, a progressive visual defect, conjunctivitis, sensorineural deafness later in life, and, in a few cases, amyloidosis. The severity is influenced only partly by the underlying mutation; unknown modifier genes and environmental factors are other possible influences. In 1999, FCAS and MWS were first linked to the CIAS1 gene. The encoded protein, cryopyrin, is a member of the pyrin and NACHT domain–containing family of proteins, which contain three domains, a PyD, a specific nucleotide-binding fold (the NACHT domain), and several tandem copies of leucine-rich repeats. Heterozygous missense mutations in the CIAS1 gene were found later in patients with the NOMID/CINCA syndrome [98]. Aksentijevich et al [97] increased the total number of known germline mutations in CIAS1 to 20, explaining a spectrum of diseases ranging from FCUS to MWS to NOMID/CINCA syndrome. Dode et al

[59] identified identical CIAS1 mutations in families with MWS and in families with FCUS of different ethnic origins, thereby demonstrating that a single CIAS1 mutation may cause both syndromes and suggesting that modifier genes are involved in determining either an MWS or an FCUS phenotype. The finding of the mutations in asymptomatic individuals further emphasizes the importance of a modifier gene (or genes) in determining disease phenotype. No CIAS1 mutation has yet been identified in the N-terminal PyD of cryopyrin. This 90–amino acid motif also is found in pyrin encoded by the FMF gene. It has recently been shown that cryopyrin interacts with ASC, leading to NF-kappa B activation, and through this pathway CIAS1 mutations may have an anti-apoptotic effect. No nuclear localization signals were identified, and no clear transmembrane regions were found, suggesting that cryopyrin is a signaling protein involved in the regulation of apoptosis.

Neonatal-onset multisystem inflammatory disease/chronic infantile neurologic cutaneous and articular syndrome

The triad of cutaneous rash, chronic meningitis, and arthropathy characterizes CINCA syndrome, also known as NOMID syndrome. It was been first described by Prieur and Griscelli [85] in 1981 and was known to the pediatric rheumatologists long before it was genetically associated with the hereditary autoimmune fever syndromes. It is a disease of chronic inflammation, often starting at birth, which lasts the entire lifetime. Long-term prognosis is poor, with progressive deafness, visual impairment, and worsening of the central nervous system manifestations in many, but not all, patients. Attempts at therapy have been disappointing [85,99,100], although recently there have been reports of success with the IL-1 receptor antagonist anakinra [101]. Twenty years after its first description, NOMID/CINCA syndrome was linked to mutations in the CIAS1 gene on chromosome 1q44 [98]. Approximately 100 cases have been identified worldwide [100]. The course of the disease is characterized by chronic inflammation with recurrent flares; no permanent remission has yet been reported. Progressive growth retardation is observed in most patients. Fever and rash are dominant symptoms. Lymphadenopathy and hepatosplenomegaly are often present during flares, but skin rash is persistent. Skin manifestations are observed in all cases, and in 75% of cases these manifestations are present at birth. The rash is nonpruritic migratory urticaria. It can be confused with a systemic juvenile idiopathic arthritis rash but is more pronounced, persisting for the life of the patient. Skin biopsies show normal epidermis, with mild inflammation and perivascular mononuclear infiltration in the dermis. Immunofluorescence studies show no immunoglobulins or complement deposits in the skin lesion. Central nervous system involvement is not always suspected during the first years. Headaches, seizures, transient episodes of hemiplegia, and spasticity of the legs are characteristic of the syndrome. Neurologic features reflect chronic aseptic meningitis with polymorphonuclear infiltration of the meninges.

Extensive evaluations for viral, fungal, or bacterial agents have been negative, and no immune deficiency has been documented. Intellectual development may remain normal, but in some patients a low IQ can occur with time. Skull anomalies include increased cranial volume, frontal bossing, and late closure of the anterior fontanelle. Brain imaging often reveals mild ventricular dilatation, prominent sulci, and increased extra-axial fluid spaces. Calcification of the falx and dura can be seen in the oldest patients, perhaps reflecting the chronic inflammation of the meninges [99,100]. Cranial morphology demonstrates a peculiar aspect consisting of overall enlargement and frontal bossing (Fig. 6). Eye involvement can lead to a progressive visual defect and to blindness in the most severely affected cases. Optic disc edema, pseudopapilledema, and optic atrophy are most common. Chronic anterior uveitis is seen in half of the cases, but neither synechia nor glaucoma is evident. Progressive perceptive deafness, in varying degrees, increase with age. Hoarseness is frequent. A saddle-nose deformity is frequent.

Musculoskeletal abnormalities are characteristic. Shortening of the hands and feet with clubbing of the fingers is seen; sometimes the palms and soles appear wrinkled. These common morphologic features create a sibling-like resemblance among patients from various geographic areas [100]. Joint symptoms vary from arthralgia with transient swelling to severe deforming arthropathy. In children with a severe arthropathy, the progression of the bony lesions can lead to sig-

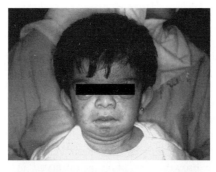
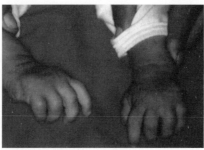

Fig. 6. A 3-year-old girl with NOMID/CINCA syndrome. Note the markedly deformed hands, rash, frontal bossing, and large head.

nificant deformity that impairs function. Symmetrical patellar overgrowth and epiphyseal and metaphyseal abnormalities often link with cartilage overgrowth, resulting in bony enlargement without synovial thickening. Joint effusions can occur, probably in association with a local, nonspecific reaction to the epiphyseal disturbances. A typical arthropathy with unique radiologic changes in the bones and joints is observed in about half of the cases. The most distinctive changes occur in the metaphyses and epiphyses at the ends of the long bones, affecting the knees, ankles, wrists, and elbows. Premature patellar ossification with subsequent patellar overgrowth is frequent. Epiphyses are large with irregular *en mie de pain* ("bread-crumb") ossification, often resulting in an overgrown and markedly deformed extremity. Growth plate histology shows a complete disorganization of the cartilage cell columns, irregular metachromasia of the cartilage substance, and no inflammatory cell infiltrates. The serum from affected patients is toxic to normal human growth cartilage cells in culture, suggesting that cartilage is a target in this disease. Hips, shoulders, and spine seem to be relatively unaffected [85,99,100].

Hypochromic anemia, leukocytosis with a predominance of polymorphonuclear neutrophils and eosinophils, high platelet counts, elevated ESR, and high levels of acute-phase reactants are often found. Secondary amyloidosis has been reported in some patients, probably as a consequence of chronic inflammation [99]. Leone et al [102] found a significantly increased expression of CD10 in some patients with NOMID/CINCA syndrome and postulated that it can serve as a useful marker of the inflammation in these patients.

Mutations in CIAS1 have been found in only approximately 50% of the cases identified clinically as NOMID/CINCA syndrome, raising the possibility of genetic heterogeneity [97]. Because CIAS1 is expressed in chondrocytes, genetic heterogeneity could explain the peculiar arthropathy of NOMID/CINCA syndrome. There were also substantial increases in IL-3 and IL-5 message, which may account for the peripheral eosinophilia observed in some patients with NOMID/CINCA syndrome. NOMID/CINCA syndrome CIAS1 is also expressed at high levels in leukocytes, predominantly in monocytes, granulocytes, and T lymphocytes. In addition to the potential proinflammatory effect of alterations in NF-kappa B signaling in white blood cells, cryopyrin has recently been shown to regulate IL-1 beta production.

The differential diagnosis comprises other childhood febrile diseases, Kawasaki disease, infantile cortical hyperostosis (Caffey 's disease), Sweet's syndrome, and Weber–Christian disease. Systemic-onset juvenile idiopathic arthritis shares many features with NOMID/CINCA syndrome but is rare in the first 6 months of life. The other hereditary autoinflammatory disorders associated with fever must be considered.

NSAIDs can relieve the pain but have no effect on the inflammatory features. Glucocorticosteroids reduce fever and pain without any effect on skin lesions, central nervous system disease, or joint manifestations. Attempts with more aggressive medications such as slow-acting anti-rheumatic drugs or cytotoxics have been disappointing [100]. Recently, favorable response to the recombinant human IL-1 receptor antagonist anakinra has been reported in three patients [101]. Some cases of death have been reported secondary to infection, vasculitis, and amyloidosis [100].

Muckle–Wells syndrome

Urticaria-deafness-amyloidosis syndrome

In 1962, Muckle and Wells described a dominantly inherited syndrome of urticaria, progressive perceptive deafness, and amyloidosis. The first manifestations of MWS usually start during infancy and consist of nonpruritic urticaria, low-grade fever, and often arthritis and conjunctivitis. Neurosensory hearing loss begins during adolescence and slowly evolves into deafness. Absent organ of Corti, atrophy of the cochlear nerve, and amyloid infiltration of the kidneys have been found on autopsy. The severity of the disease resides in the development of AA amyloidosis [59]. Additional features reported to be associated with the syndrome are buccal and genital aphthosis, cystinuria and ichthyosis, polyarthralgia, periodic abdominal pain, and microscopic hematuria. The histologic findings of cold air–induced lesions are similar to those described for other different types of physical urticaria: marked dilatation of vessels and the dermal edema, intense infiltrate of neutrophils admixed with mononuclear cells and eosinophils, and sometime leukocytoclastic vasculitis or amyloid deposits in the skin. Recently, patients with MWS have been treated successfully with anakinra. [103]. Whether this treatment proves effective in preventing amyloidosis remains to be seen; at present, there is no effective treatment to prevent the attacks or the development of amyloidosis.

Familial cold autoinflammatory syndrome

FCAS, formerly known as familial cold urticaria, is a rare autosomal dominant syndrome characterized by fever, rash, and arthralgias brought on by exposure to cold. It was first reported in 1940; since then only 20 families have been described worldwide. This disorder is often confused with acquired cold urticaria (ACU). These are distinct and unrelated entities; FCAS is related more closely to the hereditary periodic fevers, and ACU is a true physical urticaria. Diagnostically, these two disorders are distinguished by their clinical history, by dermatologic examination, and by an ice cube challenge. After exposure to cold, the patient develops urticarial wheals, pain and swelling of joints, chills, and fever [104]. The onset of symptoms after cold challenge is delayed by 30 minutes to 6 hours. Urticaria is maximal in early adult life, but others have reported cases with onset in infancy [105]. Leukocytosis is common during an attack. Systemic amyloidosis is a complication of this condition, and amyloid nephropathy is a frequent cause of death. The clinical phenotype varies largely, and some patients never experience urticaria, induction of fever by cold, conjunctivitis, severe joint

Table 3
Summary of periodic fever syndromes

Disease	Inheritance	Gene location	Protein	Clinical presentation	Amyloidosis	Treatment
FMF	*AR	MEFV (16p13)	Pyrin	Recurrent attacks of fever and peritonitis, arthritis, pleuritis, pericarditis and erysipelas-like erythema	Yes	colchicine
PFAPA	sporadic	-		Periodic episodes of fever accompanied by aphthous stomatitis, pharyngitis, and cervical adenitis	No	glucocorticosteroids
TRAPS	AR	TNFRSF1A (12p13)	TNF receptor 1	Recurrent attacks of fever, conjunctivitis, abdominal pain, rush, myalgia, pleurisy, and arthritis.	Rarely	glucocorticosteroids, etanercept
HIDS	AR	MVK (12p24)	Mevalonate kinase	Periodic attacks of fever, lymphadenopathy, abdominal pains, vomiting, diarrhea, headache, and rush	No	No effective treatment (simvastatine, etanercept, thalidomide trials)
CINCA/NOMID	#AD	CIAS1 (1q44)	NALP3	Triad of cutaneous rash, chronic meningitis, and arthropathy. Fever, deforming arthritis, hepatosplenomegaly, and prolonged course.	Yes	glucocorticosteroids, MTX, etanercept, anakinra
MWS and FCUS	AD	CIAS1 (1q44)	NALP3	Fever, chills, rigors, malaise, urticaria (cold induced), progressive perceptive deafness, polyarthralgia, myalgia, periodic abdominal pain	Yes	anakinra, stanozolol

Abbreviations: AD, autosomal dominant; AR, autosomal recessive; CINCA, chronic infantile neurologic cutaneous and articular syndrome; FCUS, familial cold urticaria syndrome, FMF, familial Mediterranean fever; HIDS, Hyperimmunoglobulinemia D and periodic fever syndrome; MTX, methotrexate; MWS, Muckle-Wells syndrome; NOMID, neonatal-onset multisystem inflammatory disease; PFAPA, periodic fever, adenopathy, pharyngitis, aphthae) syndrome; TNF, Tumor necrosis factor; TRAPS, tumor necrosis factor receptor–associated periodic syndrome.

inflammation, neurologic symptoms, or amyloidosis. Instead, a very regular periodic fever, irregular severe febrile episodes, relatively mild arthralgia, dry cough, inflammatory cardiomyopathy and nephropathy, and euthyroid thyroiditis were observed [105]. Current management of patients with this syndrome consists of education, movement to warmer climates, and warming treatments. Anti-inflammatory agents, anabolic steroids, high-dose corticosteroids, and colchicine have variable effect in these parents. Antihistamines are generally not effective. Three patients responded favorably to treatment with stanozolol [106], and anakinra has also been reported to be effective [101].

Summary

Human autoinflammatory diseases (except for PFAPA) are a heterogeneous group of genetically determined diseases characterized by seemingly unprovoked inflammation, in the absence of autoimmune or infective causes (Table 3). The last decade has witnessed tremendous advances in the understanding of these disorders. These advances have allowed therapeutic interventions, resulting in improvement in the short-term and long-term morbidity of all of these diseases. Future research into the molecular mechanisms underlying these inflammatory diseases will probably lead to a better understanding of inflammatory diseases in general and, it is hoped, to better and more targeted therapies.

References

[1] Kastner DL, O'Shea JJ. A fever gene comes in from the cold. Nat Genet 2001;29(3):241–2.
[2] Stehlik C, Reed JC. The PYRIN connection: novel players in innate immunity and inflammation. J Exp Med 2004;200(5):551–8.
[3] Liepinsh E, Barbals R, Dahl E, et al. The death-domain fold of the ASC PYRIN domain, presenting a basis for PYRIN/PYRIN recognition. J Mol Biol 2003;332(5):1155–63.
[4] Manji G, Wang L, Geddes B, et al. PYPAF1, a PYRIN-containing Apaf1-like protein that assembles with ASC and regulates activation of NF-kappa B. J Biol Chem 2002;277:11570–5.
[5] Miceli-Richard C, Lesage S, Rybojad M, et al. CARD15 mutations in Blau syndrome. Nat Genet 2001;29:19–20.
[6] Sohar E, Gafhi J, Pras M, et al. Familial Mediterranean fever. A survey of 470 cases and review of the literature. Am J Med 1967;43:227–53.
[7] La Regina MNG, Diaco M, Procopio A, et al. Familial Mediterranean fever is no longer a rare disease in Italy. Eur J Hum Genet 2004;12(2):85–6.
[8] Konstantopoulos K, Kanta A, Deltas C, et al. Familial Mediterranean fever associated pyrin mutations in Greece. Ann Rheum Dis 2003;62(5):479–81.
[9] Kotone-Miyahara Y, Takaori-Kondo A, Fukunaga K, et al. E148Q/M694I mutation in 3 Japanese patients with familial Mediterranean fever. Int J Hematol 2004;79(3):235–7.
[10] Heller H, Sohar E, Kariv I, et al. Familial Mediterranean fever. Harefuah 1955;48:91–4.
[11] Cattan R, Mamou H. 14 cas de Maladie periodique de dont 8 compliques de nephropathies. Semaine Hop Paris 1952;28:1062–70.
[12] Retmann HA, Moadie J, SemerdJian S, et al. Periodic peritonitis—heredity and pathology. Report of seventy-two cases. JAMA 1954;154:1254–9.

[13] Sohar E, Pras M, Heller J, et al. Genetics of familial Mediterranean fever. Arch Intern Med 1961;07:529–38.

[14] Heller H, Gafni J, Michaeli D, et al. The arthritis of familial Mediterranean fever (FMF). Arthritis Rheum 1966;9:1–17.

[15] Goldfinger SE. Colchicine for familial Mediterranean fever. N Engl J Med 1972;287(25):1302.

[16] Zemer D, Revach M, Pras M, et al. A controlled trial of colchicine in preventing attacks of familial Mediterranean fever. N Engl J Med 1974;291:932–44.

[17] Pras E, Aksentijevich I, Gruberg L, et al. Mapping of a gene causing familial Mediterranean fever to the short arm of chromosome 16. N Engl J Med 1992;326:1509–13.

[18] The International FMF Consortium. Ancient missense mutations in a new member of the RoRet gene family are likely to cause familial Mediterranean fever. Cell 1997;90:797–807.

[19] The French FMF Consortium. A candidate gene for familial Mediterranean fever. Nat Genet 1997;17:25–31.

[20] Michaeli D, Pras M, Rozen N. Intestinal strangulation complicating familial Mediterranean fever. BMJ 1966;2:30–1.

[21] Rabinovitch O, Zemer D, Kukia E, et al. Colchicine treatment in conception and pregnancy: two hundred thirty-one pregnancies in patients with familial Mediterranean fever. Am J Reprod Immunol 1992;28:245–6.

[22] Majeed HA, Ghandour K, Shahin HM. The acute scrotum in Arab children with familial Mediterranean fever. Pediatr Surg Int 2000;16(1–2):72–4.

[23] Saatci U, Ozen S, Ozdemir S, et al. Familial Mediterranean fever in children: report of a large series and discussion of the risk and prognostic factors of amyloidosis. Eur J Pediatr 1997; 156:619–23.

[24] Kees S, Langevitz P, Zemer D, et al. Tel Aviv: pericarditis as a rare manifestation of familial Mediterranean fever (FMF). In: Sohar E, Gafni J, Pras M, editors. Familial Mediterranean fever. Tel Aviv, Israel: Freund Publishing House; 1997. p. 129–31.

[25] Sneh E, Pras M, Michaeli D, et al. Protracted arthritis in familial Mediterranean fever. Rheumatol Rehab 1977;16:102–6.

[26] Salai M, Langevitz P, Blankstein A, et al. Total hip replacement in familial Mediterranean fever. Bull Hosp Jt Dis 1993;53:25–8.

[27] Langevitz P, Zemer D, Livneh A, et al. Protracted febrile myalgia in patients with familial Mediterranean fever. Rheumatology 1994;21:1708–9.

[28] Azizi E, Fisher BK. Cutaneous manifestations of familial Mediterranean fever. Arch Dermatol 1976;l–2:364–6.

[29] Barzilai A, Langevitz P, Goldberg I, et al. Erysipelas-like erythema of familial Mediterranean fever: clinicopathologic correlation. J Am Acad Dermatol 2000;42(5 Pt 1):791–5.

[30] Pras E, Livneh A, Balow Jr JE, et al. Clinical differences between North African and Iraqi Jews with familial Mediterranean fever. Am Med Genet 1998;75:216–9.

[31] Schlesinger M, Rubinow A, Vardy PA. Henoch-Schonlein purpura and familial Mediterranean fever. Isr J Med Sci 1985;21(1):83–5.

[32] Sachs D, Langevitz P, Morag B, et al. Polyarteritis nodosa in familial Mediterranean fever. Br J Rheumatol 1987;26(2):139–41.

[33] Said R, Hamzeh Y, Said S, et al. Spectrum of renal involvement in familial Mediterranean fever. Kidney Int 1992;41:414–9.

[34] Oner A, Erdogan O, Demircin G, et al. Efficacy of colchicine therapy in amyloid nephropathy of familial Mediterranean fever. Pediatr Nephrol 2003;18(6):521–6.

[35] Gillmore JD, Lovat LB, Persey MR, et al. Amyloid load and clinical outcome in AA amyloidosis in relation to circulating concentration of serum amyloid A protein. Lancet 2001; 358(9275):24–9.

[36] Ozkaya N, Yalcinkaya F. Colchicine treatment in children with familial Mediterranean fever. Clin Rheumatol 2003;22:314–7.

[37] Fradkin A, Yahav J, Zemer D, et al. Colchicine-induced lactose malabsorption in patients with familial Mediterranean fever. Isr J Med Sci 1995;31(10):616–20.

[38] Ben-Chetrit E, Levy M. Reproductive system in familial Mediterranean fever: an overview. Ann Rheum Dis 2003;62(10):916-9.

[39] Lidar M, Kedem R, Langevitz P, et al. Intravenous colchicine for treatment of patients with familial Mediterranean fever unresponsive to oral colchicine. J Rheumatol 2003;30(12): 2620-3.

[40] Tunca M, Tankurt E, Akbaylar Akpinar H, et al. The efficacy of interferon alpha on colchicine-resistant familial Mediterranean fever attacks: a pilot study. Br J Rheumatol 1997; 36(9):1005-8.

[41] Pras M. Familial Mediterranean fever: from clinical syndrome to the cloning of the Pyrin gene. Scand J Rheumatol 1998;27:92-7.

[42] Guijarro C, Egido J. Transcription factor-kappa B (Nf-kappa B) and renal disease. Kidney Int 2001;59:415-24.

[43] Ray A, Ray B. Persistent expression of serum amyloid A during experimentally induced chronic inflammatory condition in rabbit involves differential activation of SAF, Nf-kappa B, and C/Ebp transcription factors. J Immunol 1999;163:2143-50.

[44] Lawrence T, Gilroy GW, Colville-Nash PR, et al. Possible new role for NF-kappa B in the resolution of inflammation. Nat Med 2001;7:1291-7.

[45] Livneh A, Langevitz P, Shinar Y, et al. MEFV mutation analysis in patients suffering from amyloidosis of familial Mediterranean fever. Amyloid 1999;6:1-6.

[46] Shinar Y, Livneh A, Villa Y, et al. Common mutations in the familial Mediterranean fever gene associate with rapid progression to disability in non-Ashkenazi Jewish multiple sclerosis patients. Genes Immun 2003;4(3):197-203.

[47] Padeh S, Shinar Y, Pras E, et al. Clinical and diagnostic value of genetic testing in 216 Israeli children with familial Mediterranean fever. J Rheumatol 2003;30(1):185-90.

[48] Brik R, Riva MD, Shinaw M, et al. Familial Mediterranean fever: clinical and genetic characterization in a mixed pediatric population of Jewish and Arab patients. Pediatrics 1999; 103(5):1025-6.

[49] Shinar Y, Livneh A, Langevitz P, et al. Genotype-phenotype assessment of common genotypes among patients with familial Mediterranean fever. J Rheumatol 2000;27:1703-7.

[50] Kone Paut I, Dubuc M, Sportouch J, et al. Phenotype-genotype correlation in 91 patients with familial Mediterranean fever reveals a high frequency of mucocutaneous features. Rheumatology 2000;39:1275-9.

[51] Dewalle M, Domingo C, Rozenbaum M, et al. Phenotype-genotype correlation in Jewish patients suffering from familial Mediterranean fever. Eur J Hum Genet 1998;6:95-7.

[52] Cazeneuve C, Sarkisian T, Pecheux C, et al. MEFV-gene analysis in Armenian patients with familial Mediterranean fever: diagnostic value and unfavorable renal prognosis of the M694V homozygous genotype—genetic and therapeutic implications. Am J Hum Genet 1999;65:88-97.

[53] Shohat M, Magal N, Shohat T, et al. Phenotype-genotype correlation in familial Mediterranean fever: evidence for an association between Met694Val and amyloidosis. Eur J Hum Genet 1999;7:287-92.

[54] Booth DR, Gillmore JD, Lachmann HJ, et al. The genetic basis of autosomal dominant familial Mediterranean fever. Q J Med 2000;93:217-21.

[55] Livneh A, Aksentijevich I, Langevitz P, et al. A single mutated MEFV allele in Israeli patients suffering from familial Mediterranean fever and Behcet's disease (FMF–BD). Eur J Hum Genet 2001;9:191-6.

[56] Thomas KT, Feder Jr HM, Lawton AR, et al. Periodic fever syndrome in children. J Pediatr 1999;135:15-21.

[57] Padeh S, Brezniak N, Zemer D, et al. Periodic fever, aphthous stomatitis, pharyngitis, and adenopathy syndrome: clinical characteristics and outcome. J Pediatr 1999;135:98-101.

[58] Knockaert DC, Vanneste LJ, Bobbaers HJ. Recurrent or episodic fever of unknown origin: review of 45 cases and survey of the literature. Medicine (Baltimore) 1993;72:184-96.

[59] Dode C, Le Du N, Cuisset L, et al. New mutations of CIAS1 that are responsible for Muckle-

Wells syndrome and familial cold urticaria: a novel mutation underlies both syndromes. Am J Hum Genet 2002;70:1498–506.

[60] Miller LC, Sisson BA, Tucker LB, et al. Prolonged fevers of unknown origin in children: patterns of presentation and outcome. J Pediatr 1996;129:419–23.

[61] Marshall GS, Edwards KM, Butler J, et al. Syndrome of periodic fever, pharyngitis, and aphthous stomatitis. J Pediatr 1987;110:43–6.

[62] Marshall GS, Edwards KM. PFAPA syndrome [letter]. Pediatr Infect Dis J 1989;8:658–9.

[63] Cabral DA, Tucker LB. Malignancies in children who initially present with rheumatic complaints. J Pediatr 1999;134(1):53–7.

[64] Rosen FS, Cooper MD, Wedgewood RJP. The primary immunodeficiencies [medical progress]. N Engl J Med 1995;333:431–40.

[65] Shyur S-D, Hill HR. Immunodeficiency in the 1990s. Pediatr Infect Dis J 1991;10:595–611.

[66] DiSanto JP, Bonnefoy Y, Gauchat JF, et al. CD40 ligand mutations in X-linked immunodeficiency with hyper-IgM. Nature 1993;361:541–3.

[67] Grimbacher B, Holland SM, Gallin JI, et al. Hyper-IgE syndrome with recurrent infections— an autosomal dominant multisystem disorder. N Engl J Med 1999;340:692–702.

[68] Yang K, Hill HR. Assessment of neutrophil function disorders: practical and preventive interventions. Pediatr Infect Dis J 1994;13:906–19.

[69] Grose C, Schnetzer JR, Ferrante A, et al. Children with hyperimmunoglobulinemia D and periodic fever syndrome. Pediatr Infect Dis J 1996;15(1):72–5.

[70] Feder Jr HM. Cimetidine treatment for periodic fever associated with aphthous stomatitis, pharyngitis, and cervical adenitis. Pediatr Infect Dis J 1992;11:318–21.

[71] Abramson JS, Givner LB, Thompson JN. Possible role of tonsillectomy and adenoidectomy in children with recurrent fever and tonsillopharyngitis. Pediatr Infect Dis J 1989;8:119–20.

[72] Wright DG, Dale DC, Fauci AS, et al. Human cyclic neutropenia: clinical review and long-term follow-up of patients. Medicine (Baltimore) 1981;60:1–13.

[73] Dale DC, Hammond WP. Cyclic neutropenia: a clinical review. Blood Rev 1988;2:178–85.

[74] Engervall P, Andersson B, Bjorkholm M. Clinical significance of serum cytokine patterns during start of fever in patients with neutropenia. Br J Haematol 1995;91:838–45.

[75] Horwitz M, Benson KF, Person RE, et al. Mutations in ELA2, encoding neutrophil elastase, define a 21-day biological clock in cyclic haematopoiesis. Nat Genet 1999;23(4):433–6.

[76] Long SS. Syndrome of periodic fever, aphthous stomatitis, pharyngitis, and adenitis (PFAPA)— what it isn't. What is it? J Pediatr 1999;135(1):1–5.

[77] Williamson LM, Hull D, Mehta R, et al. Familial Hibernian fever. Q J Med 1982;51:469–80.

[78] McDermott MF, Aksentijevich I, Galon J, et al. Germline mutations in the extracellular domains of the 55 kDa TNF receptor, TNFR1, define a family of dominantly inherited autoinflammatory syndromes. Cell 1999;97:133–44.

[79] Derre J, Kemper O, Cherif D, et al. The gene for the type 1 tumor necrosis factor receptor (TNF-R1) is localized on band 12p13. Hum Genet 1991;87:231–3.

[80] Drewe E, Powell PT, Isaacs JD, et al. Prospective study of anti-tumor necrosis factor superfamily 1a and 1b fusion proteins in tumor necrosis factor associated periodic syndrome (TRAPS): clinical and laboratory findings in a series of six patients. Rheumatology (Oxford) 2003;42(2):235–9.

[81] Hull KM, Drewe E, Aksentijevich I, et al. The TNF receptor-associated periodic syndrome (TRAPS): emerging concepts of an autoinflammatory disorder. Medicine (Baltimore) 2002; 81(5):349–68.

[82] Van der Meer JWM, Vossen JM, Radl J, et al. Hyperimmunoglobulinemia D and periodic fever: a new syndrome. Lancet 1984;i:1087–90.

[83] Reeves WG, Mitchell JRA. Hyperimmunoglobulinemia D and periodic fever. Lancet 1984;i: 1463–4.

[84] Scolozzi R, Boccafogli A, Vicentini L. Hyper-IgD syndrome and other hereditary periodic fever syndromes. Reumatismo 2004;56(3):147–55.

[85] Prieur AM, Griscelli C. Nosologic aspects of systemic forms of very early onset juvenile arthritis. Apropos of 17 cases. Ann Pediatr (Paris) 1983;30(8):565–9.

[86] Drenth JPH, Powell RJ. Hyperimmunoglobulinemia D syndrome: conference. Lancet 1995; 345:445–6.

[87] Drenth JP, Cuisset L, Grateau G, et al. Mutations in the gene encoding mevalonate kinase cause hyper-IgD and periodic fever syndrome. International Hyper-IgD Study Group. Nat Genet 1999;22:178–81.

[88] McDermott M, Ogunkolade BW, McDermott EM, et al. Linkage of familial Hibernian fever to chromosome 12p13. Am J Hum Genet 1998;62:1446–51.

[89] Drenth JP HC, van der Meer JW. Hyperimmunoglobulinemia D and periodic fever syndrome. The clinical spectrum in a series of 50 patients. International Hyper-IgD Study Group. Medicine (Baltimore) 1994;73(3):133–44.

[90] Drenth JP, Boom BW, Toonstra J, et al. Cutaneous manifestations and histologic findings in the hyperimmunoglobulinemia D syndrome. International Hyper IgD Study Group. Arch Dermatol 1994;130(1):59–65.

[91] Livneh A, Drenth JP, Klasen IS, et al. Familial Mediterranean fever and hyperimmuno-globulinemia D syndrome: two diseases with distinct clinical, serologic, and genetic features. Rheumatology 1997;24(8):1558–63.

[92] Drenth JP, Vonk AG, Simon A, et al. Limited efficacy of thalidomide in the treatment of febrile attacks of the hyper-IgD and periodic fever syndrome: a randomized, double-blind, placebo-controlled trial. J Pharmacol Exp Ther 2001;298(3):1221–6.

[93] Simon A, Drewe E, van der Meer JW, et al. Simvastatin treatment for inflammatory attacks of the hyperimmunoglobulinemia D and periodic fever syndrome. Clin Pharmacol Ther 2004; 75(5):476–83.

[94] Takada K, Aksentijevich I, Mahadevan V, et al. Favorable preliminary experience with eta-nercept in two patients with the hyperimmunoglobulinemia D and periodic fever syndrome. Arthritis Rheum 2003;48(9):2645–51.

[95] Hoffmann GF, Charpentier C, Mayatepek E, et al. Clinical and biochemical phenotype in 11 patients with mevalonic aciduria. Pediatrics 1993;91:915–21.

[96] Hoffman H, Mueller J, Broide D, et al. Mutation of a new gene encoding a putative pyrin-like protein causes familial cold autoinflammatory syndrome and Muckle-Wells syndrome. Nat Genet 2001;29:301–5.

[97] Aksentijevich I, Nowak M, Mallah M, et al. De novo CIAS1 mutations, cytokine activation, and evidence for genetic heterogeneity in patients with neonatal-onset multisystem inflam-matory disease (NOMID): a new member of the expanding family of pyrin-associated auto-inflammatory diseases. Arthritis Rheum 2002;46(12):3340–8.

[98] Feldmann J, Prieur A-M, Quartier P, et al. Chronic infantile neurological cutaneous and articular syndrome is caused by mutations in CIAS1, a gene highly expressed in polymorpho-nuclear cells and chondrocytes. Am J Hum Genet 2002;71:198–203.

[99] Prieur AM, Griscelli C, Lambert F, et al. A chronic, infantile, neurological, cutaneous and articular (CINCA) syndrome. A specific entity analysed in 30 patients. Scand J Rheumatol 1987;66(Suppl):57–68.

[100] Prieur AM. A recently recognised chronic inflammatory disease of early onset characterised by the triad of rash, central nervous system involvement and arthropathy. Clin Exp Rheu-matol 2001;19(1):103–6.

[101] Frenkel J, Wulffraat NM, Kuis W. Anakinra in mutation-negative NOMID/CINCA syndrome: comment on the articles by Hawkins et al and Hoffman and Patel. Arthritis Rheum 2004; 50(11):3738–9.

[102] Leone V, Presani G, Perticarari S, et al. Chronic infantile neurological cutaneous articular syndrome: CD10 over-expression in neutrophils is a possible key to the pathogenesis of the disease. Eur J Pediatr 2003;162(10):669–73.

[103] Hawkins PN, Lachmann HJ, Aganna E, et al. Spectrum of clinical features in Muckle-Wells syndrome and response to anakinra. Arthritis Rheum 2004;50(2):607–12.

[104] Derbes VJ, Coleman WP. Familial cold urticaria. Ann Allergy 1972;30:335–41.

[105] Porksen G, Lohse P, Rosen-Wolff A, et al. Periodic fever, mild arthralgias, and reversible

moderate and severe organ inflammation associated with the V198M mutation in the CIAS1 gene in three German patients—expanding phenotype of CIAS1 related autoinflammatory syndrome. Eur J Haematol 2004;73(2):123–7.

[106] Ormerod AD, Smart L, Reid TMS, et al. Familial cold urticaria: investigation of a family and response to stanozolol. Arch Dermatol 1993;129:343–6.

ELSEVIER
SAUNDERS

PEDIATRIC CLINICS
OF NORTH AMERICA

Pediatr Clin N Am 52 (2005) 611–639

Pediatric Pain Syndromes and Management of Pain in Children and Adolescents with Rheumatic Disease

Kelly K. Anthony, PhD[a], Laura E. Schanberg, MD[b],*

[a]*Division of Medical Psychology, Department of Psychiatry and Behavioral Sciences, Duke University Medical Center, DUMC Box 3527, Durham, NC 27710, USA*
[b]*Division of Pediatric Rheumatology, Department of Pediatrics, Duke University Medical Center, DUMC 3212, Durham, NC 27710, USA*

Increasingly, pediatric rheumatologists are faced with the challenge of assessing, diagnosing, and managing pain in children and adolescents. Recent research suggests that musculoskeletal pain may be the most common complaint for which children are referred to a pediatric rheumatologist and is present in approximately 50% of all new patients [1]. A small percentage of these patients will be diagnosed with a form of juvenile idiopathic arthritis (JIA), which is marked by clinically significant pain. A larger percentage will be diagnosed with a musculoskeletal pain syndrome. Research indicates that approximately 25% of new patients presenting to pediatric rheumatology clinics are diagnosed with a pain syndrome such as fibromyalgia, complex regional pain syndrome, localized pain syndrome, or low back pain.

Given the frequency of musculoskeletal pain as a presenting complaint, understanding the nature of chronic musculoskeletal pain in children is advantageous for both the general pediatric practitioner and the subspecialist. This understanding includes familiarity with the pain experience of healthy children

Dr. Schanberg has received support for related work from the Arthritis Foundation and the Office of Research on Women's Health in conjunction with the National Institute of Arthritis and Musculoskeletal and Skin Diseases. Dr. Anthony has received support for related work from the Arthritis Foundation.

* Corresponding author. Department of Pediatrics, Division of Pediatric Rheumatology, Duke University Medical Center Box 3212, Durham, NC 27710.

E-mail address: schan001@mc.duke.edu (L.E. Schanberg).

and with the range of factors that influence pain reporting in healthy children and in children with chronic disease. In addition, a clinician should understand how to use pain-assessment instruments and be able to recognize and treat pain syndromes and disease-related pain. It is now well recognized that pain is multi-dimensional and is best understood within the context of a biopsychosocial model that incorporates biologic, environmental, and cognitive behavioral mechanisms in the development and maintenance of pain (Fig. 1). Awareness of this model enhances a clinician's ability to manage pain in children by increasing recognition of the factors influencing pain perception and highlighting the full range of pharmacologic and nonpharmacologic treatment methods available to treat pediatric pain.

This article introduces important issues related to pain in children with musculoskeletal pain syndromes and rheumatic disease, using juvenile primary fibromyalgia syndrome (JPFS) and JIA as models. A brief summary of the prevalence of pain in healthy children is followed by a summary of existing pain-assessment techniques. The remainder of the article describes the pain experience of children with JPFS and JIA and discusses issues related to pain management.

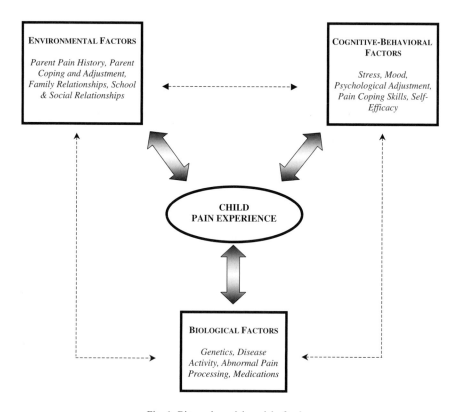

Fig. 1. Biopsychosocial model of pain.

Musculoskeletal pain in healthy children

Health care professionals often underestimate the prevalence of musculo-skeletal pain in healthy children although it is a relatively common presenting complaint to general pediatricians [2–4]. Estimates of the epidemiologic prevalence of musculoskeletal pain in general pediatric populations range from 5% to 20% [5–9], with a few studies reporting prevalence estimates as high as approximately 32% [10,11]. Almost all complaints of musculoskeletal pain in children and adolescents are benign in nature with symptoms mainly attributable to trauma (30%), overuse (28%), normal skeletal growth variation (18%), and growing pains (8%) [2]. Regardless of cause, chronic musculoskeletal pain occurs more commonly in girls [12–18] and in older children [12,16,19–24]. In one large epidemiologic study, the prevalence of pain increased with age, whereas gender differences became apparent at or just before puberty. Teenaged girls were found to be the group most frequently affected, with a prevalence of chronic musculoskeletal pain of nearly 50% [23].

Musculoskeletal pain in otherwise healthy children can persist for several months or even years. In one study, 7% of school-aged children with low back pain reported pain symptoms lasting longer than 3 months [12]. More recently, El-Metwally and colleagues [11] demonstrated higher rates of persistence, with more than 50% of school-aged children reporting persistent musculoskeletal pain at 1-year follow-up. Of the children reporting pain at 1-year follow-up, almost 65% continued to report pain at 4 years. Persistent musculoskeletal pain, particularly pain lasting more than 3 months, has been associated with significant psychologic impairment including higher levels of depression, behavior problems, and anxiety. These impairments create functional disability including disruptions in school attendance and social relationships [12,25–28]. Multiple factors that may influence the onset and maintenance of musculoskeletal pain include genetics [29], environmental familial factors [9], anatomic factors [30], psychosocial factors, and illness or pain behavior [31–33].

Assessment of pain in children

Until relatively recently, the study of pain in children was hindered by a lack of reliable and valid instruments for pediatric pain assessment. This lack probably contributed to the general underestimation of pain in healthy children and in children with chronic disease. Currently, a variety of developmentally based pediatric pain-assessment tools exist for use in both research and clinical settings (Table 1). These tools include self-reporting measures such as the Varni/Thompson Pediatric Pain Questionnaire (PPQ), the Oucher facial scale, and 100-mm visual analogue scales as well as more objective measures of pain including behavioral observation. The PPQ is a comprehensive, multidimensional tool often used in pediatric rheumatology that incorporates several techniques such as visual analogue scales, a body map, and a list of pain descriptors. It is

Table 1
Summary of pediatric pain assessment tools

Assessment tool [references]	Description	Recommended age range
Comprehensive Instrument		
Varni/Thompson Pediatric Pain Questionnaire (PPQ) [34,35]	Comprehensive, multidimensional instrument incorporating a visual analogue scale, body map, and list of pain descriptors	4 to 17 years
Facial Scales		
Oucher [36–38]	Measures pain affect. Six photos of a child's face with varying degrees of discomfort alongside an 11-point numeric scale ranging from 0 to 100.	3 to 12 years
Wong-Baker FACES [41]	Six cartoon-like faces beginning with a smiling faces for "no pain" and ending with a tearful face for "worst pain." Each face is assigned a rating of 0 to 5.	3 years and older, but most reliable and valid in children over 5 years
Faces Pain Scale [39]	Seven line-drawn faces that convey increasing levels of pain intensity. Each face is assigned a rating of 0 to 6.	3 years and older, but most reliable and valid in children over 5 years
Facial Affective Scale [40]	Measures pain affect. Nine faces convey increasing levels of distress. Each face is assigned a value ranging from 0 to 1. 0 represents maximum positive affect and 1 represents maximum negative affect.	3 years and older, but most reliable and valid in children over 5 years
Visual Analogue Scales (VAS)		
Horizontal line (eg, PPQ) [34,35]	100-mm line anchored by words such as "no hurting, no discomfort, no pain" and "hurting a whole lot, very uncomfortable, severe pain." Children mark though line to indicate pain intensity.	Most reliable and valid in children aged 5 years and above
Vertical line/Pain thermometer [42–44]	100-mm line (or thermometer) anchored by words such as "no pain at all" and "pain as bad as it can be." Children mark through the line or draw a line on the thermometer to indicate pain intensity.	3 years and above. Younger children are better able to grasp concept of VAS when line is vertical
Body Outline Figures		
Body map (eg, PPQ) [34,35,48]	Measures pain location. Children are asked to color in areas of the body that hurt. May use different colors to represent varying pain intensity.	4 years and above. Particularly useful for ages 5 to 7 years

(continued on next page)

Table 1 (*continued*)

Assessment tool [references]	Description	Recommended age range
Observation of Pain Behaviors		
Observation system for pain behavior in children with chronic arthritis [49]	Trained observers code pain behaviors while children perform a series of activities such as walking and sitting.	6 to 17 years

administered through structured interviews with parents or children. Parts of it (eg, visual analogue scales) are useful in children as young as 5 years of age [34,35]. Because it is comprehensive in scope, however, the PPQ in its entirety is cumbersome for use in a clinic setting.

More clinically useful assessment tools with demonstrated reliability and validity in many populations of children include the Oucher facial scale and a 100-mm pain thermometer. The Oucher facial scale, which is shown in Fig. 2,

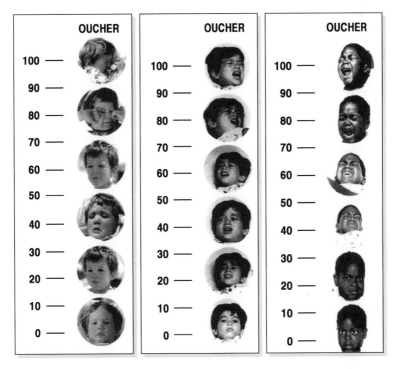

Fig. 2. Oucher Scale. (*left*) The white version of the Oucher was developed and copyrighted by Judith E. Beyer, PhD, RN, (University of Missouri-Kansas City), 1983. (*center*) The Hispanic version was developed and copyrighted by Antonia M. Villarruel, PhD, RN, and Mary J. Denyes, PhD, RN, 1990. (*right*) The African-American version was developed and copyrighted by Mary J. Denyes, PhD, RN, (Wayne State University), and Antonia M. Villarruel, PhD, RN, (University of Michigan) at Children's Hospital of Michigan, 1990. Cornelia P. Porter, PhD, RN, and Charlotta Marshall, RN, MSN, contributed to the development of the scale. All three Oucher scales are printed with permission from Judith E. Beyer, PhD.

has been demonstrated to be a measure of pain affect. It consists of six photographs of a child's face displaying varying degrees of discomfort alongside an 11-point, 0-to-100 numeric scale [36,37].White, African-American, and Hispanic versions are available [37,38]. Children are asked to select a rating that corresponds with their own levels of discomfort. Other facial scales validated for use with children include those developed by Bieri [39], McGrath [40], and Wong [41]. An example, the Wong-Baker FACES scale is shown in Fig. 3. As with the Oucher scale, these facial scales have been shown to reflect pain affect, and not solely pain intensity. For example, a child may report less pain if asked while sitting on the mother's lap than when the mother is out of the room and the child is feeling scared. On the pain thermometer, which is a variation of the visual analogue scale, the child rates current pain intensity by drawing a line on the vertical thermometer anchored by "no pain" and "pain as bad as it can be" (Fig. 4) [42–44]. Facial scales and the pain thermometer are simple to administer and understandable even by preschool-aged children over 3 years of age [45–47].

Body maps can facilitate children's report of the location of pain [34,48]. On the PPQ, children are given a simple outline with front and back views of a human body and asked to shade the areas of the body that hurt using different colors to reflect pain intensity [34]. It has been suggested that use of a body map is particularly useful with children aged 5 to 7 years, who have concrete definitions for pain consistent with their cognitive development. An example of a body map is shown in Fig. 5.

Finally, one example of a behavioral observation system for assessment of pain and pain behaviors in school-aged children and adolescents with JIA is that developed by Jaworski and colleagues [49]. In this assessment method, trained observers code pain behaviors exhibited by children while they perform a 10-minute standard video-recorded protocol of activities. The activities include sitting, walking, standing, and reclining. The validity of this method was demonstrated by a positive correlation between the frequency of a child's pain behaviors and the child's reporting of pain and by parent and physician ratings of children pain intensity [49].

In sum, a variety of tools exists to assist practitioners in assessing pain in children. These tools should be used to supplement the clinical interview during

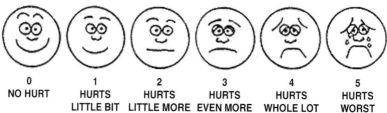

Fig. 3. Wong-Baker FACES pain rating scale. (*From* Wong, D. Whaley and Wong's nursing care of infants and children. 5th edition. St. Louis (MO): Mosby-Year Book, Inc; 1995. p. 1085; with permission.)

We would like you to draw a single line on the pain thermometer below where you usually feel pain. We are not looking for your highest level of pain, or your lowest, but how much pain you feel on average. If you put a line at the bottom of the thermometer, you would say that on average, you usually do not feel any pain. If you put a line at the top, you would say that you usually feel pain as bad as it can be.

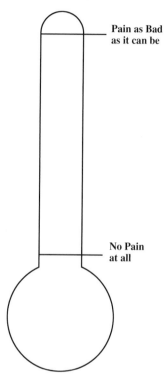

Fig. 4. Pain thermometer. (*From* Schanberg LE, Sandstrom M. Causes of pain in children with arthritis. Rheum Dis Clin North Am 1999;25:31–53; with permission.)

which information about pain characteristics such as symptom duration, intensity, alleviating and aggravating factors, progression, and radiation are obtained. Practitioners should strive to gather information from children directly in addition to interviewing parents. Direct information from the patient is particularly important in school-aged children and adolescents, because research suggests that parents may not be the most accurate reporters of a child's pain intensity, particularly at higher levels of pain [50,51].

Idiopathic musculoskeletal pain syndromes

Because of the high incidence of musculoskeletal pain in healthy children, it may be difficult for practitioners to identify which children have idiopathic

Please color in those areas where you usually feel pain.

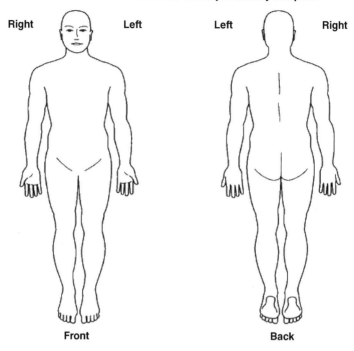

Fig. 5. Pain body map. (*From* Schanberg LE, Sandstrom M. Causes of pain in children with arthritis. Rheum Dis Clin North Am 1999;25:31–53; with permission.)

musculoskeletal pain syndromes. Moreover, these syndromes are poorly understood, with little known about cause and course [13]. Along with orthopedists and primary care physicians, rheumatologists are increasingly called upon to diagnose and manage these syndromes. Indeed, these syndromes are among the most common causes for referral to pediatric rheumatologists, compromising approximately 25% of all new patients [52]. Growing pains, complex regional pain syndrome, localized pain syndromes, low back pain, and chronic sports-related pain syndromes (eg, Osgood–Schlatter disease) are included in this group. A more comprehensive list of idiopathic pain syndromes is given in Box 1.

Complex regional pain syndrome type I (CRPS), also known as reflex sympathetic dystrophy, is characterized by burning pain, allodynia, and swelling of distal extremities along with autonomic dysfunction following injury to the extremity (Box 2) [53,54]. Although most pediatric patients with CRPS present with a history of minor trauma or repeated stress injury (eg, caused by competitive sports), many are unable to identify a precipitating event [55]. The incidence of CRPS in children is unknown, in large part because it is under-diagnosed and is often diagnosed late, with the diagnosis frequently delayed by nearly a year. The usual age of onset is between 9 to 15 years, and girls outnumber boys by as much as 6:1. Childhood CRPS differs from the adult form

Box 1. Common musculoskeletal pain syndromes in children by anatomic region

Shoulder
    Impingement syndrome
Elbow
    Little League elbow
    Panner's disease
    Avulsion fractures
    Osteochondritis dissecans
    Tennis elbow
Arm
    Complex regional pain syndrome
    Localized hypermobility syndrome
Pelvis and hip
    Avulsion injuries
    Legg–Calve–Perthes syndrome
    Slipped capital femoral epiphysis
    Congenital hip dysplasia
Knee
    Osteochondritis dissecans
    Osgood–Schlatter disease
    Sindig–Larsen syndrome
    Patellofemoral syndrome
    Malalignment syndromes
Leg
    Shin splints
    Stress fractures
    Compartment syndromes
    Growing pains
    Complex regional pain syndrome
    Localized hypermobility syndrome
Foot
    Plantar fasciitis
    Tarsal coalition
    Stress fractures
    Achilles tendonitis
    Juvenile bunion
Spine
    Musculoskeletal strain
    Spondylolisthesis
    Spondylolysis
    Scoliosis

Scheuermann disease (kyphosis)
Low back pain
Generalized
    Juvenile fibromyalgia
    Hypermobility syndrome
    Generalized pain syndrome

in that lower extremities are affected even more commonly in children [54, 56–58]. Consistent with the biopsychosocial model of pain, research has suggested that psychologic stress plays a significant role in children's disease [56,59,60], and that children may be at increased risk for development of CRPS if they have relatives with chronic pain conditions [54]. Treatment for childhood CRPS, as for other pain syndromes, seeks to improve function as much as relieve pain. These two desirable outcomes may not go hand in hand, however. It is common for children to continue to complain of pain even while they are resuming normal function. As a result, families and providers need to outline clearly the goals by which to measure treatment successes. Recommended treatment modalities include aggressive physical and occupational therapy, cognitive behavioral interventions, and sympathetic nerve blocks. Physical

Box 2. Diagnostic criteria for complex regional pain syndrome, type I [53]

A diagnosis of CRPS requires regional pain, sensory symptoms, plus two neuropathic pain descriptors and two physical signs of autonomic dysfunction.

Neuropathic descriptors

Burning
Dysesthesia
Paresthesia
Allodynia
Cold hyperalgesia

Autonomic dysfunction

Cyanosis
Mottling
Hyperhydrosis
Coolness ($\geq 3°$)
Edema

therapy, which should be started as soon as the diagnosis is made, is recommended three to four times per week, and children may need analgesic premedication at the onset. Initial treatment is limited to desensitization and moves to weight-bearing, range-of-motion, and other functional activities. On the other hand, nerve blocks are not recommended as initial therapy and should be undertaken only after other therapies have failed and only under the auspices of pediatric pain specialists. Multiple studies have shown noninvasive treatments, particularly cognitive behavioral therapy and physical therapy, are at least as efficacious as nerve blocks in children [53,55,56,59,61,62].

Fibromyalgia in children

A more common pain syndrome seen by pediatric rheumatologists is JPFS: approximately 25% to 40% of children with chronic pain syndromes fulfill criteria for JPFS [33,63]. It is characterized by widespread, persistent pain, sleep disturbance, fatigue, and the presence of multiple, discrete tender points on physical examination. JPFS is uniquely frustrating for both patients and health care providers, because children often present with high subjective distress but few objective abnormalities on standard physical examination and laboratory screening. There are limited epidemiologic data on the prevalence of JPFS. It was first described in 1985 by Yunus and Masi [63], who developed diagnostic criteria based on 33 children who suffered from persistent pain and sleep difficulties. The prevalence of JPFS has been estimated to be as high as 6% in school-aged children when less stringent diagnostic criteria for adults set forth by the American College of Rheumatology (ACR) are used [64,65]. It is diagnosed most commonly in prepubertal or adolescent girls; the average age of onset of 13 is years [33,63,66]. Symptoms may begin at an earlier age, however and also occur in young males [66]. Across the age span, the majority of children diagnosed with JPFS are white.

Because the ACR criteria have never been validated in children [67], the only reliable criteria at this time are those first set forth by Yunus and Masi (Box 3) [63]. Yunus and Masi's criteria include the presence of diffuse musculoskeletal pain in at least three areas of the body that persist for at least 3 months in the absence of an underlying condition. Results of laboratory tests are normal, and physical examination reveals at least 5 of the 18 well-defined tender points. During physical examination, patients with JPFS show few pain behaviors and move around with no evident difficulty [19], but they report high pain intensity and use words such as "miserable," "intense," and "unbearable" when describing their pain [19,68]. The Yunus and Masi [63] criteria also require that 3 of 10 minor criteria or associated symptoms be present for diagnosis. These include nonrestorative sleep (100%), fatigue (91%), chronic anxiety or tension (56%), chronic headaches (54%), subjective soft tissue swelling (61%), and pain modulated by physical activity, weather, and anxiety or stress. There is considerable overlap between the symptoms accompanying JPFS and symptoms associated with other functional disorders, including irritable bowel disease,

---

Box 3. Criteria for a diagnosis of juvenile primary fibromyalgia syndrome

Widespread musculoskeletal pain ≥ 3 months' duration, in the absence of any underlying medical condition and with normal laboratory results
Plus
Five or more well-defined tender points
    Insertion of nuchal muscles into occiput
    Upper border of trapezius — mid-portion
    Muscle attachments to upper medial border of scapula
    Anterior aspects of the C5, C7 intertransverse spaces
    Second rib space about 3 cm lateral to the sternal border
    Muscle attachments to lateral epicondyle — 2 cm below
        bony prominence
    Upper outer quadrant of gluteal muscles
    Muscle attachments just posterior to greater trochanter
    Medial fat pad of knee proximal to joint line
Plus
Three of 10 minor criteria
    Fatigue
    Sleep disturbance
    Chronic anxiety or tension
    Chronic headaches
    Irritable bowel syndrome
    Subjective soft tissue swelling
    Numbness of tingling of the extremities
    Pain modulated by stress or anxiety
    Pain modulated by weather
    Pain modulated by physical activity

---

migraines, temporomandibular joint disorder, myofascial pain syndromes, premenstrual syndrome, mood and anxiety disorders, and chronic fatigue syndrome [69]. Indeed, all these disorders may be part of a larger spectrum of related syndromes [70,71].

Course and prognosis of juvenile primary fibromyalgia syndrome

As in adults, children with fibromyalgia experience significant pain, suffering, and disability [72,73]. In addition, longitudinal studies conducted at academic centers have reported that children with JPFS continue to suffer from persistent pain and other symptoms many years following diagnosis [63,74,75]. In community samples, research has suggested better long-term outcomes [64,76,77]. These studies, however, have primarily used the ACR diagnostic criteria, that may not be applicable to children. Thus, it is generally accepted that JPFS has a chronic course that can have detrimental effects for child health and psychosocial development. As an example, adolescents with JPFS who do not receive treatment or are inadequately treated may withdraw from school and the social milieu, complicating their transition to adulthood.

Juvenile primary fibromyalgia syndrome symptoms: etiology and maintenance

Although the precise cause of JPFS is unknown, there is an emerging understanding that the development and maintenance of JPFS are related to both biologic and psychologic factors consistent with the biopsychosocial model of pain. JPFS seems to be an abnormality of pain processing characterized by disordered sleep physiology, enhanced pain perception with abnormal levels of substance P in spinal fluid, disordered mood, and dysregulation of hypothalamic-pituitary-adrenal and other neuroendocrine axes [78,79]. In addition, physiologic abnormalities have been documented in both children and adults with fibromyalgia. For example, children with JPFS have lower tender-point pain thresholds and greater pain sensitivity than seen in healthy children or in children with chronic arthritis [67,80].

The maintenance of symptoms in JPFS is clearly perpetuated by a variety of physical and psychologic factors. Children with fibromyalgia often find themselves in a vicious cycle of pain, whereby symptoms build upon one another and contribute to the onset and maintenance of new symptoms (Fig. 6). Factors likely to be included in this vicious cycle include fatigue, poor sleep, stress, anxiety, inactivity, and depressed mood. Other factors influencing symptom report and functional disability in JPFS include the child's coping mechanisms and family environment.

The majority of children with JPFS evidence sleep disturbances and psychologic distress that contribute to their level of functional disability. All the children in Yunus and Masi's [63] original sample reported waking unrefreshed, 91% reported general fatigue, and 67% reported poor sleep. In later studies, children with JPFS evidenced a higher frequency of sleep difficulties than healthy children and children with chronic arthritis, including increased sleep latency, more decreased sleep efficiency, more arousals, more intrusions on slow-wave sleep, and more morning fatigue [67,81,82]. Psychosocial distress noted in JPFS includes depression and anxiety. Estimates of anxiety disorders or major depression in children with JPFS reach 50% [63,77,83]. In addition, children with JPFS report more anxious and depressive symptoms than children with chronic arthritis or healthy controls [80]. Moreover, many children report that anxiety and stress play a significant role in the modulation of their pain [63]. Coping has been shown to predict health status in JPFS, with better health outcomes (eg, less pain, increased function, and decreased psychologic impairment) in children who evidenced greater perceived coping efficacy and less catastrophizing [68].

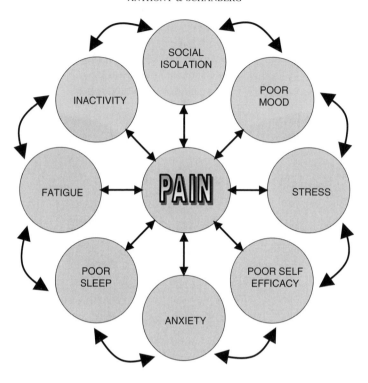

Fig. 6. Cycle of pain.

Several studies have documented familial aggregation of fibromyalgia [64,81,83]. Parents of children with JPFS also report personal histories of other chronic medical conditions including rheumatic diseases and chronic pain conditions such as low back pain, shoulder/neck pain, and migraine headaches [81,84]. In a study of the social context of pain in children with JPFS, 79% of parents of children with JPFS reported a history of at least one chronic pain condition, and 62% reported a history of two or more. In this and other studies, a more extensive pain or medical history in parents and poor parental pain coping (eg, catastrophizing) have been associated with higher global impairment and physical disability in children [67,84]. The presence of fibromyalgia and other chronic pain conditions in families of children with JPFS may indicate a genetic or biologic link in the development of JPFS; however, it might also suggest strong environmental influences, or both. Specifically, data suggest families of children with JPFS and other pain syndromes function less effectively than other families and that parents may serve as pain models for their children [80,84,85]. Overall patterns of family interaction in JPFS include less cohesion, more conflict, and decreased organization, and there may be increased parental psychologic distress [80]. Moreover, the specific nature of family relationships may be predictive of child outcomes. Schanberg and colleagues [84] demonstrated that children in families described as more active-recreational and intellectual-cultural in orientation on the Family Environment Scale reported less impairment from JPFS, whereas children in families self-described as more moral-religious and controlling in orientation reported more pain and lower levels of function. It is likely that family environments with high levels of physical disability, poor coping, and increased stress interact with a genetic or biologic predisposition to influence the expression of JPFS symptoms [79].

Treatment of juvenile primary fibromyalgia syndrome

To date, there have been no systematic, well-controlled studies of treatment in JPFS. Current treatment and management of JPFS generally follow what is advocated for adults with fibromyalgia, with modifications based on the child's age, developmental level, and social environment (eg, less medication) [66]. The major goals of treatment are to restore function and to alleviate pain. As such, treatment should address sleep as well as depression and anxiety. Treatment strategies include pharmacologic interventions, exercise-based interventions, and psychologic interventions. Drug therapies include nonsteroidal anti-inflammatory drugs (NSAIDs), tricyclic antidepressants, specific serotonin reuptake inhibitors (SSRIs), and muscle relaxants. Unfortunately, drug therapies have been largely unsuccessful. In the adult literature, studies have shown these medications provide only modest and short-term benefits [86,87]. There have been almost no studies of medication efficacy in pediatric populations. In one study with a sample of 15 children with JPFS, use of NSAIDs alone did not produce any improvement in symptoms [88]. In another study with older adolescents and adults, the combination of NSAIDs and tricyclic antidepressants was beneficial [75].

In JPS, whether treating chronic pain, comorbid anxiety, or depression, practitioners should be cautious in their use of antidepressants, particularly SSRIs. In October 2004, the United States Food and Drug Administration (FDA) issued a public health advisory regarding the use of SSRIs in children and adolescents related to the increased occurrence of suicidal thoughts in this age group (http://www.fda.gov/cder/drug/antidepressants/SSRIPHA200410.htm) with a proposed medication guide (http://www.fda.gov/cder/drug/antidepressants/SSRIMedicationGuide.htm). Results of a recent large, randomized, controlled trial studying the efficacy of fluoxetine on cognitive behavioral therapy in a sample of 439 children with depression aged 12 to 17 years indicated that fluoxetine alone (60% response rate) was significantly inferior to the combination of drug and cognitive behavioral therapy (71% response rate) but better that cognitive behavioral therapy alone [89]. In addition, there was an increased rate of suicide attempts in fluoxetine groups (6 versus 1), although no suicides were reported. There is little or no evidence supporting the use of other SSRIs (eg, sertraline) or atypical antidepressants (eg, mirtazapine, venlafaxine, and buproprion) in children and adolescents. Thus, fluoxetine should be the first antidepressant agent used, however, this and all other antidepressants should be used only with extreme caution, extensive parental education, and close, frequent monitoring for side effects. Psychiatric consultation is recommended.

In general, children with JPFS seen at tertiary care centers are encouraged to pursue a multidisciplinary treatment regimen including medication, parent and child education, graduated aggressive aerobic exercise, training in pain-coping skills, stress management, improved sleep hygiene, and psychotherapy. Indeed, in a meta-analysis of treatment studies in adult fibromyalgia, the combination of pharmacologic methods with cognitive-behavioral therapy, and exercise showed larger effect than pharmacological interventions alone [90]. These multicomponent treatment regimens are difficult to coordinate, often expensive, not fully reimbursed by insurance companies, and are poorly accepted by many families, however [74,91].

Regardless of other treatments, it is strongly recommended that children with JPFS be encouraged to return to school and resume normal activities. Parents should also be encouraged to take an active role in promoting their child's re-entry into school and other social environments [66]. As with all pain management, the goals of therapy should focus on promoting function, rather than simply alleviating pain. Moreover, the therapeutic interventions should be time limited and goal oriented with the aim of fostering self-reliance. Both the family and child need education about diagnosis as well as the interrelationships between mood, stress, poor sleep, pain, and lack of exercise in the maintenance of symptoms. Of prime importance is the establishment of a therapeutic relationship with reassurance that the pain and other symptoms the child is experiencing are indeed real and not imagined [91]. This reassurance is particularly important with pain syndromes because families are often frustrated with the medical system as the result of previous misdiagnosis or lack of diagnosis of their child's condition and perceived accusations that child is experiencing psychogenic pain or is malingering [66].

Cognitive behavioral therapy

In cognitive behavioral therapy, approaches to pain management are designed to teach children and adolescents coping skills for controlling behavioral, cognitive, and physiologic responses to pain. Cognitive behavioral therapy involves educating children and parents about mechanisms by which pain messages are transmitted and perceived as well as the role of the individual in these processes. Children then are taught various pain-coping skills with guidance in applying the skills in difficult situations. Skills taught include decreasing cognitive responses to pain and relaxation strategies such as progressive muscle relaxation, distraction, and guided imagery. Finally, children are encouraged to anticipate situations in which they are likely to experience increased pain or difficulty managing pain and to plan strategies for handling these challenges. Cognitive behavioral therapy teaches self-reliance and seeks to empower patients to be responsible for their own pain management. Cognitive behavioral therapy training has been done in individual or group formats consisting of 6 to 14 sessions. Small studies have shown the efficacy of cognitive behavioral therapy in adults and children with fibromyalgia [90,92,93] and in patients with multiple other pain conditions.

Aerobic exercise and physical therapy

Because children with JPFS are often deconditioned and are no longer participating in physical activities because of fatigue and pain, graduated aggressive aerobic exercise is another important component of treatment. Although the initiation of aerobic exercise often leads to increased pain intensity, gradual improvement follows over several weeks accompanied by a concomitant, paradoxical increase in energy level [91]. Aerobic exercise has the additional benefit of improving sleep and mood. Research has shown that it is aerobic exercise, rather than stretching, strengthening, or manipulative techniques, that is associated with symptom improvement [94,95]. Exercise and physical therapy, implemented in either an individualized or group format, can be helpful in promoting function in children with fibromyalgia [66]. Physical therapists should help children design and implement home exercise programs, enabling them to develop self-management skills and encouraging feelings of self-efficacy.

Sleep hygiene

Sleep hygiene promotes improved sleep patterns in children with fibromyalgia and other pain conditions. To improve sleep hygiene, children are encouraged to avoid napping during the day and establish a bedtime routine with consistent sleep-wake cycles even during weekends and school holidays. This is particularly important because children with fibromyalgia and other painful conditions often have disordered sleep cycles, staying awake much of the night and then sleeping during the day, resulting in more difficulty sleeping at night [66]. Improved sleep hygiene and increased aerobic activity, combined with low doses of tricyclic antidepressants, provide comprehensive treatment of sleep difficulties. Doses as low as 10 mg of either amitriptyline or nortriptyline may be efficacious. The chronic use of hypnotics should be avoided.

Research has demonstrated that children with JPFS have sleep disturbances both by history and on polysomnography. These disturbances include nonrestorative sleep, increased sleep latency, shortened total sleep time, decreased sleep efficiency, and excessive movement activity during sleep [81,82]. These findings, however, are not specific to JPFS. Children with JPFS should be treated presumptively for sleep disturbance. Generally, sleep studies are recommended only when children present with a history consistent with sleep apnea, including snoring, morning headache, and daytime sleepiness, especially in children and adolescents who are obese.

Other forms of treatment

Other suggested forms of treatment for JPFS include support groups and complementary and alternative medicine strategies. Support groups can be helpful for both children and their parents, providing social support and a sense that they are not alone in dealing with fibromyalgia. Groups should be age-specific and supervised by appropriately trained health care professionals with experience working with families of children with fibromyalgia or chronic disease. Ideally, parent groups and child groups should be conducted separately. It is also important that support groups do not foster dysfunctional behaviors that could lead to increase pain complaints [66].

Increasingly, both adults and children with JPFS, frustrated by the limitations of current therapies, have sought alternative forms of treatment including acupuncture, massage, and herbal remedies [66]. Although these treatments may be helpful for individual children with fibromyalgia, there are few data supporting their effectiveness. Moreover, some of the treatment alternatives, such as acupuncture, are not suitable for children. Future studies are needed to determine both the effectiveness and safety of these treatments for children and adults with fibromyalgia [96].

Although this discussion addresses JPFS in children, the general concepts discussed are true to some degree for all pain states. The biopsychosocial model of pain taking into account influences from the environment, cognition, and disease-specific biologic abnormalities holds true for all pain syndromes, with changes only in the relative contribution of variables. Likewise, treatment approaches are also similar but need to be individualized for every child and health condition. The following discussion of pain in JIA highlights issues pertinent to disease-related pain, again within the context of the biopsychosocial model of pain.

Pain in children with juvenile idiopathic arthritis

There is an increasing awareness by pediatric rheumatologists that pain is a clinically significant symptom for children diagnosed with JIA, requiring more attention and targeted interventions. JIA affects as many as 200,000 to 300,000 American children, making it the fifth most common childhood chronic disease [97–100]. It most commonly follows a fluctuating course characterized by unpredictable flares of disease symptoms including pain, morning stiffness, fatigue, and sleep disturbance. Children may also experience potentially painful complications including joint deformities and destruction, osteoporosis, and growth abnormalities that can lead to psychologic distress and functional disability [101,102].

Prevalence of pain in juvenile idiopathic arthritis

Advances in measures of pediatric pain in the last 15 years have enabled researchers to take a more systematic approach to the study of pain in children with JIA. The results of several studies show that pain is more prevalent in JIA than previously recognized and may persist in some patients into adulthood [103]. For example, Sherry et al [104] found that 86% of 293 children with arthritis reported pain during a routine clinic visit. In addition, data from the

Cincinnati Juvenile Arthritis Databank, which examined 462 children with arthritis, indicated that 60% of children reported joint pain at disease onset, 50% reported pain at 1-year follow-up, and 40% continued to report pain 5 years later [105]. More recent research indicates that most children with chronic arthritis experience pain on an almost daily basis and that disease flares are frequent. Using daily diary methodology, the authors demonstrated that school-aged children with chronic arthritis report pain an average of 73% of days, with the majority of children (76%) reporting pain on more than 60% of days [106]. Across studies of pain in juvenile chronic arthritis, children report average pain intensity in the mild to moderate range [34,104,105,107–109]. There is, however, considerable variability in pain ratings, with as many as 25% of the children reporting pain intensity in the higher ranges [110]. Higher levels of pain in children with chronic arthritis have been associated with poor functional outcomes including reductions in school attendance and social activities [110–112].

Predictors of pain in children with juvenile idiopathic arthritis

Although a relationship between increased disease activity and increased pain exists [34,113,114], research has consistently demonstrated limited predictive value for disease status variables. Across studies, they typically predict only a small to medium proportion of the variance in children's pain ratings (eg, 8% to 28%), with higher pain ratings in children with polyarticular disease related to more severe disease as rated by physicians [109,110,114,115]. Consequently, it has been necessary to delineate other influential factors in the pain experience of children with JIA. The most highly predictive models use a biopsychosocial approach conceptualizing pain reporting as influenced by multiple factors including disease variables, demographic variables, psychologic variables such as coping and mood, and environmental factors. For example, results of a two-part study by Thompson, Varni, and colleagues [109,111] demonstrated that scores on the Family Relationship Index of the Family Environment Scale, behavior and social subscales of the Child Behavior Checklist, and disease variables combined to predict 34% of the variance in children's present pain intensity and 72% of variance in children's ratings of their worst pain intensity. Similarly, in a sample of 56 children with chronic arthritis, Ross et al [116] reported that increased child anxiety, increased maternal distress, and increased family harmony were associated with higher child pain ratings averaged over a 1 -month time period. The role of family harmony was both surprising and contrary to study hypotheses. The authors hypothesized that increased family harmony might lend itself to increased responsiveness to the child's pain behavior, serving to reinforce both pain behavior and pain reporting in children.

The relationships between demographic variables and JIA-related pain still remain unclear. There is some suggestion that age and gender may be influential. For example, Hagglund et al [117] reported a marginally significant effect for age, with older children reporting more severe pain on a 10-cm visual analogue scale. More recently, in a large sample of 301 children with chronic arthritis, Malleson [14] reported that increased age was a significant predictor of pain in the 8- to 15-year-old age range but not for older adolescents. In other studies, age has not been a statistically significant predictor [110,113,116,118–120]. With regard to gender, several studies found no difference between the reported pain levels of boys and girls [113,114,117,118]. When differences are noted, girls report more pain than their male counterparts [119,121].

Several studies have demonstrated the role of many psychosocial variables in children's pain reporting, including emotional distress, mood, stress, and pain-coping strategies. In the authors' study investigating the interrelationships of daily stress, daily mood, and disease expression, results of multilevel random effects models indicated that day-to-day fluctuations in mood and stressful events were related to daily symptoms in children with polyarticular forms of juvenile chronic arthritis [122–124]. Specifically, worse mood and more stressful events were significantly related to increased daily pain, fatigue, and stiffness. The authors' research and that of others indicates that increased psychologic distress (eg, stress, depression, anxiety) is related to increased pain reporting as well as to poor functional outcomes such as decreased participation in school and social activities [106,116]. With regard to children's coping with pain, the use of ca-tastrophizing (eg, engaging in overly negative thinking about pain) and decreased pain-coping efficacy have been shown to predict higher pain intensity across several pain measures as well as more painful body locations, even after control-ling for demographic variables and medical status variables [110]. In a laboratory setting, catastrophizing also predicted higher pain intensity, decreased pain tolerance, and increased pain-related discomfort in children undergoing experi-mental cold pressor pain [125].

Finally, parent and family environmental variables have been shown to be related to the pain reporting of children with JIA. These variables include the nature of family relationships (eg, family harmony or conflict), increased parent psychologic distress, and parent and family pain history. For example in a sample of school-aged children with chronic arthritis, the authors [126] found that a more extensive parent and family history of pain (eg, a family history of chronic pain conditions, intensity levels of parental pain, parental pain that interfered with activities) was related to increased child self-reported pain and to higher physicians' ratings of the child's disease status. Moreover, within the context of hierarchical regression analyses, a child's catastrophizing was shown to mediate these relationships. In other words, parental and familial pain variables influ-enced the use of catastrophizing by the child, which in turn influenced the child's reporting of pain and disease activity.

Management of pain in children with juvenile idiopathic arthritis

Consistent with the biopsychosocial model of pain, a useful algorithm for the approach to treating pain in JIA is first to treat the underlying disease ag-gressively and then to combine drug treatment with nonpharmacologic modalities to treat pain. As in JPFS, goals of treatment should be to alleviate pain and to improve or preserve function in children and adolescents.

Pharmacologic management

Although no clinical trials have addressed pain management in JIA directly, the treatment of pain has focused historically on controlling the underlying disease process with medications while providing symptomatic relief with NSAIDs, acetaminophen, heat or cold, splints, adaptive devices, physical therapy, and, rarely, opioids. The mainstay of drug treatment for JIA-related pain continues to be NSAIDs with acetaminophen for acutely painful events. Moderating agents, particularly methotrexate and anti–tumor necrosis factor agents, are indicated in children with persistently active joints despite first-line treatment. Systemic steroids generally are avoided but may be useful short term to treat painful flares while other interventions are put in place. Intra-articular steroids are a safe option to manage the inflammation in monoarticular or pauciarticular arthritis but may also be useful to treat particularly symptomatic joints in a child with polyarticular arthritis. The pharmacologic management of JIA is discussed more extensively elsewhere in this issue.

Opioids are used to provide pain relief in acute situations and to maintain mobility in severely affected children. In fact, opioids may have less long-term toxicity than corticosteroids, which are used commonly for symptom management. For children with severe neck, hip, or lower extremity arthritis, the addition of opioid analgesia may make possible continued mobility, with all the associated health benefits. For children requiring opioid therapy for adequate pain management, single-agent oxycodone preparations are preferable for short-acting medication, and methadone is preferred for long-term therapy. Methadone is available in a liquid form, so it can be titrated to effect in children easily. The analgesic half-life of methadone may be increased in children and adolescents, with many needing only two or three doses per day for adequate pain relief rather than the traditional dosing every 6 hours [127,128]. Additional pediatric dosing guidelines are provided in Table 2.

As in adults, adjuvant medications are often useful for managing chronic pain in children. These medications most commonly include tricyclic antidepressants for generalized chronic pain associated with sleep disturbance. The tricyclic antidepressants, for example amitriptyline and nortriptyline, are used in low doses given at night. SSRIs should be used only with extreme caution in children and adolescents to treat mood disorders that may be comorbid. As already described, with recent FDA mandated labeling for SSRIs, these medications should only be used with close follow-up and extensive parent education about the risks of increased potential for suicide attempts.

Surgical interventions

There is no general agreement about the role of surgery in treating pain and symptoms in children with chronic arthritis, although some research suggests that children experience marked pain reduction after surgical intervention [129–131].

Table 2
Pediatric dosing guidelines for selected medications used to treat musculoskeletal pain

Medication	Daily dose	Frequency	Daily maximum
NSAIDs			
Salicylate	60–100 mg/kg	3 times/d	Serum level 20–30 mg/dL
Ibuprofen	30–40 mg/kg	3 times/d	2400 mg
Naproxen	10–20 mg	2 times/d	1000 mg
Tolectin	40 mg/kg	3 times/d	1600 mg
Nabumetone	30 mg/kg	daily	2000 mg
Etoladac SR	400–1000 mg (by age)	daily	1000 mg
Analgesics			
Acetaminophen	10–15 mg/kg/dose	Every 4 h	2–4 g
Hydrocodone	0.15 mg/kg	Every 4 h	limited by side effects
Oxycodone	0.05–0.2 mg/kg	Every 3–6 h	limited by side effects
Tramadol	25–100 mg	Every 4–6 h	300 mg
Methadone	0.2–0.4 mg/kg	Every 6–12 h	limited by side effects
Nortriptyline	10–30 mg	at bedtime	150 mg at bedtime

Abbreviation: NSAIDs, nonsteroidal anti-inflammatory agents.

Surgical interventions can include synovectomies, soft-tissue release, and arthroplasty and are generally limited to children with marked functional impairment, severe disabling pain, and deformity. Whenever possible, the age of the child should be considered, and surgery should be delayed until the growth plate has closed [132]. Surgical interventions should be performed only in specialized clinics at tertiary care centers. Given the recent pharmacologic advances in treating children with chronic arthritis, the future role of surgical interventions is unclear.

Nonpharmacologic interventions

Growing acceptance of the biopsychosocial model of pain has prompted the development and study of nonpharmacologic interventions for JIA-related pain. Research on nonpharmacologic interventions has included programs for improving physical conditioning and sleep hygiene, massage therapy, and, perhaps most importantly, cognitive behavioral therapy.

As already described, cognitive behavioral therapy aims to manage pain by improving self-reliance and facilitating normal activities through the use of coping skills, decreasing cognitive responses to pain, and using relaxation strategies including progressive muscle relaxation, distraction, and guided imagery. Two published studies have demonstrated improvements in self-reported pain ratings of children with chronic arthritis following cognitive behavioral therapy immediately after treatment and at 6-month follow-up [133,134]. Both studies, however, are limited by small sample sizes, the abbreviated scope of the cognitive behavioral therapy intervention, and the lack of functional outcome variables. Although future studies of cognitive behavioral therapy are necessary to understand fully its role in the treatment of this population, research in many other disease populations supports its applicability. Moreover, the lack of the side effects seen with pain medications and the generalizability of the skills make cognitive behavioral therapy an attractive adjunctive therapy.

As indicated, programs for improving physical conditioning and sleep hygiene in children with JIA have been advocated. Children with chronic arthritis are often less physically active than their peers as a result of disease symptoms and have decreased aerobic capacity and endurance, decreased exercise time, and decreased peak workload as compared with healthy controls [135,136]. A series of studies provides preliminary support for the safety and benefit of conditioning programs in improving symptoms in children with chronic arthritis including joint counts, cardiovascular fitness, pain, and gait efficiency [137–140]. For example, Fisher et al [140] showed that resistance exercise led to decreased pain, disability, and medication use in a sample of six children with chronic arthritis. Future studies are necessary to delineate the most appropriate exercise for children with arthritis.

Improving sleep quality is often overlooked in the treatment of pain. A recent study described frequent night waking, parasomnias, sleep anxiety, sleep-disordered breathing, and daytime fatigue in children with arthritis compared with controls [141]; disturbed sleep was also associated with increased pain in children with JIA. Thus, even simple measures to improve sleep, including use of a waterbed and sleeping in warm pajamas (eg, sweat clothes), should be recommended to children with JIA. Physical therapists can also suggest sleep positions that will maximize the child's level of comfort depending on the unique combination of active joints. Relaxation techniques such as progressive muscle relaxation or guided imagery can also be useful in improving sleep hygiene, and these strategies often are taught within the context of cognitive behavioral therapy.

Finally, one study evaluated the effectiveness of massage therapy in decreasing pain in a sample of 20 children with mild to moderate arthritis [142]. Children were assigned randomly to either a massage therapy group or a control group using relaxation techniques. Immediately after treatment, children who received massage evidenced lower levels of anxiety and decreased salivary cortisol levels. They also reported less present pain, less pain during the past week, and fewer painful locations than children in the control group.

Summary

Chronic musculoskeletal pain, whether idiopathic or disease-related, is common in childhood. Pediatric rheumatologists and other pediatric health care providers must understand the epidemiology of musculoskeletal pain as part of childhood, diagnose pain syndromes in children and rule out rheumatic disease, and be willing to initiate treatment of pain in children and adolescents. The practitioner's ability to carry out these tasks is enhanced by an awareness of the biopsychosocial model of pain, which integrates biologic, environmental, and cognitive behavioral mechanisms in describing the causes and maintenance of a child's pain. Indeed, a growing body of research in both rheumatic diseases

such as JIA and idiopathic musculoskeletal pain syndromes such as JPFS
highlights the importance of environmental and cognitive behavioral influences
in the pain experience of children in addition to the contribution of disease activity. These influences include factors innate in the child, such as emotional
distress, daily stress, coping, and mood, and familial factors, such as parental
psychologic health, parental pain history, and the nature of family interactions.
Addressing these issues while providing aggressive traditional medical management will optimize pain treatment and improve overall quality of life for children
with musculoskeletal pain.

References

[1] McGhee JL, Burks FN, Sheckles JL, et al. Identifying children with chronic arthritis based
on chief complaints: absence of predictive value for musculoskeletal pain as an indicator
of rheumatic disease in children. Pediatrics 2002;110(2):354–9.
[2] De Inocencio J. Musculoskeletal pain in primary pediatric care: analysis of 1000 consecutive
general pediatric clinic visits. Pediatrics 1998;102:e63.
[3] Schappert SM, Nelson C. National Ambulatory Medical Care Survey, 1995–1996 summary.
Vital Health Stat 1999;142(13):i–vi, 1–122.
[4] De Inocencio J. Epidemiology of musculoskeletal pain in primary care. Arch Dis Child 2004;
89:431–4.
[5] Goodman JE, McGrath PJ. The epidemiology of pain in children and adolescents: a review.
Pain 1991;46:247–64.
[6] Abu-Arafeh I, Russell G. Recurrent limb pain in school. Arch Dis Child 1996;74:336–9.
[7] McClain BC. Chronic pain in children: current issues in recognition and management. Pain
Digest 1996;6:71–7.
[8] Kristjansdottir G. Prevalence of pain combinations and overall pain: a study of headache,
stomach pain and back pain among school children. Scand J Soc Med 1997;25:58–63.
[9] Mikkelsson M, Kaprio J, Salimen JJ, et al. Widespread pain among 11-year-old Finnish twin
pairs. Arthritis Rheum 2001;44(2):481–5.
[10] Mikkelsson M, Salminen JJ, Kautiainen H. Non-specific musculoskeletal pain in preadolescents. Prevalence and 1-year persistence. Pain 1997;73:29–35.
[11] El-Metwally A, Salminen JJ, Auvinen A, et al. Prognosis of non-specific musculoskeletal pain
in preadolescents: a prospective 4-year follow-up study till adolescence. Pain 2004;110:550–9.
[12] Balague F, Dutoit G, Waldburger M. Low back pain in school-children. Scand J Rehabil Med
1988;20:175–9.
[13] Mikkelson M, Salminen JJ, Sourander A, et al. Contributing factors to the persistence of musculoskeletal pain in preadolescents: a prospective 1-year follow-up study. Pain 1998;77:67–72.
[14] Fairbank JCT, Pynsent PB, VanPoortvliet JA, et al. Influence of anthropometric factors and
joint laxity in the incidence of adolescent back pain. Spine 1984;9:461–4.
[15] Salimen JJ. The adolescent back: a field survey of 370 Finnish school children. Acta Paediatr
Scand 1984;73(Suppl 315):37–42.
[16] Viikari-Juntura E, Vuori J, Silverstein A, et al. A life-long prospective study on the role of
psychological factors in neck-shoulder and low-back pain. Spine 1991;16:1056–61.
[17] Salminen JJ, Pentti J, Terho P. Low back pain and disability in 14-year-old schoolchildren.
Acta Paediatr 1992;81:1035–9.
[18] Olsen TL, Anderson RL, Dearwater SR, et al. The epidemiology of low-back pain in an
adolescent population. Am J Public Health 1992;82:606–8.
[19] Sherry DD, McGuire T, Mellins E, et al. Psychosomatic musculoskeletal pain in childhood:
clinical and psychological analyses of 100 children. Pediatrics 1991;88:1093–9.

[20] Balague F, Nordin M, Skovron ML, et al. Non-specific low-back pain among schoolchildren: a field survey with analysis of some associated factors. J Spinal Disord 1994;7:374–9.

[21] Troussier B, Davoine P, de Gaudemaris R, et al. Back pain in school children: a study among 1178 pupils. Scand J Rehab Med 1994;26:143–6.

[22] Burton AK, Clarke RD, McClune TD, et al. The natural history of low back pain in adolescents. Spine 1996;20:2323–8.

[23] Perquin CW, Hazebroek-Kampschreur AAJM, Hunfeld JAM, et al. Pain in children and adolescents: a common experience. Pain 2000;87:51–8.

[24] Stahl M, Mikkelsson M, Kautiainen H, et al. Neck pain in adolescence. A 4-year follow-up of pain-free preadolescents. Pain 2004;110:427–31.

[25] Mikkelsson M, Sourander A, Piha J, et al. Psychiatric symptoms in preadolescents with musculoskeletal pain and fibromyalgia. Pediatrics 1997;100:220–7.

[26] Egger HL, Costello EJ, Erkanli A, et al. Somatic complaints and psychopathology in children and adolescents: stomach aches, musculoskeletal pains, and headaches. J Am Acad Child Adolesc Psychiatry 1999;38:852–60.

[27] Palermo TM. Impact of recurrent and chronic pain on child and family daily functioning: a critical review of the literature. J Dev Behav Pediatr 2000;21:58–69.

[28] Kashikar-Zuck S, Goldschneider KR, Powers SW, et al. Depression and functional disability in chronic pediatric pain. Clin J Pain 2001;17(4):341–9.

[29] Child AH. Joint hypermobility syndrome: inherited disorder of collagen synthesis. J Rheumatol 1986;13:239–43.

[30] Griegel-Morris P, Larson K, Mueller-Klaus K, et al. Incidence of common postural abnormalities in the cervical, shoulder, and thoracic regions and their association with pain in two age groups of healthy subjects. Phys Ther 1992;72:425–30.

[31] Flato B, Aasland A, Vandvik IH, et al. Outcome and predictive factors in children with chronic idiopathic musculoskeletal pain. Clin Exp Rheumatol 1997;15:569–77.

[32] McGrath PJ. Annotation: aspects of pain in children and adolescents. J Child Psychol Psychiatry 1995;36:717–30.

[33] Malleson PN, Al-Matar M, Petty RE. Idiopathic musculoskeletal pain syndromes in children. J Rheumatol 1992;19:1786–9.

[34] Varni JW, Thompson KL, Hanson V. The Varni/Thompson Pediatric Pain Questionnaire. I. Chronic musculoskeletal pain in juvenile rheumatoid arthritis. Pain 1987;28:27–38.

[35] Schanberg LE, Sandstrom MJ. Causes of pain in children with arthritis. Rheum Dis Clin North Am 1999;25:31–53.

[36] Beyer JE, Denyes MJ, Villarruel AM. The creation, validation, and continuing development of the Oucher: a measure of pain intensity in children. J Pediatr Nurs 1992;7:335–46.

[37] Beyer JE, Villaruel AM, Denyes MJ. The Oucher. The new user's manual and technical report. Denver: University of Colorado Health Science Center; 1993.

[38] Beyer JE, Knott CB. Construct validity estimation for the African-American and Hispanic versions of the Oucher scale. J Pediatr Nurs 1998;13:20–31.

[39] Bieri D, Reeve RA, Champion GD, et al. The Faces Pain Scale for the self-assessment of the severity of pain experienced by children: development, initial validation, and preliminary investigation for ratio scale properties. Pain 1990;41:139–50.

[40] McGrath PA, Seifert CE, Speechley KN, et al. A new analogue scale for assessing children's pain: an initial validation study. Pain 1996;64:435–43.

[41] Wong DL, Baker CM. Pain in children: comparison of assessment scales. Pediatr Nurs 1988; 14:9–17.

[42] Dahlquist LM, Gil KM, Armstrong FD, et al. Preparing children for medical examinations: the importance of previous medical experience. Health Psychol 1986;5:249–59.

[43] Jay SM, Ozolins M, Elliott CH, et al. Assessment of children's distress during painful medical procedures. Health Psychol 1983;2(2):133–47.

[44] Szyfelbein SK, Osgood PE, Carr DB. The assessment of pain and plasma beta-endorphin immunoactivity in burned children. Pain 1985;22:173–82.

[45] Beyer JE, Knapp TR. Methodological issues in the measurement of children's pain. J Assoc Care Child Health 1986;14:233–41.

[46] Beyer JE, Arandine CR. Convergent and discriminant validity of a self-report measure of pain intensity for children. J Assoc Care Child Health 1988;16:274–82.

[47] Aradine CR, Beyer JE, Tompkins JM. Children's pain perception before and after analgesia: a study of instrument construct validity and related issues. J Pediatr Nurs 1988;3:11–23.

[48] Savedra M, Tesler M, Holzemer WL, et al. Pain location: validity and reliability of body outline markings by hospitalized children and adolescents. Res Nurs Health 1989;12:307–14.

[49] Jaworski TM, Bradley LA, Heck LW, et al. Development of an observation method for assessing pain behaviors in children with juvenile rheumatoid arthritis. Arthritis Rheum 1995; 38:1142–51.

[50] Chambers CT, Reid GJ, Craig KD, et al. Agreement between child and parent reports of pain. Clin J Pain 1998;14:336–42.

[51] Singer AJ, Gulla J, Thode HC. Parents and practitioners are poor judges of young children's pain severity. Acad Emerg Med 2002;9:609–12.

[52] Rosenberg AM. Analysis of a pediatric rheumatology clinic population. J Rheumatol 1990; 17:827–30.

[53] Wilder RT, Berde CB, Wolohan M, Vieyra MA, et al. Reflex sympathetic dystrophy in children: clinical characteristics and follow-up of seventy patients. J Bone Joint Surg [Am] 1992; 74:910–9.

[54] Maillard SM, Davies K, Khubchandani R, et al. Reflex sympathetic dystrophy: a multidisciplinary approach. Arthritis Rheum 2004;51(2):284–90.

[55] Dangel T. Chronic pain management in children. Part II: reflex sympathetic dystrophy. Paediatr Anaesth 1998;8:105–12.

[56] Bernstein BH, Singsen BH, Kent JT, et al. Reflex neurovascular dystrophy in childhood. J Pediatr 1978;93:211–5.

[57] Veldman PH, Reynen HM, Arntz IE, et al. Signs and symptoms of reflex sympathetic dystrophy: prospective study of 829 patients. Lancet 1993;342:1012–6.

[58] Stanton RP, Malcolm JR, Wesdock KA, et al. Reflex sympathetic dystrophy in children: an orthopedic perspective. Orthopedics 1993;16:773–9.

[59] Sherry DD, Weisman R. Psychological aspects of childhood reflex neurovascular dystrophy. Pediatrics 1988;81:572–8.

[60] Silber TJ, Majd M. Reflex sympathetic dystrophy syndrome in children and adolescents. Am J Dis Child 1988;142:1325–30.

[61] Sherry DD, Wallace CA, Kelley C, et al. Short- and long-term outcomes of children with complex regional pain syndrome type 1 treated with exercise therapy. Clin J Pain 1999;15(3): 218–23.

[62] Lee BH, Scharff L, Sethna NF, et al. Physical therapy and cognitive-behavioral treatment for complex regional pain syndromes. J Pediatr 2002;141(1):135–40.

[63] Yunus MB, Masi AT. Juvenile primary fibromyalgia syndrome: a clinical study of thirty-three patients and matched normal controls. Arthritis Rheum 1985;28:138–45.

[64] Buskila D, Press J, Gedalia A, et al. Assessment of nonarticular tenderness and prevalence of fibromyalgia in children. J Rheumatol 1993;20:368–70.

[65] Wolfe F, Smythe HA, Yunus MB, et al. The American College of Rheumatology 1990 criteria for the classification of fibromyalgia. Arthritis Rheum 1990;33:160–72.

[66] Kimura Y. Fibromyalgia syndrome in children and adolescents. J Musculoskel Med 2000; 17:142–58.

[67] Reid GJ, Lang BA, McGrath PJ. Primary juvenile fibromyalgia: psychological adjustment, family functioning, coping, and functional disability. Arthritis Rheum 1997;40:752–60.

[68] Schanberg LE, Keefe FJ, Lefebvre JC, et al. Pain coping strategies in children with juvenile primary fibromyalgia syndrome: correlation with pain, physical function, and psychological distress. Arthritis Care Res 1996;9:89–96.

[69] Bell D, Bell K, Cheney P. Primary juvenile fibromyalgia syndrome and chronic fatigue syndrome in adolescents. Clin Infect Dis 1994;18:S21–3.

[70] Winfield B. Pain in fibromyalgia. Rheum Dis Clin North Am 1999;25:55–79.

[71] Breau LM, McGrath PM, Ju LH. Review of juvenile primary fibromyalgia syndrome and chronic fatigue syndrome. J Dev Behav Pediatr 1999;20:278–88.

[72] Granges G, Zilko P, Littlejohn GO. Fibromyalgia syndrome: assessment of the severity of the condition two years after diagnosis. J Rheumatol 1994;21:523–9.

[73] Ledingham J, Doherty S, Doherty M. Primary fibromyalgia syndrome: an outcome study. Br J Rheumatol 1993;32:139–42.

[74] Rabinovich CE, Schanberg LE, Stein LD, et al. A follow-up study of pediatric fibromyalgia patients [abstract]. Arthritis Rheum 1990;33(Suppl 9):S146.

[75] Siegel DM, Janeway D, Baum J. Fibromyalgia syndrome in children and adolescents: clinical features at presentation and follow-up. Pediatrics 1998;101:377–82.

[76] Buskila D, Neumann L, Hershman E, et al. Fibromyalgia syndrome in children: an outcome study. J Rheumatol 1995;22:525–8.

[77] Mikkelsson M. One year outcome of preadolescents with fibromyalgia. J Rheumatol 1999;26: 674–82.

[78] Simms R. Fibromyalgia syndrome: current concepts in pathophysiology, clinical features and management. Arthritis Care Res 1996;9:315–28.

[79] Kashikar-Zuck S, Graham TB, Huenefeld MD, et al. A review of biobehavioral research in juvenile primary fibromyalgia syndrome. Arthritis Care Res 2000;13(6):388–97.

[80] Conte PM, Walco GA, Kimura Y. Temperament and stress response in children with juvenile primary fibromyalgia syndrome. Arthritis Rheum 2003;48(10):2923–30.

[81] Roizenblatt S, Tufik S, Goldenberg J, et al. Juvenile primary fibromyalgia: clinical and polysomnographic aspects. J Rheumatol 1997;24:579–85.

[82] Tayag-Kier CE, Keenan GF, Scalzi LV, et al. Sleep and periodic limb movement in sleep in juvenile fibromyalgia. Pediatrics 2000;106(5):E70.

[83] Vandvik IH, Forseth KO. A bio-psychosocial evaluation of ten adolescents with fibromyalgia. Acta Paediatr 1994;83:766–71.

[84] Schanberg LE, Keefe FJ, Lefebvre JC, et al. Social context of pain in children with juvenile primary fibromyalgia syndrome: parental pain history and family environment. Clin J Pain 1998;14:107–15.

[85] Walker LS, Zeman JL. Parental responses to child illness behavior. J Pediatr Psychol 1992;17: 49–71.

[86] Goldenberg DL, Felson D, Dinerman H. A randomized, controlled trial of amitriptyline and naproxen in the treatment of fibromyalgia. Arthritis Rheum 1986;29:1371–7.

[87] Leventhal L. Management of fibromyalgia. Ann Intern Med 1999;131:850–8.

[88] Romano TJ. Fibromyalgia in children: diagnosis and treatment. W V Med J 1991;87:112–4.

[89] March J, Silva S, Petrycki S, Curry J, et al. Treatment for Adolescents With Depression Study (TADS) Team. Fluoxetine, cognitive-behavioral therapy, and their combination for adolescents with depression: Treatment for Adolescents With Depression Study (TADS) randomized controlled trial. JAMA 2004;292(7):807–20.

[90] Rossy LA, Buckelew SP, Dorr N, et al. A meta-analysis of fibromyalgia treatment interventions. Ann Behav Med 1992;21:180–91.

[91] Kulas DT, Schanberg LE. Musculoskeletal pain. In: Schechter NL, Berde CB, Yaster M, editors. Pain in infants, children and adolescents. 2nd edition. Philadelphia: Lippincott Williams & Wilkins; 2003.

[92] Sandstrom MJ, Keefe FJ. Self-management of fibromyalgia: the role of formal coping skills training and physical exercise training programs. Arthritis Care Res 1999;11:432–47.

[93] Walco GA, Ilowite NT. Cognitive-behavioral intervention for juvenile primary fibromyalgia syndrome. J Rheumatol 1992;19:1617–9.

[94] Sherry DD. Musculoskeletal pain in children. Curr Opin Rheumatol 1997;9:465–70.

[95] Sherry DD. An overview of amplified musculoskeletal pain syndromes. J Rheumatol 2000; 27:44–8.

[96] Berman BM, Swyers JP. Complementary medicine treatments for fibromyalgia syndrome. Best Pract Res Clin Rheumatol 1999;13:487–92.

[97] Bowyer S, Roettcher P, and the members of the Pediatric Rheumatology Database Research Group. Pediatric rheumatology clinic populations in the United States: results of a 3 year survey. J Rheumatol 1996;23:1968–74.

[98] Cassidy JT, Nelson AM. The frequency of juvenile arthritis. J Rheumatol 1988;15:535–6.

[99] Gewanter HT, Roghmann KJ, Baum J. The prevalence of juvenile arthritis. Arthritis Rheum 1983;26:599–603.

[100] Towner SR, Michet CJJ, O'Fallon WM, et al. The epidemiology of juvenile arthritis in Rochester, Minnesota 1960–1979. Arthritis Rheum 1983;26:1208–13.

[101] Hull RG. Outcome in juvenile arthritis. J Rheumatol 1988;27:66–71.

[102] Ivey J, Brewer E, Giannini E. Psychosocial functioning in children with JRA. Arthritis Rheum 1981;24:S100.

[103] Flato B, Lien G, Smerdel A, et al. Prognostic factors in juvenile rheumatoid arthritis: a case-control study revealing early predictors and outcome after 14.9 years. J Rheumatol 2003;30(2): 386–93.

[104] Sherry DD, Bohnsack J, Salmonson K, et al. Painless juvenile rheumatoid arthritis. J Pediatr 1990;116:921–3.

[105] Lovell DJ, Walco GW. Pain associated with juvenile rheumatoid arthritis. Pediatr Clin North Am 1989;36:1015–27.

[106] Schanberg LE, Anthony KK, et al. Daily pain and symptoms in children with polyarticular arthritis. Arthritis Rheum 2003;48(5):1390–7.

[107] Petty RE, Cassidy JT. Juvenile rheumatoid arthritis. In: Cassidy JT, Petty RE, editors. Textbook of pediatric rheumatology. 4th edition. Philadelphia: W.B. Saunders; 2001. p. 240–1.

[108] Gragg RA, Rapoff MA, Danovsky MB, et al. Assessing chronic musculoskeletal pain associated with rheumatic disease: further validation of the Pediatric Pain Questionnaire. J Pediatr Psychol 1996;21:237–50.

[109] Thompson KL, Varni JW, Hanson V. Comprehensive assessment of pain in juvenile rheumatoid arthritis: an empirical model. J Pediatr Psychol 1987;12:241–5.

[110] Schanberg LE, Lefebvre JC, Keefe FJ, et al. Pain coping and the pain experience in children with juvenile chronic arthritis. Pain 1997;73:181–9.

[111] Varni JW, Wilcox KT, Hanson V, et al. Chronic musculoskeletal pain and functional status in juvenile rheumatoid arthritis. Pain 1988;32:1–7.

[112] Oen K, Reed M, Malleson PN, et al. Radiologic outcome and its relationships to functional disability in juvenile rheumatoid arthritis. J Rheumatol 2003;30:832–40.

[113] Vandvik IH, Eckblad G. Relationship between pain, disease severity and psychosocial function in patients with juvenile chronic arthritis. Scand J Rheumatol 1990;19:295–302.

[114] Malleson PN, Oen K, Cabral DA, et al. Predictors of pain in children with established juvenile rheumatoid arthritis. Arthritis Rheum 2004;51(2):222–7.

[115] Ilowite NT, Walco GW, Pochaczevsky R. Assessment of pain in patients with juvenile rheumatoid arthritis: relation between pain intensity and degree of joint inflammation. Ann Rheum Dis 1992;51:343–6.

[116] Ross CK, Lavigne JV, Hayford JR, et al. Psychological factors affecting reported pain in juvenile rheumatoid arthritis. J Pediatr Psychol 1993;18:561–73.

[117] Hagglund KJ, Schopp LM, Alberts KR, et al. Predicting pain among children with juvenile rheumatoid arthritis. Arthritis Care Res 1995;8:36–42.

[118] Abu-Saad HH, Uiterwijk M. Pain in children with juvenile rheumatoid arthritis: a descriptive study. Pediatr Res 1995;38:194–7.

[119] Benestad B, Vinje O, Veirod B, et al. Quantitative and qualitative assessments of pain in children with juvenile chronic arthritis based on the Norwegian version of the Pediatric Pain Questionnaire. Scand J Rheumatol 1996;25:293–9.

[120] Baildam EM, Holt PJL, Conway SC, et al. The association between physical function and psychological problems in children with juvenile chronic arthritis. Brit J Rheum 1995;34: 470–7.

[121] Schanberg LE, Maurin E, Anthony KK, et al. Girls with polyarticular arthritis report more disease symptoms than boys. Arthritis Rheum 2001;44(Suppl):S691.

[122] Schanberg LE, Gil KM, Anthony KK, et al. Mood and stressful events predict daily fluctuations in disease symptoms in juvenile polyarticular arthritis. Arthritis Rheum 2000; 43(Suppl 9):S328.

[123] Schanberg LE, Sandstrom MJ, Starr K, et al. The relationship of daily mod and stressful events to symptoms in juvenile rheumatic disease. Arthritis Care Res 2000;13:33–41.

[124] Schanberg LE, Gil KM, Anthony KK, et al. Pain, stiffness, and fatigue in juvenile polyarticular arthritis: contemporaneous stressful events and mood as predictors. Arthritis Rheum In press.

[125] Thastum M, Zachariae R, Scholer M, et al. Cold pressor pain: comparing responses of juvenile rheumatoid arthritis patients and their parents. Scan J Rheumatol 1997;26:272–9.

[126] Schanberg LE, Anthony KK, Gil KM, et al. Parental pain history predicts child health status in children with chronic rheumatic disease. Pediatrics 2001;108:e47.

[127] Berde CB, Beyer JE, Bournaki M, et al. Comparison of morphine and methadone for prevention of postoperative pain in 3- to 7-year-old children. J Pediatr 1991;119(1):136–41.

[128] Shir Y, Rosen G, Zeldin A, et al. Methadone is safe for treating hospitalized patients with severe pain. Can J Anesth 2001;48(11):1109–13.

[129] Haber D, Goodman SB. Total hip arthroplasty in juvenile chronic arthritis. J Arthroplasty 1998; 13:259–65.

[130] Lonner JH, Stuchin SA. Synovectomy, radial head excision, and anterior capsular release in stage III inflammatory arthritis of the elbow. J Hand Surg [Am] 1997;22:279–85.

[131] Witt JD, McCullough CJ. Anterior soft-tissue release of the hip in juvenile chronic arthritis. J Bone Joint Surg [Br] 1994;73:770–3.

[132] American Pain Society. Guidelines for the management of pain in osteoarthritis, rheumatoid arthritis, and juvenile chronic arthritis. 2nd edition. Glenview (IL): American Pain Society; 2002. p. 119–30.

[133] Lavigne JV, Ross CK, Berry SL, et al. Evaluation of a psychological treatment package for treating pain in children with juvenile rheumatoid arthritis. Arthritis Care Res 1992;5: 101–9.

[134] Walco GW, Varni JW, Ilowite NT. Cognitive-behavioral pain management in children with juvenile rheumatoid arthritis. Pediatrics 1992;89:1075–9.

[135] Giannini MJ, Protas EJ. Aerobic capacity in juvenile rheumatoid arthritis and healthy children. Arthritis Care Res 1991;4:131–5.

[136] Klepper SE, Darbee J, Effgen SK, et al. Physical fitness levels in children with polyarticular juvenile rheumatoid arthritis. Arthritis Care Res 1992;5:93–100.

[137] Klepper SE. Effects of an eight-week physical conditioning program on disease signs and symptoms in children with chronic arthritis. Arthritis Care Res 1999;12:52–60.

[138] Feldman BM, Wright FV, Bar-Or O, et al. Rigorous fitness training and testing for children with polyarticular arthritis: a pilot study. Arthritis Rheum 2000;43(Suppl 9):S324.

[139] Wright FV, Raman S, Bar-Or O, et al. Pilot evaluation of the feasibility of fitness training for children with juvenile rheumatoid arthritis. Arthritis Rheum 2000;43(Suppl 9):S615.

[140] Fisher NM, Venkatraman JT, O'Neil KM. Effects of resistance exercise on children with juvenile arthritis. Arthritis Rheum 1999;42(Suppl 9):S1950.

[141] Bloom BJ, Owens JA, McGuinn M, et al. Sleep and its relationship to pain, dysfunction, and disease activity in juvenile rheumatoid arthritis. J Rheumatol 2002;29(1):169–73.

[142] Field T, Hernadez-Reif M, Seligman S, et al. Juvenile rheumatoid arthritis: benefits from massage therapy. J Pediatr Psychol 1997;22:607–17.

ELSEVIER
SAUNDERS

PEDIATRIC CLINICS
OF NORTH AMERICA

Pediatr Clin N Am 52 (2005) 641–652

Transition of the Adolescent Patient with Rheumatic Disease: Issues to Consider

Lori B. Tucker, MD*, David A. Cabral, MBBS

Division of Pediatric Rheumatology, Centre for Community Child Health Research, British Columbia Children's Hospital, 4880 Oak Street, Room K4-120, Vancouver, BC V6H 3V4, Canada

The topic of transition of youth with childhood-onset rheumatic diseases to adult health care is increasingly important, because, most of these patients will continue to have active disease or significant sequelae of their rheumatic disease into their adult lives.

This article discusses the definitions of transition and models for providing transition care to youth and young adults with rheumatic diseases in the context of differing cultural and health care systems. Issues and questions relating to pediatric rheumatology transition programming are outlined, and a model program of pediatric rheumatology transition is presented.

Defining transition

Transition for patients with chronic diseases that have begun in childhood and persisted into adulthood means different things to different people. A useful description of this developmental phase for the patient is provided by Viner [1], who describes the process of transition from pediatric to adult health care providers as one part of a wider transition, or developmental process, in which the child moves from being a dependent child to an independent adult. The American Society for Adolescent Medicine describes transition as an active medical process, "the purposeful, planned movement of adolescents and young

---

* Corresponding author.
  E-mail address: ltucker@cw.bc.ca (L.B. Tucker).

0031-3955/05/$ – see front matter © 2005 Elsevier Inc. All rights reserved.
doi:10.1016/j.pcl.2005.01.008

adults with chronic physical and medical conditions from child-centered to adult-oriented health care systems" [2]. Both of these definitions point out that transition involves a fluid movement in a continuum, rather than an administrative event in which the patient moves from the pediatric or adolescent clinic to the adult rheumatologist's office.

The issues and definitions of transition may differ substantially, based on cultural background. For example, in some countries, children are considered adults at the age of 13 years; all adolescents older than 13 years are cared for by adult health care providers, and there is no tradition of adolescent medicine. In these countries, the processes and issues surrounding transition would have to be considered in a completely different context than in European or North American systems. To date, there has been little research on or discussion of how the transition from pediatric to adult rheumatology care differs between cultures.

Why is transition important for youth with rheumatic diseases?

Juvenile idiopathic arthritis (JIA), systemic lupus erythematosus (SLE), juvenile dermatomyositis (JDM), and other rheumatic diseases often continue to cause problems for patients into their adult years. Current research suggests that approximately one third of youth with JIA will continue to have active disease well into adulthood. These patients will require on-going medical treatment, and many will have significant disability [3–8]. Several additional studies that span many years and span several major therapeutic advances (such as the use of methotrexate) describe the outcomes of not-quite-comparable groups of patients (ie, patients with juvenile rheumatoid arthritis, juvenile chronic arthritis, JIA, or other entities) [9–13]. In spite of their unavoidable limitations, the results of all of these studies demonstrate the significant and life-long impact of childhood-onset arthritis. A series of studies published by Packham and Hall [9–12] examine long-term outcomes of a large, well-documented cohort of adults who had juvenile arthritis. In this group of 246 patients (mean age, 35.4 years), a large number of patients continued to have persisting pain and active disease requiring medications; functional disability, mood disturbance and unemployment were also common. Foster et al [13] reviewed 16 studies of outcome of juvenile arthritis in patients followed from 1 to more than 20 years between 1962 and 2002. Approximately one third of patients had disability as measured by Steinbrocker classification [14], and a significant number (between 10% and 45%) had persistent disease activity long into their adult lives. Foster's own work examining the outcome of 82 adults with JIA (disease duration, median 21 years; range, 3–61 years) confirms these results and also examines the health-related quality of life of these patients using standardized patient-report questionnaires [13]. The patients had poor health-related quality of life in all physical domains as compared with healthy peers and impaired scores in social and emotional functioning. The patients had significant functional disability as measured by the

Health Assessment Questionnaire: adults aged 31 to 45 years had a mean score of 1.3, and adults older than 45 years had a mean score of 2.2. These scores suggest that, rather than diminishing as patients enter adulthood, the impact of JIA becomes more significant as patients get older.

The long-term outcome for young adults with other chronic rheumatic diseases such as SLE, JDM, and vasculitis has not been well studied. One can anticipate that virtually all youth with SLE will continue to require rheumatologic care in adulthood, and many already have significant damage from active disease in their childhood years. Recent studies have been published using the Systemic Lupus International Collaborating Clinics/American College of Rheumatology Damage Index to determine damage in youth with childhood-onset SLE [15,16]. In three studies, most patients had accumulated significant organ system damage 3 to 5 years after onset of disease [17–19].

The long-term outcome for childhood-onset JDM has not been documented in the literature. One small review by Peloro et al [20] reviewed 16 patients seen over a 30-year period in one center. Six patients were reported to be in long-term remission of their disease, with average follow-up of 3 to 4.5 years, and six patients had disease flares requiring additional treatment. Another small review by Chalmers et al [21] in 1982 studied 18 adults an average of 18.5 years after diagnosis of JDM. The majority of the patients did well, with only three having significant residual disability. These subjects enjoyed a good level of educational and employment attainment. The impact of the JDM on patients' functional abilities or quality of life later in life has not been assessed in any large, recent patient cohorts.

Why is transition a challenge for youth with rheumatic disease?

The developmental tasks of late adolescence and early adulthood are monumental even in the best of circumstances (Box 1), and having a chronic rheumatic disease during this period complicates the trajectory. There is a risk for parental

---

Box 1. Developmental tasks of adolescence

Independence and assertiveness
    Independent health behaviors
    Self-advocacy
Development of peer relationships
Focus on education, vocation
Development of sexual identity
Health and lifestyle

overprotection of children with a chronic disease, and this protection may frustrate the adolescent's pursuit of independence and ultimately self-advocacy. The inability to participate fully in usual activities (eg, sports, shopping, parties) may further isolate youth with rheumatic disease and delay development of effective peer relationships and supports that are integral to gaining independence from parents. Adolescents with rheumatic disease may not receive adequate or timely counseling about important issues such as sexual health [22].

Inevitably, youth who have had chronic rheumatic disease throughout childhood become weary of the constant intrusion of medications, doctors appointments, and the continual feeling of being different from peers, and they often reject their treatments. They may become severely noncompliant with medications and appointments and also may engage in risk-taking behaviors that pose a danger to their health (eg, a patient taking methotrexate who binge drinks with friends). By 18 years of age, at the latest, most of these grown-up children will need to make the transition to adult-oriented health services. This transition is recognized as a period of high risk for dropping out of the health care system [23]; therefore an attempt to impose a strict time of transfer to adult health care during this period increases the risk that the patient will develop a severe disease flare or complications.

What is the current availability of transition programming in pediatric rheumatology clinics? What barriers exist to providing transition services?

The level of transition programming in pediatric rheumatology clinics is variable and depends on many factors that often are related to the local health care system and health care funding. Informal survey of North American pediatric rheumatologists at meetings and through Internet discussions reveals no standard approach to transition issues and considerable variability in practice. Commonly expressed barriers to developing transition programming are funding, staff, and resources.

The British Pediatric Rheumatology Group, led by J. E. McDonagh and colleagues [24,25], has studied the issues around adolescent rheumatology care in the United Kingdom through an extensive series of surveys of various health care providers, patients, and parents. They reported that 18% of rheumatology units in the UK treating children with rheumatic diseases had a dedicated adolescent treatment unit [25]. Many health professionals, however, reported low level of comfort in dealing with the issues of suicidal risk, sexual health screening, drug use, risk-taking behaviors, and psychiatric complaints. Barriers to providing adolescent-oriented care were lack of adolescent teaching materials, inadequate clinic time, and limited training in dealing with adolescent issues [26]. Lack of integration among service providers (between regional and local hospitals and among health providers, social services, and community services) was cited as a significant barrier as well.

Barriers to well-integrated transition can be related to issues involving the patient, the family, the pediatric rheumatologist and team, or the adult rheumatologist (Box 2) [1,26]. These issues are not rheumatology-specific; similar difficulties are found in transitioning youth with other chronic illnesses such as diabetes [22] and cystic fibrosis [27].

Box 2. Barriers to successful transition for youth with rheumatic disease

Patient-related

> Burn out
> Poor adherence
> Limited knowledge about disease and treatments
> Limited insight about long-term impact of poor adherence
> Inadequate self-advocacy skills
> Reluctance to leave known and trusted staff

Parent-related

> Reluctance to relinquish control
> Reluctance to leave known and trusted staff

System-related

> Gaps in health care financing as patient moves through education and early career
> Lack of appropriate health care services for youth
> Difficulty in providing smooth transfer of records between old and new care providers

Pediatric providers

> Difficulty in 'letting go'
> Limited options for adult rheumatology care

Adult providers

> Limited knowledge of childhood onset rheumatic disease, outcomes, and adolescent developmental trajectory
> Inadequate coordination or support for these complex patients
> Limited availability of multiple service providers

Models of transition

There are relatively few well-described models for transition of pediatric rheumatology patients into adult rheumatology care, and there are virtually no data of the process of transition for these patients. Sawyer and colleagues [28] describe three general models for transition care for adolescents with chronic illness: (1) disease-focused transition from pediatric care to an adult subspecialist, (2) primary care–coordinated care spanning adolescent to adult care, and (3) generic adolescent health services, with care coordinated by adolescent care providers. In practical terms, a primary care–based model is not generally feasible because of the many barriers that prevent primary care doctors from providing the complex care required by most youth with rheumatic disease: lack of time, lack of knowledge of these rare diseases and their treatment, and lack of specific knowledge about the impact of rheumatic disease on adolescent development. Well-developed adolescent medicine services are not universally available across North America or Europe. Therefore, the most common and practical model for transitional health care services for youth with rheumatic disease is a disease-focused transition from pediatric to adult rheumatology services.

When does transition begin and end?

When transition should begin and end remains controversial. Some transition programs suggest beginning early transition planning when the patient is 10 to 12 years old [29]. From a practical standpoint, many programs aim toward transition from pediatric health care services at the common social transition of high school completion, and frequently this transition may be dictated by administrative rules of the local health care system. One study from the United Kingdom examining transition programs for youth with type I diabetes in four districts in Oxford found that transition to adult health care services occurred between the ages of 13 to 22 years; the mean age of transition was 18 years [30].

The approach to transition currently adopted by a number of groups in North America, including the authors' program in Vancouver, begins to integrate some transition discussions with parents and children in mid-adolescence. Adolescents aged 15 years and older are generally seen alone by the physician and nurse for at least part of the clinic visit. Their parents join the patient for the portion of the visit that encompasses decision-making. Issues of independence in taking medications, communicating with the medical care team, school and vocation concerns, and lifestyle are addressed as part of the usual care for adolescents in the pediatric rheumatology clinic. At age 18 years, the rheumatology care of adolescents is transferred to a collaborative young adult transition clinic. A final transfer of rheumatology care to adult rheumatologist is individualized, depending on achievement of transition goals.

What goals should be adopted for a pediatric rheumatology transition program?

Transition clinics or programs can be an effective strategy to deliver targeted health care together and to prepare youth and young adults with childhood-onset rheumatic diseases for transfer to adult health care. This model of care provision is supported by the Canadian Pediatric Society Adolescent Medicine Committee [31].

The identification of clear goals for a pediatric rheumatology transition program can help assure that all participants recognize the scope of their responsibilities. Sharing the goals for the transition program with parents and youth helps define their expectations and their own responsibilities during this process. Box 3 shows the set of goals used in the authors' transition program, the Young Adults with Rheumatic Diseases (YARD) Clinic. The goals were developed to reflect the developmental tasks of adolescents as well as to promote successful transfer to adult rheumatology care.

The Vancouver model for providing transition care to youth with rheumatic diseases: the Young Adults with Rheumatic Disease Clinic

The YARD Clinic was developed in Vancouver, BC, to address the need for providing developmentally appropriate rheumatology specialty care to youth over age 18 years with childhood-onset rheumatic diseases and to facilitate successful transfer of rheumatology care to the adult clinic. Many youth with rheumatic diseases are not prepared at age 18 years to have their rheumatology care transferred to the adult clinic, because they are still working through major

---

Box 3. Goals of a pediatric rheumatology transition program

1. Education
   Knowledge about disease, medications, and roles of health care providers
   Skills in communication with health care providers
2. Assist with separation from parents with respect to medical issues
3. Encourage adherence to medical recommendations
4. Provide assistance/guidance with issues of education, jobs/career, finances/health care coverage, independent living, and relationships outside the family
5. Implement final transfer to adult health care providers (rheumatologist and others as necessary), providing adequate records to new care providers

developmental issues. Therefore, the YARD Clinic provides a supportive environment and education in advocacy and independence skills aimed at eventual transfer to adult care at age 22 to 24 years.

The model for this clinic is shared clinical care by pediatric and adult rheumatologists in the same clinic setting, with a clinical nurse specialist, a social worker, established links with physiotherapy, occupational therapy, vocational and sexual counseling services, and a developing network of youth-friendly adult medicine subspecialists. The YARD Clinic has been functioning in its current format since 1995. The clinic is an integral part of the pediatric rheumatology program but is located at a different site.

The YARD Clinic functions with a set of principles that have been developed by the staff and modified as found necessary. The YARD clinic was developed to accept patients who have a definite diagnosis of a childhood-onset rheumatic disease and who have been followed in the pediatric rheumatology program at the British Columbia Children's Hospital. Patients are not accepted for new diagnostic evaluations, and patients over 17 years of age who are newly diagnosed with a rheumatic disease are generally not accepted. This decision was based on two considerations: (1) the limitations the available resources placed on the clinic's capacity, and (2) the belief that young adults aged 17 to 19 years who have lived with a childhood rheumatic disease have issues that are fundamentally different from those of patients with a new diagnosis at this age.

The move to the YARD Clinic is one important step in a process that begins in the pediatric rheumatology clinic several years earlier. At approximately age 14 or 15 years, the adolescent patients begin to spend a small amount of time alone with the pediatric rheumatologist and nurse. This time gives the clinic staff an opportunity for confidential discussions with the patient regarding adolescent health issues including sexual health, risk-taking behaviors, family problems, and vocational issues. Families are informed of the YARD Clinic as the patient reaches the age of 16 years. Transfer to the clinic generally occurs when the patient is 18 years old; for many patients, this is the year of graduation from high school.

One of the most important and often difficult issues in promoting a youth's independence during transition is the role and involvement of parents in their teen's health care. Most parents of children with a chronic rheumatic disease have spent many years organizing physician appointments, ensuring that medications are taken on time and regularly, getting medication renewals, performing or promoting physiotherapy and occupational therapy, and dealing with school and other community care providers. Many adolescents reach the age of 18 years without being able to name accurately their disease or medications; although they may have been given this information many times in the clinic, they are happy to let their parents take care of matters and have little incentive to assume responsibility themselves. Taking on independent health care responsibility is a late priority among the other areas of developing independence in their lives.

To smooth the transition from the parent-focused pediatric rheumatology program into the patient-focused YARD program, parents are invited to attend a portion of their teen's first visit to the YARD Clinic, if the teen agrees. In the authors' experience, most transitioning adolescents attend their first visits completely on their own. After the first visit, parents are not invited to the clinic visits. Parents are actively discouraged from taking a coordinating role in the teen's on-going health care (eg, making or changing appointments, requesting prescription refills, or taking a leading role in medication decision-making). Indeed, the physician will not discuss any aspects of their child's care or progress without express permission of the patient, and parents are encouraged to obtain the information directly from the patient. For some parents, this transition is difficult. A clinical nurse specialist and social worker work with the young adult and, if necessary, the parent to provide support for the patient and family.

When is the final transfer to adult rheumatology?

Patients are generally followed in the YARD program for 3 to 5 years. This time allows the patient to have the additional supports of the YARD program during the critical period when the patient is engaged in making educational and vocational decisions, establishing strong independent peer relationships, and, for many young adults, leaving home and establishing independent living. The timing of the patient's final transfer to an adult rheumatology physician is individualized. Box 4 shows the general goals used to assess readiness for transfer. At each YARD Clinic appointment after the age of 20 years, the team discusses the patient's readiness to transfer to adult care to identify areas that need further development.

Not all patients will have a successful transition from the pediatric rheumatology clinic through the YARD Clinic to adult rheumatology care. In the authors' experience, if the patient has not reached the transitional goals by 23 years, continuing in the program is unlikely to be of any benefit, and care

---

Box 4. Determining patient's readiness to transfer care to an adult rheumatologist

1. Patient has relatively stable disease.
2. Patient has adequate understanding of the disease and its treatments.
3. Patient has demonstrated ability to make and attend appointments and take care of medication needs.
4. Patient has developed an independent adult relationship with the health care providers in the YARD clinic.
5. Patient has a family doctor in the community and demonstrates the ability to use the family doctor appropriately.

is transferred. There are patients who have developmental delays, and their adolescent development may last late into adulthood. For some families, an enmeshed psychologic relationship between a parent and adolescent prevents the adolescent from developing independent health care behaviors.

What role can the pediatrician or primary care provider play in transition?

Frequently, the role of the pediatrician or primary health care provider is not well developed in considering issues of transition for youth with rheumatic diseases. In the model of the medical home promoted by the American Academy of Pediatrics [32], pediatric health care for children and adolescents should be a collaboration between parents and health care providers to provide accessible, community-based, coordinated health care. For youth with rheumatic disease, health care should incorporate the primary health care providers (pediatrician or family doctor, community based therapists), the subspecialty team (pediatric rheumatologist, nurse, subspecialty therapist, social worker, psychologist, and others), parents, school, and patient.

The primary health care provider should play an important supportive role for the family and patient by promoting a future planning perspective from an early stage [33].

Visits to the family doctor or pediatrician can provide an important opportunity for the adolescent to practice speaking to the doctor alone. These opportunities promote independence and the development of advocacy skills in an environment that feels safe and comfortable for the adolescent and the parents.

If the patient is followed by a pediatrician for primary health care, the transition to a primary care doctor (internist or family doctor) should be discussed and encouraged. This transition should take into account the needs of the young adult: does the patient prefer a male or female doctor, a group practice or solo practice? The young adult's choice of primary health care provider should be an integral part of the transition plan, because acquiring the skills to use a primary doctor properly is part of transition teaching.

Summary

The goals of pediatric rheumatologists are to ensure the best possible medical, functional, and social outcomes for their patients. Transition from pediatric to adult rheumatology care is a critical component of comprehensive care for adolescents and young adults with rheumatic disease. In the past few years, there has been increasing interest in the transition phase of pediatric rheumatology care and acknowledgment that best-quality services are not available to all patients. Improving transition care for youth with childhood-onset rheumatic diseases requires collaboration between pediatric and adult rheumatologists and between rheumatologists and primary care providers. Providers of transition care must recognize that young adults with rheumatic diseases present complex medical and psychologic needs.

Acknowledgments

The authors acknowledge the support and contributions of the staff involved with the Young Adults with Rheumatic Diseases Clinic in Vancouver, BC: Angela How, MD, Stephanie Ensworth, MD, Glenda Avery, Paul Adams, and Susie Goundar.

References

[1] Viner R. Transition from paediatric to adult care. Bridging the gaps or passing the buck? Arch Dis Child 1999;81:271–5.

[2] Blum RW, Garell D, Hodgman CH, et al. Transition from child-centered to adult health-care systems for adolescents with chronic conditions. A position paper of the Society for Adolescent Medicine. J Adolesc Health 1993;14(7):570–6.

[3] Duffy CM. Health outcomes in pediatric rheumatic diseases. Curr Opin Rheumatol 2004;16: 102–8.

[4] Andersson Gare B, Fasth A. The natural history of juvenile chronic arthritis: a population based cohort study. II Outcome. J Rheumatol 1995;22:308–19.

[5] Minden K, Niewerth M, Listing J, et al. Long-term outcome in patients with juvenile idiopathic arthritis. Arthritis Rheum 2002;46(9):2392–401.

[6] Flato B, Aasland A, Vinje O, et al. Outcome and predictive factors in juvenile rheumatoid arthritis and juvenile spondyloarthropathy. J Rheumatol 1998;25:366–73.

[7] David J, Cooper C, Hickey L, et al. The functional and psychological outcomes of juvenile chronic arthritis in young adulthood. Br J Rheumatol 1994;33:876–81.

[8] Oen K, Malleson PN, Cabral DA, et al. Disease course and outcome of juvenile rheumatoid arthritis in a multicenter cohort. J Rheumatol 2002;29:1989–99.

[9] Packham JC, Hall MA, Pimm TJ. Long-term follow-up of 246 adults with juvenile idiopathic arthritis: predictive factors for mood and pain. Rheumatology (Oxford) 2002;41(12):1444–9.

[10] Packham JC, Hall MA. Long-term follow-up of 246 adults with juvenile idiopathic arthritis: social function, relationships and sexual activity. Rheumatology (Oxford) 2002;41(12):1440–3.

[11] Packham JC, Hall MA. Long-term follow-up of 246 adults with juvenile idiopathic arthritis: education and employment. Rheumatology (Oxford) 2002;41(12):1436–9.

[12] Packham JC, Hall MA. Long-term follow-up of 246 adults with juvenile idiopathic arthritis: functional outcome. Rheumatology (Oxford) 2002;41(12):1428–35.

[13] Foster HE, Marshall N, Myers A, et al. Outcome of adults with juvenile idiopathic arthritis. Arthritis Rheum 2003;48(3):767–75.

[14] Steinbrocker I, Traeger CH, Batterman RC. Criteria for determination of progression of rheumatoid arthritis and of functional capacity of patients with disease. JAMA 1949;140:209.

[15] Gladman DD, Urowitz MB, Goldsmith CH, et al. The reliability of the Systemic Lupus International Collaborating Clinics/American College of Rheumatology Damage Index in patients with systemic lupus erythematosus. Arthritis Rheum 1997;40(5):809–13.

[16] Gladman D, Ginzler E, Goldsmith C, et al. The development and initial validation of the SLICC/ACR damage index for SLE. Arthritis Rheum 1996;39:363–9.

[17] Brunner HI, Silverman ED, To T, et al. Risk factors for damage in childhood-onset systemic lupus erythematosus: cumulative disease activity and medication use predict disease damage. Arthritis Rheum 2002;46(2):436–44.

[18] Ravelli A, Duarte-Salazar C, Buratti S, et al. Assessment of damage in juvenile-onset systemic lupus erythematosus: a multicenter cohort study. Arthritis Rheum 2003;49(4):501–7.

[19] Miettunen PM, Ortiz-Alvarez O, Petty RE, et al. Gender and ethnic origin have no effect on long term outcome of childhood onset systemic lupus erythematosus. J Rheumatol 2004;31(8): 1650–4.

[20] Peloro TM, Miller OF, Hahn TF, et al. Juvenile dermatomyositis: a retrospective review of a 30-year experience. J Am Acad Dermatol 2001;45(1):28–34.

[21] Chalmers A, Sayson R, Walters R. Juvenile dermatomyositis: medical, social, and economic status in adulthood. Can Med Assoc J 1982;126(1):31–3.

[22] Britto MT, Rosenthal SL, Taylor J, et al. Improving rheumatologists' screening for alcohol use and sexual activity. Arch Pediatr Adolesc Med 2000;154(5):478–83.

[23] McGill M. How do we organize smooth, effective transfer from pediatric to adult diabetes care? Horm Res 2002;57(Suppl 1):66–8.

[24] Shaw KL, Southwood TR, McDonagh JE, et al. Developing a programme of transitional care for adolescents with juvenile idiopathic arthritis: results of a postal survey. Rheumatol 2004;43: 211–9.

[25] McDonagh JE, Southwood TR, Shaw KL, British Paediatric Rheumatology Group. Unmet education and training needs of rheumatology health professionals in adolescent health and transition care. Rheumatology 2004;43:737–43.

[26] Fox A. Physicians as barriers to successful transitional care. Int J Adolesc Med Health 2002; 14(1):3–7.

[27] Nasr S, Campbell C, Howatt W. Transition program from pediatric to adult care for cystic fibrosis patients. J Adolesc Health 1992;13:682–5.

[28] Sawyer S, Blair S, Bowes G. Chronic illness in adolescents: transfer or transition to adult services? J Paediatr Child Health 1997;33:88–90.

[29] Youth Health Program BC Children's Hospital. On TRAC—taking responsibility for adolescent/adult care. Vancouver (BC): Children's Hospital; 2000. Available at: http://infosource.cw.bc.ca/cw_yhlth/content/prgOnTrac.asp. Accessed November 1, 2004.

[30] Kipps S, Bahu T, Ong K, et al. Current methods of transfer of young people with type I diabetes to adult services. Diabet Med 2002;19:649–54.

[31] Adolescent Medicine Committee. (Canadian Pediatric Society). Care of the chronically ill adolescent. Canadian Journal of Pediatrics 1994;4:124–7.

[32] Medical Home Initiatives for Children with Special Needs Project Advisory Committee. The medical home. Pediatrics 2002;110:184–6.

[33] Olsen DG, Swigonski NL. Transition to adulthood: the important role of the pediatrician. Pediatrics 2004;113:e159–62.

ELSEVIER
SAUNDERS

PEDIATRIC CLINICS
OF NORTH AMERICA

Pediatr Clin N Am 52 (2005) 653–667

Index

Note: Page numbers of article titles are in **boldface** type.

A

Abciximab, for Kawasaki disease, 563

Abdominal pain
in familial Mediterranean fever, 580–581
in tumor necrosis factor receptor–
associated periodic syndrome, 594

Acetaminophen
for Henoch-Schönlein purpura, 555
for juvenile idiopathic arthritis, 631

Acute hemorrhagic edema of infancy, versus
Henoch-Schönlein purpura, 554–555

Adalimumab, for juvenile idiopathic
arthritis, 435

Adaptive immune system, in juvenile
idiopathic arthritis, 340–347

Adhesion molecules, in inflammatory
myopathies, 499

Adolescents, with rheumatic disease, transition
to adult care. *See* Rheumatic diseases,
transition to adult care.

Alopecia, in systemic lupus
erythematosus, 447

Alternative medicine, for fibromyalgia, 628

American College of
Rheumatology classification
of juvenile idiopathic arthritis, 413
of juvenile systemic sclerosis, 521–522
of systemic lupus erythematosus,
443–444

Amyloidosis
in familial cold autoinflammatory
syndrome, 602–604
in familial Mediterranean fever, 584
in juvenile idiopathic arthritis, 349
in urticaria-deafness-amyloidosis
syndrome, 602

Amyopathic juvenile dermatomyositis, 510

Anakinra, for juvenile idiopathic arthritis, 436

Anemia
in antiphospholipid antibody
syndrome, 479
in juvenile systemic sclerosis, 527–528
in Kawasaki disease, 559
in systemic lupus erythematosus,
459–460

Aneurysms
in Kawasaki disease, 398–399, 558, 560,
562–563
in polyarteritis nodosa, 399–400,
563–565

Angiography
cerebral
in polyarteritis nodosa, 399–400
in Wegener's granulomatosis, 401
coronary, in Kawasaki disease, 398–399
in Takayasu's arteritis, 401–402, 565

Ankylosis spondylitis, arthritis in, 419

Anticardiolipin antibodies
in antiphospholipid antibody syndrome,
469, 471–472, 485
in juvenile localized scleroderma, 536
in systemic lupus erythematosus,
462–463

Anticoagulants, for antiphospholipid antibody
syndrome, 486–488

Antidepressants
for fibromyalgia, 625–626
for juvenile idiopathic arthritis, 631

Antigen-presenting cells, in juvenile idiopathic
arthritis, 343

Anti-neutrophil cytoplasmic antibodies
in Churg–Strauss syndrome, 568–569
in microscopic polyangiitis, 568
in Wegener's granulomatosis, 566–568

Antinuclear antibodies
in juvenile localized scleroderma, 536
in juvenile systemic sclerosis, 528
in systemic lupus erythematosus,
462–463

Changing Your Address?

Make sure your subscription changes too! When you notify us of your new address, you can help make our job easier by including an exact copy of your Clinics label number with your old address (see illustration below.) This number identifies you to our computer system and will speed the processing of your address change. Please be sure this label number accompanies your old address and your corrected address—you can send an old Clinics label with your number on it or just copy it exactly and send it to the address listed below.

We appreciate your help in our attempt to give you continuous coverage. Thank you.

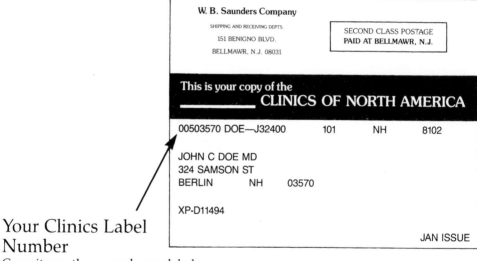

Your Clinics Label Number
Copy it exactly or send your label along with your address to:
W.B. Saunders Company, Customer Service
Orlando, FL 32887-4800
Call Toll Free 1-800-654-2452

Please allow four to six weeks for delivery of new subscriptions and for processing address changes.